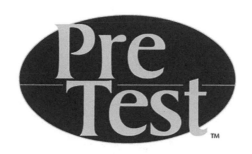

Pathology

PreTest™ Self-Assessment and Review

Notice

Medicine is an ever-changing science. As new research and clinical experience broaden our knowledge, changes in treatment and drug therapy are required. The authors and the publisher of this work have checked with sources believed to be reliable in their efforts to provide information that is complete and generally in accord with the standards accepted at the time of publication. However, in view of the possibility of human error or changes in medical sciences, neither the authors nor the publisher nor any other party who has been involved in the preparation or publication of this work warrants that the information contained herein is in every respect accurate or complete, and they disclaim all responsibility for any errors or omissions or for the results obtained from use of the information contained in this work. Readers are encouraged to confirm the information contained herein with other sources. For example, and in particular, readers are advised to check the product information sheet included in the package of each drug they plan to administer to be certain that the information contained in this work is accurate and that changes have not been made in the recommended dose or in the contraindications for administration. This recommendation is of particular importance in connection with new or infrequently used drugs.

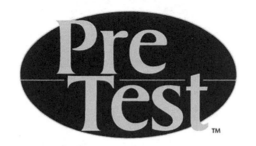

Pathology
PreTest™ Self-Assessment and Review
Twelfth Edition

Earl J. Brown, MD
Associate Professor
Department of Pathology
Quillen College of Medicine
Johnson City, Tennessee

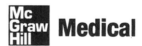 **Medical**

New York   Chicago   San Francisco   Lisbon   London   Madrid   Mexico City
Milan   New Delhi   San Juan   Seoul   Singapore   Sydney   Toronto

The McGraw·Hill Companies

Pathology: PreTest™ Self-Assessment and Review, Twelfth Edition

1 2 3 4 5 6 7 8 9 0 DOC/DOC 0 9 8 7

ISBN-13: 978-0-07-147182-4
ISBN-10:   0-07-147182-0

This book was set in Berkeley by International Typesetting and Composition.
The editors were Catherine A. Johnson and Regina Y. Brown.
The production supervisor was Sherri Souffrance.
Project management was provided by International Typesetting and Composition.
The cover designer was Maria Scharf.
Cover photo: Red Blood Cells: © Image Source / Alamy (RF)
RR Donnelley was printer and binder.

This book is printed on acid-free paper.

Library of Congress Cataloging-in-Publication Data

Pathology: PreTest self-assessment and review / [edited by] Earl J. Brown.—12th ed.
    p. ; cm.
  Includes bibliographical references and index.
  ISBN-13: 978-0-07-147182-4 (pbk. : alk. paper)
  ISBN-10: 0-07-147182-0 (pbk. : alk. paper)
  1. Pathology—Examinations, questions, etc. I. Brown, Earl, 1956-.
  [DNLM: 1. Pathology—Examination Questions. QZ 18.2 P297   2007]
RB31.P325 2007
616.07076—dc22   2006033367

Contents

Urinary System

Reproductive Systems

Endocrine System

Skin

Musculoskeletal System

Nervous System

Student Reviewers

Amy S. Arrington, PhD
Baylor College of Medicine
Class of 2007

Silke Heinisch
Temple University School of Medicine
Class of 2010

Farrant Sakaguchi
University of Utah
Class of 2008

Dedication

To Steve and Luke, who showed me that the race is not always won by the young and swift, but sometimes by those who persevere and keep on running, and to Karen, who reminded me that running fast is so much better than running slowly.

Laboratory Values

Substance	Source	Normal
Albumin	Serum	3.2–4.5 g/dL
Alkaline phosphatase	Serum	20–130 IU/L
Bicarbonate	Plasma	21–28 mM
Bilirubin, direct (conjugated)	Serum	<0.3 mg/dL
Bilirubin, indirect (unconjugated)	Serum	0.1–1.0 mg/dL
Bilirubin, total	Serum	0.1–1.2 mg/dL
BUN	Serum	8–23 mg/dL
Calcium	Serum	9.2–11.0 mg/dL (4.6–5.5 meq/L)
Chloride	Serum	95–103 meq/L
Cholesterol	Serum	150–250 mg/dL
Creatinine	Serum	0.6–1.2 mg/dL
GGT (γ-glutamyltransferase)	Serum	5–40 IU/L
Glucose (fasting)	Serum	70–110 mg/dL
Insulin	Plasma	4–24 μIU/mL
Iron	Serum	60–150 μg/dL
Iron saturation	Serum	20–55%
Osmolality	Serum	280–295 mosm/L
Phosphorus	Serum	2.3–4.7 mg/dL
Potassium	Plasma	3.8–5.0 meq/L
Protein	Serum	6.0–7.8 g/dL
Sodium	Plasma	136–142 meq/L
T_3 resin uptake	Serum	25–38 relative % uptake
Thyrotropin (TSH)	Serum	0.5–5 μIU/mL
Thyroxine, free (FT$_4$)	Serum	0.9–2.3 ng/dL
Thyroxine, total (T$_4$)	Serum	5.5–12.5 μg/dL
Triiodothyronine (T$_3$)	Serum	80–200 mg/dL

Hematology

Platelet count		150,000–450,000/μL
White cell count		4,440–11,000/μL
Lymphocyte count		1,000–4,800/μL (about 34%)
Mean corpuscular volume (MCV)		80–96 μm^3
Mean corpuscular hemoglobin (MCH)		27.5–33.2 pg
Mean corpuscular hemoglobin concentration (MCHC)		33.4–35.5%
Hemoglobin	Whole blood	Female 12–16 g/dL Male 13.5–18 g/dL

Preface

The study of pathology, a science so basic to clinical medicine, has been abbreviated sadly in many medical schools in recent years, and that too at a time when explosive growth is occurring in the science. Recent advances in immunopathology, diagnosis of bacterial and viral diseases including AIDS, and detection of infectious agents such as papillomavirus in cervical dysplasia are proceeding at a tremendous rate. The eleventh edition of *Pathology: PreTest™ Self-Assessment and Review* includes such new subject areas as predictive values in the interpretation of laboratory data, the importance of cytokines, the molecular basis of genetic and other disease processes, and molecular biology techniques as these apply to lymphoproliferative disorders and other tumors.

The medical student must feel submerged at times in the flood of information—occasionally instructors may have similar feelings. This edition is not intended to cover all new knowledge in addition to including older anatomic and clinical pathology. It is, rather, a serious attempt to present important facts about many disease processes in the hope that the student will read much further in major textbooks and journals and will receive some assistance in passing medical school, licensure, or board examinations.

Introduction

Each *PreTest™ Self-Assessment and Review* allows medical students to comprehensively and conveniently assess and review their knowledge of a particular basic science, in this instance pathology. The 500 questions parallel the format and degree of difficulty of the questions found in the United States Medical Licensing Examination (USMLE) Step 1. Practicing physicians who want to hone their skills before USMLE Step 3 or recertification may find this to be a good beginning in their review process. Each question is accompanied by an answer, a paragraph explanation, and a specific page reference to an appropriate textbook or journal article. A bibliography listing sources can be found following the last chapter of this text.

Each multiple-choice question in this book contains four or more possible answer options. In each case, select the ONE BEST ANSWER to the question.

An effective way to use this PreTest™ is to allow yourself one minute to answer each question in a given chapter. As you proceed, indicate your answer beside each question. By following this suggestion, you approximate the time limits imposed by the Step 1 exam.

After you finish going through the questions in the section, spend as much time as you need verifying your answers and carefully reading the explanations provided. Pay special attention to the explanations for the questions you answered incorrectly—but read every explanation. The author of this material has designed the explanations to reinforce and supplement the information tested by the questions. If you feel you need further information about the material covered, consult and study the references indicated.

The High-Yield Facts added for this edition are provided to facilitate rapid review of pathology topics. It is anticipated that the reader will use the High-Yield Facts as a "memory jog" before proceeding through the questions.

High-Yield Facts
in Pathology

I. CELL INJURY

a. Reversible Cell Injury

- swelling of cell organelles and entire cell
- dissociation of ribosomes from endoplasmic reticulum
- decreased energy production by mitochondria
- increased glycolysis → decreased pH → nuclear chromatin clumping

b. Irreversible Cell Injury

- irreversible damage to cell membranes and mitochondria
- influx of calcium into mitochondria; forms dense bodies (flocculent densities in heart)
- release of cellular enzymes (e.g., SGOT, LDH, and CPK after MI)
- nuclear degeneration (pyknosis, karyolysis, karyorrhexis)
- cell death

2. FATTY CHANGE OF THE LIVER (STEATOSIS; FATTY METAMORPHOSIS)

a. Mechanisms

1. Increased delivery of free fatty acids to liver
   - starvation
   - corticosteroids
   - diabetes mellitus

2. Increased formation of triglycerides
   - alcohol (note: NADH > NAD)

3. Decreased formation of apoproteins
   - carbon tetrachloride
   - protein malnutrition (kwashiorkor)

3. CELL DEATH

a. Apoptosis

1. Characteristics
   - "programmed" cell death
   - single cells (not large groups of cells)
   - cells shrink → form apoptotic bodies
   - gene activation → forms endonucleases
   - peripheral condensation of chromatin with DNA ladder
   - no inflammatory response

2. Mechanisms/phases
   a) initiation phase → caspases are activated
   b) execution phase → cell death occurs
      i. two distinct pathways
         i) extrinsic → receptor-mediated pathway
            - mediated by cell surface death receptors → type 1 TNF receptor (TNFR1) and Fas (CD95)
         ii) intrinsic (or mitochondrial) pathway
            - increased permeability of mitochondria → example is cytochrome c released into cytoplasm via bax channels

3. Examples of apoptosis:
   a) physiologic
      - involution of thymus
      - cell death within germinal centers of lymph nodes
      - fragmentation of endometrium during menses
      - lactating breast during weaning
   b) pathologic
      - viral hepatitis
      - cytotoxic T cell–mediated immune destruction (type IV hypersensitivity)

b. Necrosis

1. Characteristics
   - cause → hypoxia or toxins (irreversible injury)
   - many cells or clusters of cells
   - cells swell
   - inflammation present

2. Examples of necrosis:
- coagulative necrosis → ischemia (especially of the heart and kidney but not the brain)
- liquefactive necrosis → bacterial infection (and brain infarction)
- fat necrosis → pancreatitis and trauma to the breast
- caseous necrosis → tuberculosis
- fibrinoid necrosis → autoimmune disease (type III hypersensitivity reaction)
- gangrene → ischemia to extremities → dry (mainly coagulative necrosis) or wet (mainly liquefactive necrosis due to bacterial infection)

4. TERMS

a. Cellular Adaptation
- hypertrophy → increase in the size of cells
- hyperplasia → increase in the number of cells
- atrophy → decrease in the size of an organ
- aplasia → failure of cell production
- hypoplasia → decrease in the number of cells
- metaplasia → replacement of one cell type by another
- dysplasia → abnormal cell growth

b. Abnormal Organ Development
- anlage → primitive mass of cells
- aplasia → complete failure of an organ to develop (anlage present)
- agenesis → complete failure of an organ to develop (no anlage present)
- hypoplasia → reduction in the size of an organ due to a decrease in the number of cells
- atrophy → decrease in the size of an organ due to a decrease in the size or number of preexisting cells

5. STEM CELLS (LOCATIONS ARE CALLED NICHES)
- liver → oval cells in the canals of Hering of the liver
- muscle → satellite cells in the basal lamina of myotubules
- cornea → limbus cells in the canals of Schlemm
- colon → base of the crypts
- brain → dentate gyrus of the hippocampus

6. CARDINAL SIGNS OF INFLAMMATION

- rubor → red (vasodilation)
- calor → hot (increased blood flow)
- tumor → swollen (fluid accumulation)
- dolor → pain (bradykinin, and the like.)

7. COMPLEMENT CASCADE

a. Products
- C3b → opsonin
- C5a → chemotaxis and leukocyte activation
- C3a, C4a, C5a → anaphylatoxins
- C5–9 → membrane attack complex

b. Deficiencies
- deficiency of C3 and C5 → recurrent pyogenic bacterial infections
- deficiency of C6, C7, and C8 → recurrent infections with *Neisseria* species
- deficiency of C1 esterase inhibitor → hereditary angioedema
- deficiency of decay-accelerating factor → paroxysmal nocturnal hemoglobinuria

8. THROMBOXANE VS. PROSTACYCLIN

a. Thromboxane (TxA2)
- produced by platelets
- causes vasoconstriction
- stimulates platelet aggregation

b. Prostacyclin (PGI2)
- produced by endothelial cells
- causes vasodilation
- inhibits platelet aggregation

9. GRANULOMATOUS INFLAMMATION

a. Caseating Granulomas
- aggregates of activated macrophages (epithelioid cells)
- tuberculosis

b. Noncaseating Granulomas
- sarcoidosis
- fungal infections
- foreign-body reaction

10. COLLAGEN TYPES

a. Fibrillar Collagens
- type I → skin, bones, tendons, mature scars
- type II → cartilage
- type III → embryonic tissue, blood vessels, pliable organs, immature scars

b. Amorphous Collagens
- type IV → basement membranes
- type VI → connective tissue

11. EDEMA

a. Exudates
1. Composition
   - increased protein
   - increased cells
   - specific gravity greater than 1.020
2. Cause
   - inflammation
   - increased blood vessel permeability
3. Examples
   - inflammatory edema of lung → bacterial pneumonia
   - inflammatory edema of pleural cavity → empyema

b. Transudates
1. Composition
   - no increased protein
   - no increased cells
   - specific gravity less than 1.012
2. Cause → abnormality of Starling forces
   a) increased hydrostatic (venous) pressure
   - congestive heart failure
   - portal hypertension
   b) decreased oncotic pressure → due to decreased albumin
   - liver disease
   - renal disease (nephrotic syndrome)

   c) lymphatic obstruction
- tumors or surgery
- filaria

12. CARCINOMAS

a. Squamous Cell Carcinoma
- skin cancer
- lung cancer
- esophageal cancer
- cervical cancer

b. Adenocarcinoma
- lung cancer
- colon cancer
- stomach cancer
- prostate cancer
- endometrial cancer

c. Transitional Cell Carcinoma
- urinary bladder cancer
- renal cancer (renal pelvis)

d. Clear Cell Carcinoma
- renal cortex
- vaginal cancer (associated with DES)

e. Signet Cell Carcinoma → stomach cancer

13. NEOPLASMS

a. Benign
- grow slowly
- remain localized
- may have well-developed fibrous capsule
- do not metastasize
- well differentiated histologically

b. Malignant
- grow rapidly
- locally invasive

- irregular growth; no capsule
- capable of metastasis
- variable degrees of differentiation (well differentiated, moderately differentiated, poorly differentiated)

14. ONCOGENE EXPRESSION

a. Growth Factors

1. *c-sis*
   - β chain of platelet-derived growth factor
   - astrocytomas and osteogenic sarcomas

b. Growth Factor Receptors

1. *c-erb B1*
   - receptor for epidermal growth factor
   - breast cancer and squamous cell carcinoma of the lung

2. *c-neu*
   - receptor for epidermal growth factor
   - breast cancer

3. *c-fms*
   - receptor for colony-stimulating factor (CSF)
   - leukemia

c. Abnormal Membrane Protein Kinase

1. *c-abl*
   - membrane tyrosine kinase
   - chronic myelocytic leukemia (CML); on chromosome 9 → t(9;22)

d. GTP-Binding Proteins

1. *c-ras*
   - product is p21 (protein)
   - adenocarcinomas

e. Nuclear Regulatory Proteins

- *c-myc* → Burkitt's lymphoma; on chromosome 8 → t(8;14)
- *N-myc* → neuroblastoma
- *L-myc* → small cell carcinoma of the lung
- *c-jun*
- *c-fos*

15. CHROMOSOMES AND CANCER

a. Point Mutations
- *c-ras* → adenocarcinomas

b. Translocations
- *c-abl* on chromosome 9 → CML → t(9;22)
- *c-myc* on chromosome 8 → Burkitt's lymphoma → t(8;14)
- *bcl-2* on chromosome 18 → nodular lymphoma → t(14;18)
- *bcl-1*-PRAD1, cyclin D1) on chromosome 11 → mantle cell lymphoma → t(11;14)
- RAR (retinoic acid receptor) → acute promyelocytic leukemia (M3 AML) → t(15;17)
- EWS gene on chromosome 22 → Ewing's sarcoma → t(11;22) forms fusion gene EWS-FLI1

c. Gene Amplification
- *N-myc* → neuroblastoma
- *c-neu* → breast cancer
- *c-erb B2* → breast cancer

16. ANTIONCOGENES

a. Tumor Suppressor Genes
- Rb → retinoblastoma and osteogenic sarcoma (osteosarcoma)
- p53 → many tumors and the Li-Fraumeni syndrome
- WT1 → Wilms' tumor and aniridia
- NF1 → neurofibromatosis type 1
- NF2 → neurofibromatosis type 2; product of NF2 is merlin

17. CARCINOGENS

a. Chemicals
1. Initiators
   - tobacco smoke → many tumors
   - alkylating agents (anti-cancer drugs) → many tumors
   - benzene → leukemias
   - vinyl chloride → angiosarcomas of the liver
   - beta-naphthylamine → cancer of the urinary bladder
   - azo dyes → tumors of the liver
   - aflatoxin → hepatoma

- asbestos → mesotheliomas and lung tumors
- arsenic → skin cancer

2. Promoters
   - saccharin → bladder cancer in rats
   - hormones (estrogen)

b. Viruses

1. RNA Viruses
   - acute-transforming viruses
   - slow-transforming viruses
   - HTLV-1 → adult T-cell leukemia/lymphoma

2. DNA Viruses
   a. HPV (histologically see koilocytosis)
      - cervical neoplasia (types 16 and 18)
      - condyloma (types 6 and 11)
      - verruca vulgaris
   b. EBV
      - African Burkitt's lymphoma
      - carcinoma of the nasopharynx
      - B cell immunoblastic lymphoma
   c. Hepatitis B and hepatitis C
      - liver cancer
   d. HHV 8 (Kaposi sarcoma-associated herpesvirus)
      - Kaposi sarcoma
   e. *H. pylori*
      - stomach cancer and lymphoma

c. Radiation

- UV radiation (UVB) produces pyrimidine (thymine) dimers in DNA
- ionizing radiation (x-rays and gamma rays) cause breaks in nucleic acids
- radon is associated with lung cancer in non-smokers

18. DNA REPAIR DEFECTS (CHROMOSOME INSTABILITY SYNDROMES)

a. Xeroderma Pigmentosa

- decreased endonuclease causing defect in repairing pyrimidine (thymidine) dimers caused by UV light
- individuals develop multiple skin cancers in sun exposed skin

b. Ataxia Telangiectasia
- sensitive to x-rays (increased risk lymphoid malignancies and leukemia)
- recurrent infections (due to decreased IgA levels), oculocutaneous telangiectasia, cerebellar ataxia

c. Fanconi Anemia
- increased sensitivity to DNA cross-linking agents (increased risk of leukemia)
- hypoplastic thumbs and radii, anemia with mental retardation, small eyes, small genitalia, and renal abnormalities

d. Bloom Syndrome
- severe immunodeficiency, growth retardation, and increased sensitivity to radiation
- short stature, "parrot"-beak nose, and facial ("butterfly") rash
- cell cultures → quadriradial configurations and increased sister chromatid exchange

19. PARANEOPLASTIC SYNDROMES

- Cushing's syndrome (increased cortisol) → lung cancer
- carcinoid syndrome (increased serotonin) → lung cancer or carcinoid tumor of the small intestine
- syndrome of inappropriate ADH secretion (SIADH) → lung cancer and intracranial neoplasms
- hypercalcemia → lung cancer or multiple myeloma
- hypocalcemia → medullary carcinoma of the thyroid (secretes procalcitonin; stains as amyloid)
- hypoglycemia → liver cancer and tumors of the mesothelium (mesotheliomas)
- polycythemia (erythropoietin) → kidney tumors, liver tumors, and cerebellar vascular tumors

20. TUMOR MARKERS

a. α-Fetoprotein (AFP)
- liver cancer (hepatocellular carcinoma)
- germ cell tumors (e.g., yolk sac tumors, embryonal carcinoma, NOT seminoma)

b. β-HCG (Human Chorionic Gonadodotropin)
- gestational trophoblastic disease (e.g., choriocarcinoma, hydatidiform mole)
- dysgerminoma
- seminoma (10% of cases)

c. Prostate-Specific Antigen (PSA) and Prostatic Acid Phosphatase (PAP)
- adenocarcinoma of prostate

d. Carcinoembryonic Antigen (CEA)
- adenocarcinomas of colon, pancreas, stomach, and breast (nonspecific marker)

e. CA-125
- ovarian cancer

f. S-100
- melanoma
- neural tumors

21. PROTEIN-ENERGY MALNUTRITION (PEM)

a. Kwashiorkor
- dietary protein deficiency (without calorie deficiency)
- anasarca (generalized edema)
- fatty liver (due to decreased apoproteins and decreased VLDL synthesis)
- abnormal skin and hair
- defective enzyme formation → malabsorption (hard to treat)

b. Marasmus
- dietary calorie deficiency (without protein deficiency)
- generalized wasting ("skin and bones")

22. NUTRITIONAL DEFICIENCIES

a. Lipid Soluble
1. Vitamin A
   - night blindness
   - dry eyes and dry skin
   - recurrent infections

2. Vitamin D
   - decreased calcium
   - bone → decreased calcification, increased osteoid
   - children → rickets
   - adults → osteomalacia

3. Vitamin E
   - degeneration of posterior columns of spinal cord

4. Vitamin K
   - decreased vitamin K–dependent factors → II, VII, IX, X, and proteins C and S
   - increased bleeding
   - increased PT and PTT

b. **Water Soluble**

1. Vitamin B_1 (Thiamine)
   - beriberi → wet (cardiac) or dry (neurologic)
   - Wernicke-Korsakoff syndrome (lesions of mammillary bodies)

2. Vitamin B_3 (Niacin)
   - pellagra → 3Ds → dermatitis, dementia, diarrhea (and death)

3. Vitamin B_{12} (Cobalamin)
   - megaloblastic (macrocytic) anemia
   - hypersegmented neutrophils (>5 lobes)
   - subacute combined degeneration of the spinal cord

4. Vitamin C (Ascorbic Acid)
   - scurvy
   - defective collagen formation → poor wound healing (wounds reopen)
   - bone → decreased osteoid
   - perifollicular hemorrhages ("corkscrew" hair)
   - bleeding gums and loose teeth

5. Folate
   - megaloblastic (macrocytic) anemia
   - hypersegmented neutrophils
   - associated with neural tube defects in utero

6. Iron→ microcytic hypochromic anemia (with increased TIBC)

23. INHERITANCE PATTERNS

a. Autosomal Dominant (AD)

- disease produced in heterozygous state
- no skipped generations → parents affected (unless new mutation or reduced penetrance)
- father-to-son transmission possible
- males and females affected equally
- recurrence risk is 50% (one parent usually affected and one normal)

b. Autosomal Recessive (AR)

- disease produced in homozygous state
- heterozygous individuals are carriers
- generations may be skipped (not affected)
- father-to-son transmission possible
- males and females affected equally
- recurrence risk is 25% (both parents are usually heterozygous carriers)

c. X-Linked Dominant (XD)

- no skipped generations
- no male-to-male transmission
- females affected twice as often as males

d. X-Linked Recessive (XR)

- skipped generations
- no male-to-male transmission
- males affected more frequently than females

e. Y Inheritance

- only males affected
- only male-to-male transmission
- all males affected

f. Mitochondrial

- males and females equally affected
- only females transmit the disease

24. EXAMPLES OF XR

a. Hematology Diseases
- glucose-6-phosphate dehydrogenase (G6PD) deficiency
- hemophilia A (deficiency of factor VIII)
- hemophilia B (deficiency of factor IX)

b. Immunodeficiency Diseases
- Bruton agammaglobulinemia
- chronic granulomatous disease
- Wiskott-Aldrich syndrome

c. Storage Diseases
- Fabry's disease
- Hunter's syndrome

d. Muscle Diseases
1. Duchenne's muscular dystrophy
   - defective dystrophin gene (muscle breakdown)
   - pseudohypertrophy of calf muscles
   - Gower maneuver (using hands to rise from floor)
2. Becker's muscular dystrophy

e. Metabolic Diseases
- diabetes insipidus
- Lesch-Nyhan syndrome

f. Other Diseases
- red-green color blindness
- fragile X syndrome
- Menkes "kinky hair" syndrome → inability to transport copper within cells

25. CHROMOSOMES

a. Terms
- haploid → number of chromosomes in germ cells (23)
- diploid → number of chromosomes found in nongerm cells (46)
- euploid → any exact multiple of the haploid number
- aneuploid → any nonmultiple of the haploid number

- triploid → three times the haploid number (69)
- tetraploid → four times the haploid number (92)
- trisomy → three copies of the same chromosome

26. AUTOSOMAL TRISOMIES

a. Trisomy 13 (Patau's Syndrome)
- mental retardation
- microcephaly and microphthalmia
- holoprosencephaly (fused forebrain)
- fused central face ("cyclops")
- cleft lip and palate
- heart defects

b. Trisomy 18 (Edwards' Syndrome)
- mental retardation
- micrognathia
- heart defects
- rocker-bottom feet
- clenched fist with overlapping fingers

c. Trisomy 21 (Down Syndrome)
- most cases due to maternal nondisjunction during meiosis I (associated with increased maternal age)
- minority of cases due to Robertsonian (balanced) translocation
- mental retardation (most common familial cause)
- oblique palpebral fissures with epicanthal folds
- horizontal palmar crease
- heart defects (endocardial cushion defect is most common)
- acute lymphoblastic leukemia (first 2 years of life)
- Alzheimer's disease (almost 100% incidence after age 35)
- duodenal atresia ("double-bubble" sign on x-ray)
- increased susceptibility to infections

27. CHROMOSOMAL DELETIONS

a. 5p- (Cri du Chat)
- high-pitched cry
- mental retardation
- heart defects and microcephaly

b. 11p- → WT1 Gene (Wilms' tumor)
- WAGR syndrome → Wilms' tumor, aniridia, genital abnormalities, and mental retardation
- Denys-Drash syndrome → Wilms' tumor, gonadal dysgenesis and renal failure

c. 13q- → retinoblastoma

d. 15q- (Imprinted gene is inactivated, usually by methylation)

1. Maternal deletion (paternal gene is imprinted) → Angelman's syndrome
   - deletion involves maternal UBE3A gene
   - stiff, ataxic gait with jerky movements
   - inappropriate laughter ("happy puppets")
   - may be due to two copies of paternal 15 chromosome (paternal uniparental disomy)

2. Paternal deletion (maternal gene is imprinted) → Prader-Willi syndrome
   - mental retardation
   - short stature and obesity
   - small hands and feet
   - hypogonadism
   - may be due to two copies of maternal 15 chromosome (paternal uniparental disomy)

28. PAX (PAIRED BOX) GENES
- PAX-2 → "renal-coloboma" syndrome
- PAX-3 → Waardenburg syndrome (white forelocks of hair; eye colors don't match)
- PAX-5 → lymphoplasmacytoid lymphoma
- PAX-6 → aniridia and Wilms' syndrome
- PAX-8 → follicular thyroid carcinoma
- PAX-9 → congenital absence of teeth

29. HYPOGONADISM
a. Klinefelter's Syndrome
- most common genotype is 47,XXY
- male hypogonadism
- testicular dysgenesis → small, firm, atrophic testes

- decreased testosterone
- increased FSH, LH, estradiol
- decreased secondary male characteristics
- tallness, gynecomastia, and female distribution of hair
- infertility

b. Turner's Syndrome

- most common genotype is 45,XO
- female hypogonadism
- ovarian dysgenesis → streak ovaries (due to lack of two X chromosomes)
- decreased estrogen
- increased LH, FSH
- primary amenorrhea
- decreased secondary female characteristics (due to decreased estrogen)
- skeletal abnormalities → short stature; haploinsufficiency of the short stature homeobox (SHOX) gene
- web neck (cystic hygroma)

30. AMBIGUOUS SEXUAL DEVELOPMENT

a. True Hermaphrodite

- ovaries and testes both present

b. Female Pseudohermaphrodite (XX Individual)

1. Congenital Adrenal Hyperplasia (in an XX Individual)
   - development of ovaries (due to two X chromosomes)
   - Müllerian duct development (due to lack of MIF)
   - Wolffian duct regression (due to lack of local testosterone production)
   - external male (due to excess systemic formation of DHT)

c. Male Pseudohermaphrodite (XY Individual)

1. Isolated deficiency of MIS (Mullerian Inhibiting Substance)
   - phenotypic male with inguinal hernia and impalpable contralateral gonad
   - uterus and fallopian tube in the hernia sac
   - normal levels of testosterone; bilateral vas deferens present

2. Androgen Insensitivity Syndrome (XY Individual)
   - testicular feminization
   - Müllerian duct regression (due to MIF)
   - Wolffian duct regression (due to lack of testosterone receptors)
   - phenotypic female (due to lack of receptors for DHT)
3. Decreased 5-alpha-Reductase (XY Individual)
   - formation of testes (due to presence of Y chromosome)
   - Müllerian duct regression (due to MIF)
   - Wolffian duct development (due to testosterone)
   - decreased DHT (due to lack of 5-alpha-reductase)
   - variable external genitalia (due to decreased DHT)

31. DISORDERS OF TRINUCLEOTIDE REPEATS

a. Fragile X Syndrome → CGG repeats
   - mental retardation (second most common familial cause; trisomy 21 is first)
   - long face with large ears
   - large testes (macroorchidism)
   - trinucleotide sequence expanded in females, not males

b. Huntington's Syndrome → CAG repeats

c. Myotonic Dystrophy → GCT repeats

d. Friedreich Ataxia → expansion of frataxin gene

e. Spinal-Bulbar Muscular Atrophy → CAG repeats

32. LYMPHOCYTES

a. B Cells
   - form plasma cells that secrete immunoglobulin
   - surface antigen receptor composed of immunoglobulin
   - rearrange immunoglobulin genes from germ line configuration
   - CD19 → pan–B cell marker
   - CD20 → pan–B cell marker, also called L26
   - CD21 → pan–B cell marker, receptor for EBV
   - CD22 → pan–B cell marker

b. **T Cells**
- secrete lymphokines
- surface antigen receptor (TCR) is attached to CD3
- rearrange genes for T-cell receptor
- CD2 → receptor for sheep erythrocyte (E rosette)
- CD3 → attached to T-cell receptor
- CD4 → helper T cells, bind with MHC class II antigens
- CD5 → pan–T-cell marker
- CD7 → pan–T-cell marker
- CD8 → cytotoxic T cells, bind with MHC class I antigens

c. **Natural Killer Cells**
- large granular lymphocytes
- do not need previous sensitization
- CD16 → receptor for Fc portion of IgG

33. IMMUNOGLOBULINS

a. **IgM**
- large molecule (pentamer)
- secreted early in immune response (primary response)
- cannot cross the placenta
- can activate complement
- contains a J chain

b. **IgG**
- most abundant immunoglobulin in serum
- secreted during second antigen exposure →secondary or amnestic response)
- can cross the placenta
- can activate complement
- can function as opsonin

c. **IgE**
- allergies, asthma, parasitic infection
- found attached to the surface of basophils and mast cells
- participates in type I hypersensitivity reactions

d. IgA
- usually a dimer with a J chain and a secretory component
- found along GI tract and respiratory tract
- secretory immunoglobulin
- can activate alternate complement pathway

E. IgD
- receptor for B cells
- found on the surface of mature B cells

34. T LYMPHOCYTES

a. CD4+ Cells

1. Characteristics
   - helper T lymphocytes
   - respond to MHC class II antigens
2. Subtypes:
   a) T helper-1 (T_H1) cells
      - secrete → IL-2, IL-3, GM-CSF, δ-interferon, and lymphotoxin (β-TNF)
      - stimulate cell-mediated immune reactions → fight intracellular organisms
   b) T helper-2 (T_H2) cells
      - secrete → IL-3, IL-4, IL-5, IL-6, IL-10, and GM-CSF
      - stimulate antibody production → fight extracellular organisms

b. CD8+ Cells
- cytotoxic T lymphocytes
- respond to MHC class I antigens

35. MAJOR HISTOCOMPATIBILITY COMPLEX (MHC)

a. Class I Antigens
- found on all nucleated cells
- transmembrane α-glycoprotein chain with β2-microglobulin
- react with antibodies and CD8-positive lymphocytes
- fight virus-infected cells and transplants

b. Class II Antigens

- found on antigen-presenting cells, B cells, and T cells
- transmembrane α chain and β chain
- react with CD4-positive lymphocytes
- fight exogenous antigens that have been processed by antigen-presenting cells

36. DISEASES ASSOCIATED WITH HLA TYPES

- ankylosing spondylitis → HLA-B27
- primary hemochromatosis → HLA-A3
- 21-hydroxylase deficiency → HLA-BW47
- rheumatoid arthritis → HLA-DR4
- insulin-dependent (type I) diabetes mellitus → HLA-DR3/DR4
- systemic lupus erythematosus → HLA-DR2/DR3

37. HYPERSENSITIVITY REACTIONS

a. Type I

- binding of antigen to previously formed IgE bound to mast cells and basophils
- release of histamine and leukotrienes C4 and D4
- urticaria (hives)
- anaphylaxis

b. Type II

- antibody (IgG or IgM) binds to antigens in situ
- cells destroyed by complement or cytotoxic cells (antibody-dependent cell-mediated cytotoxicity)
- linear immunofluorescence (IF)
- transfusion reactions, Goodpasture's disease, Pemphigus vulgaris, and the like.

c. Type III

- antibody (IgG or IgM) binds to antigens forming immune complexes
- granular IF
- systemic → serum sickness
- local reaction → Arthus reaction

d. Type IV

1. Delayed type hypersensitivity
   - CD4 lymphocytes
   - extrinsic antigen associated with class II MHC
   - formation of activated macrophages (epithelioid cells) → granulomas
   - PPD skin test
   - contact dermatitis (poison ivy, poison oak)

2. Cell-mediated immunity
   - CD8 lymphocytes
   - intrinsic antigen associated with class I MHC
   - viral infections and transplant rejection

38. AUTOANTIBODIES

a. Nuclear

- diffuse (homogenous) → DNA (many diseases), histones (drug-induced SLE)
- rim (peripheral) → double-stranded DNA (SLE)
- speckled (non-DNA extractable nuclear proteins) → Smith (SLE), SS-A and SS-B (Sjögren syndrome), Scl-70 (progressive systemic sclerosis)
- nucleolar (RNA) → many (e.g., progressive systemic sclerosis)
- centromere → CREST syndrome

b. Cytoplasmic

- mitochondria → primary biliary cirrhosis

c. Cells

- smooth muscle → lupoid hepatitis (autoimmune chronic active hepatitis)
- neutrophils → Wegener's granulomatosis and microscopic polyarteritis
- parietal cell and intrinsic factor → pernicious anemia
- microvasculature of muscle → dermatomyositis

d. Proteins

- immunoglobulin → rheumatoid arthritis
- thyroglobulin → Hashimoto's thyroiditis
- GM-CSF → pulmonary alveolar proteinosis (PAP)

e. Structural Antigens

- lung and glomerular basement membranes → Goodpasture's disease
- intercellular space of epidermis → pemphigus vulgaris
- epidermal basement membrane → bullous pemphigoid

f. Receptors
- acetylcholine receptor → myasthenia gravis
- thyroid hormone receptor → Graves' disease
- insulin receptor → diabetes mellitus

39. ANTINEUTROPHIL CYTOPLASMIC ANTIBODIES (ANCAs)

a. C-ANCAs (cytoplasmic)
- proteinase 3 → Wegener's granulomatosis

b. P-ANCAs (perinuclear)
- myeloperoxidase → microscopic polyarteritis

40. AMYLOIDOSIS

a. Amyloid
- any protein having β-pleated sheet tertiary configuration
- apple-green birefringence with Congo red stain

b. Systemic Deposition
- multiple myeloma → deposits of amyloid light (AL) protein
- chronic inflammatory diseases → deposits of amyloid-associated (AA) protein
- hemodialysis → deposits of β2-microglobulin (a component of MHC class I antigens)

c. Localized Deposition
- senile cardiac disease → deposits of amyloid transthyretin (ATTR)
- Alzheimer's disease → deposits of β2-amyloid protein
- medullary carcinoma of thyroid → deposits of procalcitonin
- non–insulin-dependent diabetes mellitus (type II) → deposits of AIAPP (islet amyloid peptide) in islets of Langerhans of pancreas

41. DEFECTS IN INFLAMMATION OR IMMUNITY

a. Chédiak-Higashi Syndrome
- autosomal recessive
- defective polymerization of microtubules
- giant lysosomes in leukocytes
- recurrent infections
- albinism (abnormal formation of melanin)

b. **Chronic Granulomatous Disease**
   - defective NADPH oxidase (enzyme on membrane of lysosomes)
   - recurrent infections with catalase-positive organisms
   - abnormal nitroblue tetrazolium dye test

c. **Severe Combined Immunodeficiency (SCID)**
   1. General
      - decrease involves both T cells and B cells
      - infections with viruses, fungi, and bacteria
   2. X-linked form
      - mutation in common gamma chain subunit of cytokine receptors
      - cytokine receptor that is mainly responsible for this defect is the receptor for interleukin-7
   3. Autosomal recessive forms
      a) Swiss type
         - lack of adenosine deaminase
         - prenatal diagnosis and gene therapy possible
      b) Omenn syndrome
         - mutations in the RAG-1 and RAG-2 genes
         - inability to rearrange the VDJ regions in the T-cell and B-cell receptors

d. **X-Linked Agammaglobulinemia of Bruton (XLA)**
   - mutation involving cytoplasmic Bruton tyrosine kinase (BTK)
   - defective maturation of B lymphocytes past the pre-B stage
   - absence of germinal centers and plasma cells
   - bacterial infections begin at the age of 9 months (loss of maternal antibody)
   - therapy with immunoglobulin injections

e. **Common Variable Immunodeficiency (CVID)**
   - variable clinical presentation
   - recurrent infections → especially bacteria and Giardia
   - hyperplastic B cell areas
   - therapy with immunoglobulin injections

f. Isolated Deficiency of IgA
- probably the most common form of immunodeficiency
- most patients are asymptomatic
- may develop anti–IgA antibodies
- risk of anaphylaxis with transfusion

g. DiGeorge's Syndrome
- defective development of pharyngeal pouches 3 and 4
- deletion of chromosome 22
- lack of thymus → no T cells (recurrent viral and fungal infections)
- lack of parathyroid glands → hypocalcemia and tetany
- think "CATCH-22": Cardiac abnormalities, Abnormal facies (hypertelorism, low set ears, prominent nose), T-cell defects (secondary to abnormal development of the thymus), Cleft palate, Hypocalcemia (secondary to primary hypoparathyroidism)

h. Wiskott-Aldrich Syndrome (WAS)
- mutation in gene that codes for the Wiskott-Aldrich syndrome protein (WASP)
- recurrent pyogenic infections, eczema, and thrombocytopenia
- progressive loss of T-cell function and decreased IgM

i. Acquired Immunodeficiency Syndrome (AIDS)
- cause → HIV infection
- infection of CD4 T lymphocytes
- inversion of CD4/CD8 ratio (normal is 2:1)
- decreased humoral and cell-mediated immunity → recurrent infections
- increased incidence of malignancy (Kaposi's sarcoma and immunoblastic lymphoma)

42. VIRAL CHANGES
a. Giant Cells
- herpes simplex virus (HSV)
- cytomegalovirus (CMV)
- measles (Warthin-Finkeldey giant cells)
- respiratory syncytial virus
- HIV → in brain due to fusion of microglial cells

b. Inclusions
- herpes simplex virus (Cowdry A bodies)
- smallpox virus (Guarnieri's bodies)
- rabies virus (Negri bodies)
- molluscum contagiosum (molluscum bodies)

c. Ground-Glass Change
- nucleus → herpes simplex virus
- cytoplasm (of hepatocytes) → hepatitis B

d. Atypical Cells
- atypical lymphocytes → Epstein-Barr virus
- smudge cells → adenovirus (respiratory epithelial cells)
- koilocytosis → human papillomavirus (HPV)

43. SYSTEMIC MYCOSES

a. Candidiasis
- *Candida albicans*
- pseudohypha
- white plaques (thrush)

b. Histoplasmosis
- *Histoplasma capsulatum*
- found within the cytoplasm of macrophages
- bird droppings; bat guano in caves
- Ohio and Mississippi valleys

c. Aspergillosis
- *Aspergillus* species
- septate hyphae with acute-angle branching
- fruiting bodies (when exposed to air → fungus ball in lung cavity)

d. Blastomycosis
- *Blastomyces dermatitidis*
- broad-based budding
- eastern United States

e. Coccidioidomycosis
- *Coccidioides immitis*
- large spherules filled with many small endospores
- southwestern United States (San Joaquin Valley)

f. Cryptococcosis
- *Cryptococcus neoformans*
- CNS infection in immunosuppressed patients
- mucicarmine-positive capsule
- India ink stain of CSF

g. Mucormycosis
- nasal infection in diabetic patients
- broad, nonseptate hyphae with right-angle branching

44. FAMILIAL HYPERLIPIDEMIA

a. Type I Hyperlipoproteinemia
- familial hyperchylomicronemia
- mutation in lipoprotein lipase gene
- increased serum chylomicrons

b. Type II Hyperlipoproteinemia
- familial hypercholesterolemia
- mutation involving LDL receptor
- increased serum LDL
- increased serum cholesterol

c. Type III Hyperlipidemia
- floating or broad beta disease
- mutation in apolipoprotein E
- increased chylomicron remnants and IDL
- increased serum triglycerides and cholesterol

d. Type IV Hyperlipidemia
- familial hypertriglyceridemia
- unknown mutation
- increased serum VLDL
- increased serum triglycerides and cholesterol

e. Type V Hyperlipidemia
- mutation in apolipoprotein CII
- increased serum chylomicrons and VLDL
- increased serum triglycerides and cholesterol

45. ANEURYSMS

a. Atherosclerotic Aneurysms
- cause → atherosclerosis
- location → abdominal aorta (between renal arteries and bifurcation of the aorta)
- pulsatile mass
- may rupture → sudden, severe abdominal pain in male older than 55
- treat with surgery when diameter is >5 cm

b. Luetic Aneurysms
- cause → syphilis (treponema) infection
- obliterative endarteritis (plasma cells around small blood vessels)
- location → ascending (thoracic) aorta
- may produce aortic regurgitation or rupture

c. Dissecting Aneurysms
1. Due to cystic medial necrosis of aorta
   - hypertension
   - Marfan's syndrome → due to defect in fibrillin gene
2. "Double-barrel" aorta on x-ray

d. Berry Aneurysms
- location → bifurcation of arteries in circle of Willis
- most commonly bifurcation of anterior communicating artery
- subarachnoid hemorrhage
- associated with polycystic renal disease

46. CARDIAC HYPERTROPHY

a. Concentric Hypertrophy
- response to pressure overload (e.g., hypertension or aortic stenosis)
- sarcomeres proliferate in parallel
- increased ventricular thickness
- no change in size of ventricular cavity

b. Eccentric Hypertrophy
- response to volume overload
- sarcomeres proliferate in series
- no increase in ventricle thickness
- increase in size of ventricular cavity

47. CONGENITAL HEART DEFECTS

a. Left-to-Right Shunts
1. Ventricular septal defect (VSD) → most common congenital cardiac anomaly
2. Atrial septal defect (ASD)
3. Patent ductus arteriosus (PDA)
   - "machine-like" heart murmur
   - indomethacin closes PDA

b. Right-to-Left Shunts
1. Tetralogy of Fallot (TOF) → most common cause of congenital cyanotic heart disease
   - pulmonary stenosis
   - ventricular septal defect
   - dextropositioned (overriding) aorta
   - right ventricular hypertrophy

c. No Shunts
1. Coarctation of the aorta
   - infantile type (preductal)
   - adult type (postductal) → rib notching, increased BP in upper extremities, decreased BP in lower extremities
2. Transposition of the great vessels
   - need shunt to be present in order to survive (e.g., PDA)
   - PGE keeps ductus open

48. ATROPHY OF THE STOMACH

a. Type A → Autoimmune Gastritis
- autoantibodies to parietal cells and intrinsic factor → pernicious anemia
- decreased vitamin B_{12} → megaloblastic anemia
- increased serum gastrin levels
- histologic changes found in fundus of stomach

b. **Type B** → **Environmental**
- no autoantibodies present
- associated with *Helicobacter pylori* (urease breath test is positive)
- decreased serum gastrin levels
- histologic changes found in antrum of stomach

49. INFLAMMATORY BOWEL DISEASE (IBD)

a. **Ulcerative Colitis**
- crypt abscesses (microabscesses) and crypt distortion
- disease begins in rectum and extends proximally (no skip lesions)
- does not involve small intestines
- superficial mucosal involvement (not transmural)
- increased risk of colon cancer and toxic megacolon

b. **Crohn's Disease**
- granulomas
- segmental involvement (skip lesions)
- may involve small intestines (regional enteritis or ileitis)
- transmural involvement → fissures, fistulas, and obstruction

50. GALLSTONES

a. **Cholesterol Stones**
- yellow stones
- risk factors → Fs → fat, female, fertile, forty, fifty
- increased incidence in Native Americans

b. **Bilirubin (Pigment) Stones**
- black stones
- risk factors → chronic hemolysis and infections of biliary tract
- increased incidence in Asians

51. CONGENITAL ADRENAL HYPERPLASIA (CAH)

a. **21-Hydroxylase Deficiency**
- decreased cortisol → increased ACTH
- decreased aldosterone
- sodium loss in the urine → salt-wasting form of CAH
- hyperkalemic acidosis
- virilism in females

b. 11-Hydroxylase Deficiency
- decreased cortisol → increased ACTH
- decreased aldosterone
- increased DOC and 11-deoxycortisol → increased mineralocorticoid effects
- sodium retention → hypertensive form of CAH
- hypokalemic alkalosis
- virilism in females

c. 17-Hydroxylase Deficiency
- decreased cortisol → increased ACTH
- no decreased aldosterone
- decreased sex hormones
- females → primary amenorrhea
- males → pseudohermaphrodites

52. MULTIPLE ENDOCRINE ABNORMALITIES

a. Multiple Endocrine Neoplasia (MEN)
1. Type 1 (Wermer's Syndrome)
   - parathyroid
   - pituitary
   - pancreas
2. Type 2 (Sipple's Syndrome)
   - parathyroid
   - medullary carcinoma of thyroid
   - pheochromocytoma
3. Type 3 (MEN 2B)
   - medullary carcinoma of thyroid
   - pheochromocytoma
   - mucosal neuromas
   - Marfanoid habitus

b. Autoimmune Polyendocrine Syndromes (APS)
1. Type I (APS1)
   - autoimmune adrenitis plus chronic mucocutaneous candidiasis and abnormalities of the skin, nails, and teeth (ectodermal dystrophy)

- also called APECED = autoimmune polyendocrinopathy, candidiasis, and ectodermal dystrophy
- mutations in AIRE-1 (autoimmune regulator) gene
- may also develop autoimmune hypoparathyroidism, idiopathic hypogonadism, and pernicious anemia

2. Type II (APS2)
   - autoimmune adrenalitis plus autoimmune thyroiditis (Hashimoto's thyroiditis) or type 1 diabetes mellitus

53. RENAL (GLOMERULAR) SYNDROMES
a. Nephrotic Syndrome

1. Characteristics
   - marked proteinuria → hypoalbuminemia and edema
   - increased cholesterol → oval fat bodies in the urine
2. Examples (nonproliferative glomerular disease):
   a) Minimal change disease (lipoid nephrosis)
      - normal light microscopy
      - EM reveals fusion of foot processes of podocytes
   b) Focal segmental glomerulosclerosis (FSGS)
      - may be associated with mutation of NPHS2 gene which codes for podocin
   c) Membranous glomerulonephropathy (MGN)
      - thickening of basement membrane ("spikes and domes")
      - uniform subepithelial deposits
   d) Diabetes mellitus

b. Nephritic Syndrome

1. Characteristics
   - hematuria (red blood cells and red blood cell casts in urine)
   - variable proteinuria and oliguria
   - retention of salt and water (hypertension and edema)
2. Examples (proliferative glomerular disease):
   a) Focal segmental glomerulonephritis (FSGN)
      - mesangial deposits of IgA
      - Berger's disease

b) Acute (diffuse) proliferative glomerulonephritis (DPGN)
  i. post-streptococcal glomerulonephritis
    • large, irregular subepithelial deposits
  ii. type IV lupus nephritis
    • subendothelial deposits form "wire-loop" lesions
c) Membranoproliferative glomerulonephritis (MPGN)
  • subendothelial deposits → type I MPGN
  • intramembranous deposits → type II MPGN (dense deposit disease)
  • splitting of basement membrane by mesangium → "tram-track" appearance
d) Rapidly progressive glomerulonephritis (RPGN)

54. GLOMERULAR DEPOSITS

a. Subepithelial
  • diffuse proliferative glomerulonephritis (DPGN) → irregular and large
  • membranous glomerulonephropathy (MGN) → uniform and small

b. Intramembranous (Basement Membrane)
  • membranoproliferative glomerulonephritis (MPGN), type II

c. Subendothelial
  • membranoproliferative glomerulonephritis, type I
  • SLE (WHO type IV)

d. Mesangial
  • focal segmental glomerulonephritis (FSGN)
  • Henoch-Schönlein purpura

55. RAPIDLY PROGRESSIVE GLOMERULONEPHRITIS (RPGN)

a. Linear Immunofluorescence
  • antimembrane antibody
  • Goodpasture's disease

b. Granular Immunofluorescence
  • immune complexes
  • other glomerular or systemic disease

c. **Minimal or Negative Immunofluorescence**
  - pauci-immune disease
  - Wegener's granulomatosis
  - microscopic polyarteritis nodosa

56. CEREBRAL HEMORRHAGE

a. **Epidural Hematoma (above the dura)**
  - severe trauma
  - arterial bleeding (middle meningeal artery)
  - symptoms occur rapidly

b. **Subdural Hematoma (below the dura)**
  - minimal trauma in elderly
  - venous bleeding (bridging veins)
  - symptoms occur slowly

c. **Subarachnoid Hemorrhage**
  - rupture of berry aneurysm
  - "worst headache ever"
  - bloody or xanthochromic spinal tap

57. INFECTIONS OF THE MENINGES

a. **Bacterial Infections**
  - increased neutrophils and protein in CSF
  - decreased glucose in CSF
  - life-threatening

Age	Organism
Neonates	*Escherichia coli*
6 months to 6 years	*Streptococcus pneumoniae*
6 years to 16 years	*Neisseria meningitidis* (meningococcus)
Older than 16 years	*Streptococcus pneumoniae*
Epidemics	*Neisseria meningitidis*

b. Viral Infections
- increased lymphocytes in CSF
- normal glucose in CSF
- mild and self-limited

58. ATROPHY OF THE NERVOUS SYSTEM

a. Alzheimer's Disease
- diffuse atrophy of cerebral cortex
- dementia (most common cause in elderly)
- senile plaques (with β-amyloid core)
- neurofibrillary tangles (with abnormal tau protein)

b. Pick's Disease
- unilateral frontal or temporal lobe atrophy

c. Huntington's Disease
- trinucleotide repeat disorder
- atrophy of caudate and putamen → decreased GABA and acetylcholine
- progressive dementia
- choreiform movements

d. Parkinson's Disease
- substantia nigra (depigmentation)
- decreased dopamine in corpus striatum
- cogwheel rigidity and akinesia
- tremor
- treatment → dopamine agonists

59. JOINTS

a. Rheumatoid Arthritis
- rheumatoid factor (IgM antibody against antibody)
- pannus formation in synovium (hyperplastic synovium with lymphocytes and plasma cells)
- ulnar deviation of fingers
- subcutaneous rheumatoid nodules (at pressure points)
- pain worse in morning ("morning stiffness"); pain decreases with activity

b. Osteoarthritis
- degenerative joint disease ("wear and tear")
- loss of articular cartilage → smooth subchondral bone (eburnation)
- osteophyte formation (DIP → Heberden's nodes, PIP → Bouchard's nodes)
- pain worse in evening; pain increases with activity

c. Gout
- hyperuricemia → precipitation of monosodium urate crystals (needle-shaped, negatively birefringent crystals)
- first MTP joint (big toe)
- tophus formation
- increased production of uric acid → Lesch-Nyhan syndrome
- increased turnover of nucleic acid → leukemias and lymphomas
- decreased excretion of uric acid → chronic renal disease, ethanol intake, diabetes

60. STAINS

a. Routine (H&E)
1. Hematoxylin
   - blue and basic
   - stains negatively charged structures → DNA and RNA
2. Eosin
   - pink and acidophilic
   - stains positively charged structures → mitochondria

b. Special Stains
- fats → oil red O
- glycogen → PAS-positive, diastase-sensitive
- iron → Prussian blue
- hemosiderin → Prussian blue
- amyloid → Congo red
- alpha1 antitrypsin → PAS-positive, diastase-resistant
- calcium → von Kossa

61. ENZYMES/LAB TESTS

a. Aminotransferases (AST, ALT)
- myocardial infarction (AST)
- alcoholic hepatitis (AST > ALT)
- viral hepatitis (ALT > AST)

b. **Creatine Kinase (CK or CPK)**
  • myocardial infarction (CPK-MB)
  • muscle diseases (DMD)

c. **Lactate Dehydrogenase (LDH) → myocardial infarction (LDH1 > LDH2)**

d. **Amylase or Lipase → acute pancreatitis**

e. **C-reactive Protein (CRP)**
  • can be used to differentiate bacterial infection (elevated CRP) from viral infection (decreased CRP)
  • used to monitor autoimmune disorders
  • determines the risk of developing cardiovascular diseases (stroke or myocardial infarction)

f. **Atrial Natriuretic Peptide (ANP)**
  • increased in patients with hypertension and congestive heart failure
  • serial measurements may help in the clinical management of congestive heart failure

g. **TIBC → increased with iron deficiency anemia**

h. **Hemoglobin A2 → increased with beta-thalassemia**

i. **Free Erythrocyte Porphyrin (FEP) → iron deficiency anemia and lead poisoning**

62. HISTOLOGIC "BODIES"

a. **Psammoma Body:**
  • papillary carcinoma of the thyroid
  • papillary tumors of the ovary
  • meningioma

b. **Immunoglobulin**
  • Russell body → cytoplasmic or extracellular
  • Dutcher body → nucleus (Waldenström's macroglobulinemia)

c. **Councilman's Body → viral hepatitis**

d. **Mallory Body → alcoholic hyaline (composed of prekeratin intermediate filaments)**

e. **Cowdry A Body → herpes**

f. **Aschoff's Body** → **rheumatoid fever**

g. **Ferruginous Body** → **asbestos (covered with iron)**

h. **Negri Body** → **rabies**

i. **Lewy Body** → **major component is alpha-synuclein**
   - nigrostriatal → Parkinson's
   - cerebral cortex → Lewy body dementia → the third most common cause of dementia
   - sympathetic neurons → Shy-Drager syndrome

j. **Heinz Body (denatured hemoglobin)** → **G6PD deficiency**

k. **Barr Body** → **number of X chromosomes minus one**

l. **Donovan Body** → **granuloma inguinale (caused by *Calymmatobacterium donovani*)**

m. **Asteroid Body** → **sarcoidosis**

n. **Prismatic Bodies** → **metachromatic leukodystrophy**

o. **Whorled Lamellar Bodies** → **Tay-Sachs**

p. **Call-Exner Bodies** → **granulosa cell tumor of the ovary**

63. HEALING OF THE MYOCARDIUM AFTER A MYOCARDIAL INFARCTION

	Gross	Microscopy
0–12 h	None	Usually none (?wavy fibers)
12–24 h	Pallor	Coagulative necrosis
1–3 days	Hyperemic (red) border	Above + neutrophils
4–7 days	Pale yellow	Above + macrophages
7–14 days	Red-purple border	Above + granulation tissue
>2 weeks	Gray-white scar	Fibrosis (scar)

64. FAMILIAL STORAGE DISORDERS

Storage Disease	Enzyme Deficiency	Substance Accumulating
Pompe's disease	α-1,4-glucosidase (acid maltase)	Glycogen
Hurler's syndrome	α-L-iduronidase	Heparan sulfate, dermatan sulfate
Hunter's syndrome	Iduronate-2-sulfatase	Heparan sulfate, dermatan sulfate
Niemann-Pick disease	Sphingomyelinase	Sphingomyelin
Tay-Sachs disease	Hexosaminidase A	G_{M2} ganglioside
Sandhoff's disease	Hexosaminidase A and B	G_{M2} ganglioside and globoside
Gaucher's disease	Glucocerebrosidase	Glucocerebroside
Fabry's disease	α-Galactosidase A	Ceramide trihexosidase

General Pathology

Questions

DIRECTIONS: Each item below contains a question or incomplete statement followed by suggested responses. Select the **one best** response to each question.

1. A 55-year-old male alcoholic presents with symptoms of liver disease and is found to have mildly elevated liver enzymes. A liver biopsy examined with a routine hematoxylin and eosin (H&E) stain reveals abnormal clear spaces in the cytoplasm of most of the hepatocytes. Which of the following materials is most likely forming these cytoplasmic spaces?

a. Calcium
b. Cholesterol
c. Hemosiderin
d. Lipofuscin
e. Triglyceride

2. An adult patient presents with the sudden onset of massive diarrhea. Grossly, this individual's stool has the appearance of "rice-water" because of the presence of flecks of mucus. Cultures of this patient's stool grow Vibrio cholerae, a curved gram-negative rod that secretes an enterotoxin consisting of a toxic A subunit and a binding B subunit. The cholera enterotoxin causes massive diarrhea through which one of the following mechanisms?

a. Inhibiting the conversion of Gi-GDP to Gi-GTP
b. Inhibiting the conversion of Gs-GTP to Gs-GDP
c. Stimulating the conversion of Gi-GDP to Gi-GTP
d. Stimulating the conversion of Gs-GDP to Gs-GTP
e. Stimulating the conversion of Gs-GTP to Gs-GDP

3. In an evaluation of an 8-year-old boy who has had recurrent infections since the first year of life, findings include enlargement of the liver and spleen, lymph node inflammation, and a superficial dermatitis resembling eczema. Microscopic examination of a series of peripheral blood smears taken during the course of a staphylococcal infection indicates that the bactericidal capacity of the boy's neutrophils is impaired or absent. Which of the following is the most likely cause of this child's illness?

a. Defect in the enzyme NADPH oxidase
b. Defect in the enzyme adenosine deaminase (ADA)
c. Defect in the IL-2 receptor
d. Developmental defect at the pre-B stage
e. Developmental failure of pharyngeal pouches 3 and 4

4. A 24-year-old woman presents with severe pain during menses (dysmenorrhea). To treat her symptoms, you advise her to take indomethacin. This drug may reduce her pain because it interferes with the production of which one of the following substances?

a. Bradykinin
b. Histamine
c. Leukotrienes
d. Phospholipase A_2
e. Prostaglandin F_2

5. Which one of the listed cells is thought to be the source of hepatic stem cells?

a. Ito cells
b. Limbus cells
c. Oval cells
d. Paneth cells
e. Satellite cells

6. A 25-year-old woman presents with a history of losing four pregnancies in the past 5 years. She also has a history of recurrent pains in her legs secondary to recurrent thrombosis. Her symptoms are most likely due to a deficiency of which one of the following substances?

a. PA inhibitors
b. Protein C
c. Plasmin
d. Thrombin
e. C'1 inactivator

7. Individual II-2 in the associated pedigree was diagnosed with hemophilia A. Which one of the following individuals would be most at risk for developing also hemophilia A?

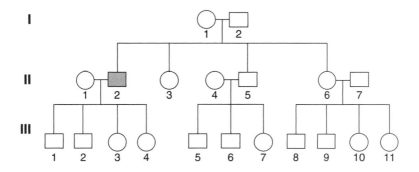

a. II-3
b. II-6
c. III-3
d. III-5
e. III-8

8. A 23-year-old woman presents with progressive bilateral loss of central vision. You obtain a detailed family history from this patient and produce the associated pedigree (dark circles or squares indicate affected individuals). Which of the following transmission patterns is most consistent with this patient's family history?

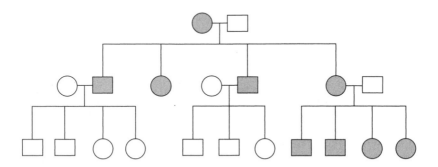

a. Autosomal recessive
b. Autosomal dominant
c. X-linked recessive
d. X-linked dominant
e. Mitochondrial

9. A 10-month-old baby is being evaluated for visual problems and motor incoordination. Examination of the child's fundus reveals a bright "cherry-red spot" at the macula. Talking to the family of this visually impaired 10-month-old infant, you find that they are Jewish and their family is from the eastern portion of Europe (Ashkenazi Jews). Based on this specific family history, which one of the following enzymes is most likely to be deficient in this infant?

a. Aryl sulfatase
b. β-glucocerebrosidase
c. Hexosaminidase A
d. Hexosaminidase B
e. Sphingomyelinase

10. A 4-year-old boy presents with mental retardation, self-mutilation, and hyperuricemia. These clinical signs are consistent with an X-linked recessive disorder that is caused by the deficiency of an enzyme that normally participates in which one of the following biochemical processes?

a. Conversion of homogentisic acid to methylacetoacetate
b. Degradation of galactocerebroside
c. Breakdown of branched-chain amino acids
d. Recycling of guanine and hypoxanthine
e. Synthesis of UMP and CTP

11. A 22-year-old man is being evaluated for infertility. Physical examination finds a tall young adult male who has gynecomastia and a female distribution of hair. Examination of the scrotum finds small, firm testes, and a testicular biopsy reveals atrophic sclerotic tubules with hyperplasia of the interstitial Leydig cells. Chromosomal analysis finds the abnormal karyotype 47,XXY. Which one of the listed sets of serum lab values is most likely to be present in this patient?

	Testosterone	Follicle-Stimulating Hormone (FSH)	Luteinizing Hormone (LH)	Estradiol
a.	Increased	Increased	Increased	Increased
b.	Increased	Decreased	Decreased	Decreased
c.	Decreased	Increased	Increased	Decreased
d.	Decreased	Increased	Increased	Increased
e.	Decreased	Decreased	Decreased	Decreased

12. A young boy is being evaluated for developmental delay, mild autism, and mental retardation. Physical examination reveals the boy to have large, everted ears and a long face with a large mandible. He is also found to have macroorchidism (large testes), and extensive workup reveals multiple tandem repeats of the nucleotide sequence CGG in his DNA. Which of the following is the most likely diagnosis?

a. Fragile X syndrome
b. Huntington's chorea
c. Myotonic dystrophy
d. Spinal-bulbar muscular atrophy
e. Ataxia-telangiectasia

13. A 55-year-old woman presents with dry eyes, a dry mouth, and difficulty swallowing solid food. Physical examination finds enlargement of her parotid glands along with marked dryness of her buccal mucosa. Laboratory examination finds the presence of both SS-A and SS-B antibodies. A biopsy of her lip is likely to show infiltration of minor salivary glands by what type of inflammatory cell?

a. Basophil
b. Eosinophil
c. Epithelioid cell
d. Lymphocyte
e. Neutrophil

14. An 8-month-old male infant is admitted to the hospital because of a bacterial respiratory infection. The infant responds to appropriate antibiotic therapy, but is readmitted several weeks later because of severe otitis media. Over the next several months, the infant is admitted to the hospital multiple times for recurrent bacterial infections. Workup finds a lack of B cells past the pre-B stage. The infant has no previous history of viral or fungal infections. Which of the following is the most likely diagnosis?

a. Agammaglobulinemia of Bruton
b. Common Variable Immunodeficiency
c. DiGeorge's syndrome
d. Isolated IgA deficiency
e. Omenn syndrome

15. A 27-year-old man presents with a testicular mass and is found to have high serum levels of α-fetoprotein (AFP). Microscopic examination of a biopsy from this mass reveals sheets of undifferentiated cells along with focal primitive glandular differentiation. The tumor cells have large and hyperchromatic nuclei. Further workup fails to reveal the presence of any metastatic disease as the tumor is confined within the testis. Based on all of these findings, which of the following best characterizes this tumor?

	Tumor Aggressiveness	Grade	Stage
a.	Benign	Low	Low
b.	Benign	Low	High
c.	Malignant	Low	Low
d.	Malignant	High	Low
e.	Malignant	High	High

16. A 35-year-old man living in a southern region of Africa presents with increasing abdominal pain and jaundice. He has worked as a farmer for many years, and sometimes his grain has become moldy. Physical examination reveals a large mass involving the right side of his liver, and a biopsy specimen from this mass confirms the diagnosis of liver cancer (hepatocellular carcinoma). Which of the following substances is most closely associated with the pathogenesis of this tumor?

a. Aflatoxin B1
b. Direct-acting alkylating agents
c. Vinyl chloride
d. Azo dyes
e. β-naphthylamine

17. A 59-year-old man is found to have a 3.5-cm mass in the right upper lobe of his lung. A biopsy of this mass is diagnosed as a moderately differentiated squamous cell carcinoma. Workup reveals that no bone metastases are present, but laboratory examination reveals that the man's serum calcium levels are 11.5 mg/dL. This patient's paraneoplastic syndrome is most likely the result of the ectopic production of which of the following substances?

a. Parathyroid hormone
b. Parathyroid hormone-related peptide
c. Calcitonin
d. Calcitonin-related peptide
e. Erythropoietin

18. A 22-year-old woman presents with the abrupt onset of a high fever, nausea, diffuse watery diarrhea, myalgia, shock, and a diffuse skin rash. Physical examination finds as fever, hypotension, and a diffuse erythroderma (sunburn-like rash) with redness of her mucosal surfaces. The rash involves her palms and soles. She states that it began on her trunk and spread to her arms and legs. Laboratory examination finds elevated serum liver and muscle enzymes, but tests for Rocky Mountain spotted fever, measles, hepatitis B, and antinuclear antibody were all negative. Which of the following is the most likely diagnosis?

a. Cellulitis caused by *Staphylococcus aureus*
b. Erysipelas caused by *Streptococcus pyogenes*
c. Impetigo cause by *Streptococcus pyogenes*
d. Secondary syphilis caused by *Treponema pallidum*
e. Toxic shock syndrome caused by *Staphylococcus aureus*

19. Several days after exploring a cave in eastern Kentucky, a 39-year-old woman develops shortness of breath and a low-grade fever. Chest x-rays reveal several irregular areas in both upper lung fields along with enlarged hilar and mediastinal lymph nodes. A biopsy of one of these lymph nodes reveals granulomatous inflammation. Multiple small yeasts surrounded by clear zones are seen within macrophages. Which one of the following organisms is most likely responsible for this individual's disease?

a. Aspergillus species
b. Blastomyces dermatitidis
c. Candida albicans
d. Histoplasma capsulatum
e. Mucor

20. A 65-year-old woman presents with several bruises on her skin and a prolonged nosebleed. She does not recall any trauma that caused the skin bruises, and she also states that her urine now appears bloody. Recently she has been taking a broad-spectrum sulfonamide for a urinary tract infection, but she says that she borrowed "a few extra pills" from her neighbor. Laboratory tests demonstrate a prolonged PT and PTT. This woman most likely has a deficiency of which one of the following vitamins?

a. Vitamin A
b. Vitamin B_1
c. Vitamin B_6
d. Vitamin C
e. Vitamin K

21. Hypoxia decreases cellular levels of adenosine 5'-triphosphate (ATP) and inhibits the normal function of the plasma membrane ouabain-sensitive Na-K-ATPase pump. Which one of the following changes will result from decreased function of this membrane ion pump?

	Sodium Ion Changes	Potassium Ion Changes
a.	Decreased sodium ions inside the cell	Decreased potassium ions outside the cell
b.	Decreased sodium ions inside the cell	Increased potassium ions outside the cell
c.	Increased sodium ions inside the cell	Increased potassium ions outside the cell
d.	Increased sodium ions outside the cell	Increased potassium ions inside the cell
e.	Increased sodium ions outside the cell	Decreased potassium ions inside the cell

22. A 54-year-old man develops a thrombus in his left anterior descending coronary artery. The area of myocardium supplied by this vessel is irreversibly injured. The thrombus is destroyed by the infusion of streptokinase, which is a plasminogen activator, and the injured area is reperfused. The patient, however, develops an arrhythmia and dies. An electron microscopic (EM) picture taken of the irreversibly injured myocardium reveals the presence of large, dark, irregular amorphic densities within mitochondria. What are these abnormal structures?

a. Apoptotic bodies
b. Flocculent densities
c. Myelin figures
d. Psammoma bodies
e. Russell bodies

23. An autopsy is performed on a 64-year-old man who died of congestive heart failure. Sections of the liver reveal yellow-brown granules in the cytoplasm of most of the hepatocytes. Which of the following stains would be most useful to demonstrate with positive staining that these yellow-brown cytoplasmic granules are in fact composed of hemosiderin (iron)?

a. Oil red O stain
b. Periodic acid–Schiff stain
c. Prussian blue stain
d. Sudan black B stain
e. Trichrome stain

24. A 48-year-old man who has a long history of excessive drinking presents with signs of alcoholic hepatitis. Microscopic examination of a biopsy of this patient's liver reveals irregular eosinophilic hyaline inclusions within the cytoplasm of the hepatocytes. These eosinophilic inclusions are composed of which one of the following substances?

a. Immunoglobulin
b. Excess plasma proteins
c. Prekeratin intermediate filaments
d. Basement membrane material
e. Lipofuscin

25. A 38-year-old woman presents with intermittent pelvic pain. Physical examination reveals a 3-cm mass in the area of her right ovary. Histologic sections from this ovarian mass reveal a papillary tumor with multiple, scattered small, round, laminated calcifications. Which of the following is the basic defect producing these abnormal structures?

a. Bacterial infection
b. Dystrophic calcification
c. Enzymatic necrosis
d. Metastatic calcification
e. Viral infection

26. A 30-year-old woman presents with malaise and increasing fatigue. Physical examination finds a yellow-tinge to her skin and sclera, and laboratory evaluation finds elevated serum liver enzymes. After further workup, the diagnosis of viral hepatitis is made. This workup included a liver biopsy, which revealed scattered, eosinophilic cells (Councilman bodies), but very little inflammation was present. These Councilman bodies were formed by an active process that characteristically lacks an inflammatory response and results from the activation of genes that forms new enzymes, such as endonucleases. These enzymes subsequently destroy the cell itself. Which of the following terms best describes this process?

a. Apoptosis
b. Autophagy
c. Heterophagy
d. Metaplasia
e. Necrosis

27. Pyogenic bacterial infections and ischemic brain infarcts most characteristically produce which one of the listed types of necrosis?

a. Caseous necrosis
b. Coagulative necrosis
c. Fat necrosis
d. Fibrinoid necrosis
e. Liquefactive necrosis

28. Which one of the listed statements best describes the mechanism through which Fas (CD95) initiates apoptosis?

a. BCL2 product blocks bax channels
b. Cytochrome c activates Apaf-1
c. FADD stimulates caspase 8
d. TNF inhibits IκB
e. TRADD stimulates FADD

29. Histologic sections of an enlarged tonsil from a 9-year-old girl reveal an increased number of reactive follicles containing germinal centers with proliferating B lymphocytes. Which of the following terms best describes this pathologic process?

a. B lymphocyte hypertrophy
b. Follicular dysplasia
c. Follicular hyperplasia
d. Germinal center atrophy
e. Germinal center metaplasia

30. A patient presents with a large wound to his right forearm that is the result of a chain saw accident. You treat his wound appropriately and follow him in your surgery clinic at routine intervals. Initially his wound is filled with granulation tissue, which is composed of proliferating fibroblasts and proliferating new blood vessels (angiogenesis). Which of the following substances is thought to be the most important growth factor involved in angiogenesis?

a. Epidermal growth factor (EGF)
b. Platelet-derived growth factor (PDGF)
c. Transforming growth factor-alpha (TGF-α)
d. Transforming growth factor-beta (TGF-β)
e. Vascular endothelial growth factor (VEGF)

31. Which one of the listed receptors is the type of receptor on leukocytes that binds to pathogen-associated molecular patterns (PAMPs) and mediates the innate immune response to bacterial lipopolysaccharide?

a. Cytokine receptor
b. G-protein-coupled receptor
c. Mannose receptor
d. Opsonin receptor
e. Toll-like receptor

32. A 4-year-old boy presents with progressive trouble breathing over the past couple of hours. Physical examination finds a young boy in moderate respiratory distress with inflamed and edematous regions involving his epiglottis and uvula. Material from his inflamed epiglottis is cultured and grow colonies of *Hemophilus influenzae*. This bacteria has increased amounts of sialic acid, which can inhibit the alternate complement system. That is, organisms with increased amounts of sialic acid, such as *Streptococcus pneumonia, H. influenzae,* and *Neisseria meningitidis,* need to be killed by the classic complement pathway. Which of the following substances is most likely to activate the classic complement pathway?

a. Aggregated IgA
b. Aggregated IgD
c. C3 nephritic factor
d. IgE bound to antigen
e. IgG bound to antigen

33. A 17-year-old boy is being evaluated for failure to have a growth spurt and the recent development of signs of premature aging. Physical examination finds the boy to be short with thin skin and muscle atrophy. The skin of his face is wrinkled and his lips appear atrophic. In the last year, he also has developed bilateral cataracts and early signs of osteoporosis. None of these signs were present in his first decade of life. Which of the following is the most likely diagnosis?

a. DiGeorge's syndrome
b. Hutchinson-Gilford syndrome
c. Leukocyte adhesion deficiency
d. Shwachman-Diamond syndrome
e. Werner syndrome

34. A 3-year-old boy presents with recurrent bacterial and fungal infections primarily involving his skin and respiratory tract. Physical examination reveals the presence of oculocutaneous albinism. Examination of a peripheral blood smear reveals large granules within neutrophils, lymphocytes, and monocytes. The total neutrophil count is found to be decreased. Further workup reveals ineffective bactericidal capabilities of neutrophils due to defective fusion of phagosomes with lysosomes. Which of the following is the most likely diagnosis?

a. Ataxia-telangiectasia
b. Chédiak-Higashi syndrome
c. Chronic granulomatous disease
d. Ehlers-Danlos syndrome
e. Sturge-Weber syndrome

35. A 29-year-old woman is being evaluated to find the cause of her urine turning a dark brown color after a recent upper respiratory tract infection. She has been otherwise asymptomatic, and her blood pressure has been within normal limits. Urinalysis finds moderate blood present with red cells and red cell casts. Immunofluorescence examination of a renal biopsy reveals deposits of IgA within the mesangium. These clinical findings suggest that her disorder is associated with activation of the alternate complement system. Which of the following serum laboratory findings is most suggestive of activation of the alternate complement system rather than the classic complement system?

	Serum C2	Serum C3	Serum C4
a.	Decreased	Normal	Normal
b.	Normal	Decreased	Normal
c.	Normal	Normal	Decreased
d.	Decreased	Normal	Decreased
e.	Decreased	Decreased	Decreased

36. A 19-year-old woman is being evaluated for recurrent facial edema, especially around her lips. She also has recurrent bouts of intense abdominal pain and cramps, sometimes associated with vomiting. Laboratory examination finds decreased C4, while levels of C3, decay-accelerating factor, and IgE are within normal limits. A deficiency of which one of the following substances is most likely to be associated with these clinical findings?

a. β_2-integrins
b. C1 esterase inhibitor
c. Decay-accelerating factor
d. Complement components C3 and C5
e. NADPH oxidase

37. Which of the following substances is produced by the action of lipoxygenase on arachidonic acid, is a potent chemotactic factor for neutrophils, and causes aggregation and adhesion of leukocytes?

a. C5a
b. Prostacyclin
c. IL-8
d. Thromboxane A_2
e. Leukotriene B_4

38. During acute inflammation, histamine-induced increased vascular permeability causes the formation of exudates (inflammatory edema). Which of the following cell types is most likely to secrete histamine and cause this increased vascular permeability?

a. Endothelial cells
b. Fibroblasts
c. Lymphocytes
d. Mast cells
e. Neutrophils

39. Histologic sections of lung tissue from a 68-year-old woman with congestive heart failure and progressive breathing problems reveal numerous hemosiderin-laden cells within the alveoli. Which of the following is the cell of origin of these "heart failure cells"?

a. Endothelial cells
b. Eosinophils
c. Lymphocytes
d. Macrophages
e. Pneumocytes

40. What type of leukocyte actively participates in acute inflammatory processes and contains myeloperoxidase within its primary (azurophilic) granules and alkaline phosphatase in its secondary (specific) granules?

a. Neutrophils
b. Eosinophils
c. Monocytes
d. Lymphocytes
e. Plasma cells

41. A 37-year-old man presents with a cough, fever, night sweats, and weight loss. A chest x-ray reveals irregular densities in the upper lobe of his right lung. Histologic sections from this area reveal groups of epithelioid cells with rare acid-fast bacilli and a few scattered giant cells. At the center of these groups of epithelioid cells are granular areas of necrosis. What is the source of these epithelioid cells?

a. Bronchial cells
b. Fibroblasts
c. Lymphocytes
d. Monocytes
e. Pneumocytes

42. A 47-year-old man presents with pain in the midportion of his chest. The pain is associated with eating and swallowing food. Endoscopic examination reveals an ulcerated area in the lower portion of his esophagus. Histologic sections of tissue taken from this area reveal an ulceration of the esophageal mucosa that is filled with blood, fibrin, proliferating blood vessels, and proliferating fibroblasts. Mitoses are easily found, and most of the cells have prominent nucleoli. Which of the following statements best describes this ulcerated area?

a. Caseating granulomatous inflammation
b. Dysplastic epithelium
c. Granulation tissue
d. Squamous cell carcinoma
e. Noncaseating granulomatous inflammation

43. A routine H&E histologic section from an irregular white area within the anterior wall of the heart of a 71-year-old man who died secondary to ischemic heart disease reveals the myocytes to be replaced by diffuse red material. This material stains blue with a trichrome stain. Which of the following statements correctly describes this material?

a. It is secreted by endothelial cells and links macromolecules to integrins
b. It is secreted by fibroblasts and has a high content of glycine and hydroxyproline
c. It is secreted by hepatocytes and is mainly responsible for intravascular oncotic pressure
d. It is secreted by monocytes and contains a core protein that is linked to mucopolysaccharides
e. It is secreted by plasma cells and is important in mediating humoral immunity

44. A 27-year-old woman presents because of trouble with her vision. Physical examination reveals a very tall, thin woman with long, thin fingers. Examining her eyes reveals the lens of her left eye to be in the anterior chamber. Her blood levels of methionine and cystathionine are within normal levels. Which of the following is the most likely cause of this patient's signs and symptoms?

a. Abnormal copper metabolism
b. Decreased levels of vitamin D
c. Decreased lysyl hydroxylation of collagen
d. Defective synthesis of fibrillin
e. Defective synthesis of type I collagen

45. Which of the following changes best describes the pathophysiology involved in the production of pulmonary edema in patients with congestive heart failure?

a. Decreased plasma oncotic pressure
b. Widespread endothelial damage
c. Increased hydrostatic pressure
d. Increased vascular permeability
e. Acute lymphatic obstruction

46. A 22-year-old second-year medical student develops a "red" face after being asked a question during lecture. Which of the following statements best describes this vascular reaction?

a. Active hyperemia
b. Acute congestion
c. Nonpalpable purpura
d. Passive hyperemia
e. Petechial hemorrhage

47. A 53-year-old man after recovering from a myocardial infarction is advised by his physician to take one "baby" aspirin every day to reduce the chance of his developing a second myocardial infarction. The theory behind this advice is that aspirin decreases the formation of thrombi within the coronary arteries by inhibiting the platelet formation of which substance?

a. Fibrinogen
b. Prostacyclin
c. Thrombomodulin
d. Thromboplastin
e. Thromboxane

48. Assuming that the levels of all of the other coagulation factors are within normal limits, which of the following laboratory findings is most consistent with an individual who is not taking any medication but has a familial deficiency of coagulation factor VII?

	Prothrombin Time (PT)	Partial Thromboplastin Time (PTT)
a.	Prolonged	Normal
b.	Normal	Prolonged
c.	Shortened	Normal
d.	Normal	Shortened
e.	Shortened	Prolonged

49. During the autopsy of a 46-year-old man who died when the motorcycle he was riding was hit by a truck, a 1.2-cm red mass is found within a branch of the left pulmonary artery. Grossly this mass is rubbery, gelatinous, and has a "chicken fat" appearance. Histologic sections reveal that this mass is not attached to the wall of the pulmonary artery, and alternating lines of Zahn are not seen. Which of the following statements best describes this intravascular mass?

a. Postmortem blood clot
b. Postmortem hematoma
c. Premortem embolic blood clot
d. Premortem non-embolic thrombus
e. Premortem non-thrombotic embolus

50. A 19-year-old offensive tackle for a major university football team fractures his right femur during the first game of the season. He is admitted to the hospital and over the next several days develops progressive respiratory problems. Despite extensive medical intervention, he dies 3 days later. At the time of autopsy oil red O–positive material is seen in the small blood vessels of the lungs and brain. Which of the following is the most likely diagnosis?

a. Air emboli
b. Amniotic fluid emboli
c. Fat emboli
d. Paradoxical emboli
e. Saddle emboli

51. A 9-year-old boy suddenly develops severe testicular pain. He is taken to the emergency room, where he is evaluated and immediately taken to surgery. There his left testis is found to be markedly hemorrhagic due to testicular torsion. Which of the following mechanisms is primarily involved in producing this type of testicular infarction?

a. Arterial occlusion
b. Septic implantation
c. Decreased collateral blood flow
d. Increased dual blood flow
e. Venous occlusion

52. A young child who presents with megaloblastic anemia is found to have increased orotate in the urine due to a deficiency of orotate phosphoribosyl transferase. This enzyme deficiency decreased the synthesis of which substance?

a. Glycogen
b. Purine
c. Pyrimidine
d. Sphingomyelin
e. Tyrosine

53. A newborn girl is being evaluated for breathing problems and is found to have a cleft palate and micrognathia. Her very small jaw caused posterior displacement of her tongue, which then obstructed both respiration and swallowing. Based on these physical findings the diagnosis of Pierre Robin sequence is made. Which of the following is the best definition of the clinical term "sequence"?

a. A defect that results from interference in a normally developing process
b. A pattern of nonrandom anomalies with an unknown mechanism
c. An alteration of a normally formed body part by mechanical forces
d. Multiple anomalies having a recognizable pattern and known pathogenesis
e. The combination of a primary defect along with its secondary structural changes

54. A 33-year-old man presents with acute, severe abdominal pain. Physical examination finds hyper-extensible skin, hypermobile joints, and prominent venous markings that are easily seen through his abnormal skin. Workup finds that his acute abdominal pain is due to spontaneous rupture of his colon. Based on these clinical findings and appropriate workup, the diagnosis of type IV Ehlers-Danlos syndrome is made. This disorder results from abnormalities involving the structural protein type III collagen. As a general rule, familial disorders such as type IV Ehlers-Danlos syndrome that result from abnormalities of structural proteins (rather than deficiencies of enzymes) and present during adulthood (rather than childhood) have what type of inheritance pattern?

a. Autosomal dominant
b. Autosomal recessive
c. Mitochondrial
d. X-linked dominant
e. X-linked recessive

55. A 5-year-old boy presents with recurrent hemarthroses and intramuscular hematomas. Laboratory tests reveal a normal bleeding time, platelet count, and PT, but the PTT is prolonged. This boy's condition results from a deficiency of coagulation factor VIII. The gene that codes for this coagulation factor is located on which one of the following chromosomes?

a. Chromosome 5
b. Chromosome 14
c. Chromosome 21
d. X chromosome
e. Y chromosome

56. A couple living in the United States has four children, three girls, and one boy, all of whom are under the age of 10. Two of the girls have been diagnosed with cystic fibrosis, but the boy, who is 7 years of age, appears normal. Neither of the parents has clinical signs of cystic fibrosis. What is the chance that this boy is a carrier for the gene that causes cystic fibrosis?

a. 0%
b. 25%
c. 50%
d. 75%
e. 100%

57. Assuming a frequency for a certain allele to be "p" and a frequency "q" of another allele at the same locus on the same autosomal chromosome in a population with random mating (panmixia), then according to the Hardy-Weinberg principle, what is the number of heterozygous carriers?

a. p * p
b. q * q
c. p * q
d. 2 * p * q
e. (p * p) + (p * q)

58. A 6-year-old girl is being evaluated for recurrent episodes of lightheadedness and sweating due to hypoglycemia. These symptoms are not improved by subcutaneous injection of epinephrine. Physical examination reveals an enlarged liver and a single subcutaneous xanthoma. An abdominal computed tomography (CT) scan reveals enlargement of the liver along with bilateral enlargement of the kidneys. Laboratory examination reveals increased serum uric acid and cholesterol with decreased serum glucose levels. Following oral administration of fructose, there is no increase in blood glucose levels. A liver biopsy specimen reveals increased amounts of glycogen in hepatocytes, which also have decreased levels of glucose-6-phosphatase. Which of the following is the most likely diagnosis?

a. Andersen's syndrome (type IV glycogen storage disease)
b. Cori's disease (type III glycogen storage disease)
c. McArdle's syndrome (type V glycogen storage disease)
d. Pompe's disease (type II glycogen storage disease)
e. von Gierke's disease (type I glycogen storage disease)

59. A 6-month-old boy is being evaluated for failure to thrive, along with persistent vomiting, seizures, and a low-grade fever. Physical examination finds a protuberant abdomen due to enlargement of both the liver and spleen, along with a "cherry-red spot" on his retina and diffuse enlarged lymph nodes. A bone marrow biopsy reveals an abnormal diffuse proliferation of foamy macrophages filled with lipid ("foam cells"). Electron microscopy reveals cytoplasmic bodies that resemble concentric lamellated myelin figures within the foamy macrophages. Rare parallel pallisading lamella ("zebra bodies") are also seen in the cytoplasm of these cells with electron microscopy. Which of the following substances is most likely to be found at abnormally high levels within these foamy macrophages?

a. Ceramide trihexose
b. Glucocerebroside
c. Heparan sulfate
d. Sphingomyelin
e. Sulfatide

60. A 9-year-old boy is being evaluated for deafness. Physical examination reveals a child with short stature, coarse facial features (low, flat nose; thick lips; widely spaced teeth; facial fullness), a large tongue, and clear corneas. Laboratory examination reveals increased urinary levels of heparan sulfate and dermatan sulfate. Metachromatic granules (Reilly bodies) are found in leukocytes from a bone marrow biopsy. These leukocytes are also found to be deficient in iduronosulfate sulfatase. Which of the following is the most likely diagnosis?

a. Hunter's disease
b. Hurler's disease
c. I cell disease
d. Metachromatic leukodystrophy
e. Wolman's disease

61. A 45-year-old man presents with severe pain in both knee joints. At the time of surgery, his cartilage is found to have a dark blue-black color. Further evaluation reveals that the patient's urine has darkened rapidly with time. Which of the following is the most likely diagnosis?

a. Hyperphenylalaninemia
b. Tyrosinemia
c. Tyrosinase-positive oculocutaneous albinism
d. Alkaptonuria
e. Maple syrup urine disease

62. A 22-year-old woman in the second month of her first pregnancy presents with lower abdominal pain and vaginal bleeding. Histologic examination of blood clots taken from the vaginal vault reveals decidualized tissue and occasional chorionic villi. Chromosomal analysis of these products of conception from her spontaneous abortion reveals a triploid karyotype. What is the total number of chromosomes present in this abnormal karyotype?

a. 23
b. 46
c. 47
d. 69
e. 92

63. A 25-year-old man presents with painless enlargement of the left side of his scrotum. Physical examination reveals a single mass involving his left testis. Laboratory examination reveals markedly increased levels of AFP. This testicular mass is resected surgically. The diagnosis of embryonal carcinoma, a germ cell tumor, is made based on microscopic finding of a poorly differentiated tumor composed of large cells in solid sheets having occasional areas of glandular differentiation. Chromosomal studies on the malignant tumor cells reveal the presence of an isochromosome of the short arm of chromosome 12, that is, i(12p). Which abnormality results in the formation of an isochromosome?

a. A deletion occurs at both ends of a chromosome with fusion of the damaged ends
b. A rearrangement involves two breaks within a single chromosome with inverted reincorporation of the segment
c. A segment of one chromosome is transferred to a different chromosome
d. A translocation occurs between two acrocentric chromosomes
e. One arm of a chromosome is lost and the remaining arm is duplicated

64. The first child of a couple has trisomy 21 (not the result of mosaicism), and they come to you wanting to know the risk of having another child with Down syndrome. The mother's age is 23, and the father's age is 25. Both appear normal and neither have had any unusual diseases. You analyze their karyotypes and find that the father's karyotype is normal, but the mother has a Robertsonian translocation involving chromosome 21 (21q21q). Which of the following percentages is the best estimate of the chance that the next living child of this couple will have Down syndrome?

a. 0%
b. 15%
c. 33%
d. 50%
e. 100%

65. A male infant dies 1 day after birth. Gross examination at the time of autopsy reveals polydactyly, a cleft lip and palate, and a single, central eye ("cyclops"). Further examination reveals holoprosencephaly, consisting of fused frontal lobes with a single ventricle. Which of the listed chromosomal abnormalities is most consistent with these findings?

a. Deletion 21
b. Deletion 22
c. Trisomy 13
d. Trisomy 18
e. Trisomy 21

66. A 2-month-old girl presents with a soft, high-pitched, mewing cry and is found to have microcephaly, low-set ears and hypertelorism, and several congenital heart defects. Which of the following abnormal karyotypes is most likely to be associated with these clinical signs?

a. 46,XX,4p⁻
b. 46,XX,5p⁻
c. 46,XX,13q⁻
d. 46,XX,15q⁻
e. 46,XX,17p⁻

67. Deletion of the maternal allele that codes for UBE3A, the product of which is an enzyme involved in the ubiquitin-proteosome proteolytic pathway, is likely to produce which one of the listed sets of clinical signs and symptoms?

a. Ataxic gait with jerky movements and inappropriate laughter
b. Exomphalos with macroglossia and gigantism
c. Growth retardation with severe hypotonia and micrognathia
d. Obesity with small hands and hypogonadism
e. Short stature with sleep disturbances and self-destructive behavior

68. A 19-year-old woman of average intelligence and short stature is being evaluated for amenorrhea. Medical history is pertinent for the fact that she has never menstruated. Physical examination reveals that she has a shield-shaped chest and her elbows turn outward when her arms are at her sides. She also has a "thick neck" and secondary female characteristics are absent. Serum estrogen levels are found to be decreased, while both FSH and LH levels are increased. Which one of the listed karyotypes would most likely produce an abnormality of the short stature homeobox (SHOX) gene and possibly be responsible for the short stature of this woman?

a. 45,X0
b. 45,XX,del(13)
c. 47,XX,+21
d. 47,XXY
e. 48,XXXX

69. A 17-year-old individual who is phenotypically female presents for workup of primary amenorrhea and is found to have an XY karyotype. Which of the following is the most likely diagnosis?

a. Androgen insensitivity syndrome
b. Deficiency of 5-α-reductase
c. Kallmann's syndrome
d. Mixed gonadal dysgenesis
e. Turner's syndrome

70. A 4-year-old boy is being evaluated for the acute development of multiple hemorrhagic areas on his skin and gums. Examination of his peripheral blood reveals a markedly increased white cell count to 50,000, the majority of which are lymphoid cells having prominent nucleoli. A bone marrow biopsy reveals the marrow to be diffusely infiltrated by these same cells and a diagnosis of acute lymphoblastic lymphoma is made. Special stains on these malignant cells demonstrate cytoplasmic staining for μ heavy chain. They lack surface immunoglobulin, but do express nuclear TdT staining and surface markers for CD19 and CD20. These malignant cells have the staining characteristics of what type of cell?

a. Lymphoid stem cell
b. Pre-pre B cell
c. Pre-B cell
d. Immature B cell
e. Virgin B cell

71. A 27-year-old woman presents with tender cervical lymphadenopathy. A biopsy of one of the enlarged lymph nodes in this area is diagnosed by the pathologist as being a "reactive lymph node with follicular hyperplasia." The associated schematic depicts the morphology of this reactive change. The majority of the proliferating cells in the area marked by the arrow labeled with an "*" are in the process of transforming into cells that eventually will secrete which substance?

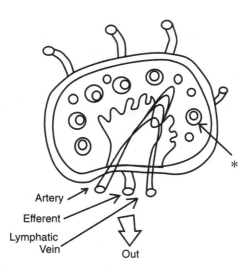

a. Erythropoietin
b. Gamma-interferon
c. Immunoglobulin
d. Interleukin-2
e. Interleukin-3

72. A 3-month-old infant born premature at 35 weeks of gestation is being evaluated for ocular problems and seizures. An x-ray of this infant's head reveals extensive cerebral calcification in the periventricular areas. Because of this combination of clinical signs, the possibility of congenital toxoplasmosis is considered. Elevated levels (titers) of which one of the following types of antibodies, if directed against Toxoplasma gondii, would best support this diagnosis?

a. IgG
b. IgM
c. IgD
d. IgE
e. IgA

73. Which one of the listed cytokines is secreted by macrophages and functions as a major mediator of acute inflammation by stimulating acute-phase reactions such as fever production along with increasing vascular permeability and stimulating fibroblasts?

a. Interleukin-1
b. Interleukin-2
c. Interleukin-3
d. Interleukin-5
e. Interleukin-12

74. A 29-year-old woman presents with anorexia, nausea, and vomiting. Physical examination reveals a slight yellow discoloration to her skin. Laboratory evaluation finds elevated liver enzymes, while a liver biopsy reveals focal acute inflammation with ballooning degeneration of the hepatocytes. A few scattered necrotic hepatocytes are seen that have the appearance of Councilman bodies. These apoptotic bodies are the result of the induction of apoptosis in viral infected hepatocytes by cytotoxic T lymphocytes. In the mechanism for this destruction of viral-infected hepatocytes, cytotoxic T lymphocytes only recognize antigens that are bound to which substance?

a. Class I antigens
b. Class II antigens
c. Class III antigens
d. C3b
e. The Fc portion of IgG

75. A 20-year-old man presents with low back pain and stiffness. Radiographic examination finds extensive calcification of the vertebral and paravertebral ligaments, producing a "bamboo spine." Rheumatoid factor is not identified in his peripheral blood. This patient's abnormalities are most likely the result of a disorder that is most closely associated with which one of the following HLA types?

a. HLA-A3
b. HLA-B27
c. HLA-BW47
d. HLA-DR3
e. HLA-DR4

76. Ten minutes after being stung by a wasp, a 30-year-old man develops multiple patches of red, irregular skin lesions over his entire body. These lesions (urticaria) are pruritic, and a new crop of lesions develops the next day. Which one of the following statements correctly describes an important component of the pathomechanism of this immune response?

a. Activated T lymphocytes stimulate smooth-muscle cells
b. IgA is attached to basophils and mast cells
c. IgA is attached to lymphocytes and eosinophils
d. IgE is attached to basophils and mast cells
e. IgE is attached to lymphocytes and eosinophils

77. After receiving incompatible blood, a patient develops a transfusion reaction in the form of back pain, fever, shortness of breath, and hematuria. Which one of the following statements best classifies this type of immunologic reaction?

a. Systemic anaphylactic reaction
b. Systemic immune complex reaction ·
c. Delayed type hypersensitivity reaction
d. Complement-mediated cytotoxicity reaction
e. T cell-mediated cytotoxicity reaction

78. A 26-year-old African American woman presents with nonspecific symptoms including fever, malaise, and increasing respiratory problems. A chest x-ray reveals enlarged hilar lymph nodes, while laboratory tests find her serum calcium level to be elevated. A transbronchial biopsy reveals scattered chronic inflammatory cells, reactive epithelial changes, and several noncaseating granulomas. The pathomechanism involved in the formation of these noncaseating granulomas involves the activation of macrophages to form epithelial cells by the action of which substance?

a. Gamma-interferon
b. Leukotriene C4
c. Interleukin-2
d. Interleukin-5
e. Interleukin-12

79. Which of the following is the definition of an allograft?

a. A graft between a human and an animal
b. A graft between two individuals of different species
c. A graft between two individuals of the same species
d. A graft between two individuals of the same inbred strain
e. A graft between identical twins

80. Minutes after a donor kidney is connected to the recipient's blood vessels, the transplanted kidney turns blue, becomes flaccid, excretes a few drops of bloody urine, and has to be removed. Histologic examination of the kidney reveals neutrophils within arterioles, glomeruli, and peritubular capillaries. Immunoglobulin and complement are found to be deposited in blood vessel walls. Which of the following mechanisms is primarily involved in this type of transplant rejection?

a. Donor cytotoxic T lymphocytes are directed against host antigens
b. Host cytotoxic T lymphocytes are directed against donor antigens
c. Donor natural killer cells are directed against host antigens
d. Preformed donor antibodies are directed against host antigens
e. Preformed host antibodies are directed against donor antigens

81. A 38-year-old woman presents with increasing fatigue and pruritus. Laboratory evaluation finds an increased serum alkaline phosphatase along with slightly elevated serum bilirubin levels. A liver biopsy reveals a marked lymphocytic infiltrate in the portal tracts along with occasional granulomas. Based on these findings, the diagnosis of primary biliary cirrhosis is made. Which of the following types of autoantibodies is most specific for this disorder?

a. Anti-IgG antibodies
b. Anti-mitochondrial antibodies
c. Anti-neutrophil cytoplasmic antibodies
d. Anti-nuclear antibodies
e. Anti-smooth-muscle antibodies

82. A 28-year-old woman presents with increasing fatigue, arthritis, shortness of breath, and a bimalar, photosensitive, erythematous rash. Biopsies from this rash reveal liquefactive degeneration of the basal layer of the epidermis with a perivascular lymphoid infiltrate. Immunofluorescence examination reveals linear deposits of IgG and complement at the dermal-epidermal junction in a granular pattern. Physical examination finds bilateral pleural effusions, the fluid from which when examined histologically reveals multiple oval amorphic eosinophilic bodies being phagocytized by phagocytic leukocytes. Which of the following is the most likely diagnosis?

a. Dermatomyositis
b. Rheumatoid arthritis
c. Sjögren's syndrome
d. Systemic amyloidosis
e. Systemic lupus erythematosus

83. A 36-year-old woman presents with increased trouble swallowing. Physical examination finds hypertension and sclerodactyly, while laboratory examination finds an autoantibody against DNA topoisomerase (anti-Scl-70). Which of the following biopsies is most characteristic of this disorder?

a. A conjunctival biopsy that reveals noncaseating granulomas
b. A peripheral nerve biopsy that reveals rare acid-fast bacteria
c. A skin biopsy that reveals dermal fibrosis with an absence of adnexal structures
d. A subcutaneous fat biopsy that reveals an infiltrate of plasma cells and eosinophils
e. A temporal artery biopsy that reveals fragmentation of the internal elastic lamina

84. A 59-year-old man presents with increasing fatigue, swelling, and bone pain. Laboratory evaluation finds increased serum protein and calcium along with markedly increased amounts of protein in his urine. Subsequently he develops signs of progressive renal failure. Microscopic examination of a renal biopsy reveals deposits of eosinophilic, Congo red–positive material in the glomeruli. When viewed under polarized light, this material displays an apple-green birefringence. What is the most likely composition of this material?

a. Light chains
b. Transthyretin
c. Beta-2-protein
d. Beta-2-microglobulin
e. Procalcitonin

85. A 7-month-old male infant is admitted to the hospital with chronic diarrhea. In his first few months of life this infant has had several episodes of bacterial pneumonia and otitis media along with oral candidiasis and a viral infection. Workup finds that the thymus is small, lymphoid tissues are hypoplastic, and both B and T lymphocytes are decreased in number in the peripheral blood. Serum calcium levels were within normal limits. Which one of the listed defects is associated with the X-linked recessive form for this infant's immunodeficiency disease?

a. Decreased production of NADPH oxidase
b. Decreased synthesis of adenosine deaminase in lymphocytes
c. Mutation in the common gamma chain subunit of cytokine receptors
d. Mutation in the gene coding for the Wiskott-Aldrich syndrome protein (WASP)
e. Mutation in the gene coding for CD40L

86. A 30-year-old man presents with unexplained weight loss and a few enlarged lymph nodes. An enzyme-linked immunoassay (ELISA) for HIV antibody detection is positive, and a confirmatory Western blot test is ordered. This test is reported as positive, as bands for p24 and gp41 are present. Which HIV gene codes for the p24 antigen?

a. *env*
b. *gag*
c. *pol*
d. *vpu*
e. *vpx*

87. A 52-year-old man presents with symptoms of gastric pain after eating. During workup, a 3-cm mass is found in the wall of the stomach. This mass is resected and histologic examination reveals a tumor composed of cells having elongated, spindle-shaped nuclei. The tumor does not connect to the overlying epithelium and is found only in the wall of the stomach. Which of the following is the cell of origin of this tumor?

a. Adipocyte
b. Endothelial cell
c. Glandular epithelial cell
d. Smooth-muscle cell
e. Squamous epithelial cell

88. A 64-year-old man presents with symptoms of anemia. On workup, you discover that the patient has been losing blood from the gastrointestinal (GI) tract secondary to a tumor mass in his colon. The pathology report from a biopsy specimen indicates that this mass is an invasive adenocarcinoma. Which of the following histologic appearances is most likely to be seen in a biopsy specimen taken from this tumor mass?

a. A uniform proliferation of fibrous tissue
b. A disorganized mass of proliferating fibroblasts and blood vessels
c. A disorganized mass of cells forming keratin
d. A uniform proliferation of glandular structures
e. A disorganized mass of cells forming glandular structures

89. A 35-year-old man presents with the new onset of a "bulge" in his left inguinal area. After performing a physical examination, you diagnose the bulge to be an inguinal hernia. You refer the patient to a surgeon, who repairs the hernia and sends the resected hernia sac to the pathology laboratory along with some adipose tissue, which he calls a "lipoma of the cord." The pathology resident examines the tissue grossly and microscopically and decides that it is not a neoplastic lipoma, but instead is nonneoplastic normal adipose tissue. Which one of the following features could best differentiate a benign well-differentiated lipoma from normal adipose tissue?

a. Cellular pleomorphism
b. Clonal proliferation
c. Numerous mitoses
d. Prominent nucleoli
e. Uniform population

90. Which one of the following numbered sequences best illustrates the postulated sequence of events that precedes the formation of an infiltrating squamous cell carcinoma of the cervix?

1 = Carcinoma in situ
2 = Invasive carcinoma
3 = Mild dysplasia
4 = Moderate dysplasia
5 = Severe dysplasia
6 = Squamous metaplasia

a. 3, then 4, then 5, then 1, then 6, then 2
b. 3, then 4, then 5, then 6, then 1, then 2
c. 5, then 4, then 3, then 1, then 6, then 2
d. 6, then 3, then 4, then 5, then 1, then 2
e. 6, then 4, then 3, then 5, then 2, then 1

91. During a routine physical examination, a 49-year-old man is found to have a 2.5-cm "coin lesion" in the upper lobe of his left lung. The lesion is removed surgically, and histologic sections reveal sheets of malignant cells with clear cytoplasm (clear cell carcinoma). Which of the following is the most likely site of origin for this metastatic lung tumor?

a. Appendix
b. Breast
c. Kidney
d. Pancreas
e. Stomach

92. A 46-year-old woman who lives in Southern Japan develops a diffuse, rapidly spreading rash. Workup finds hypercalcemia along with a mediastinal mass. Examination of the peripheral smear reveals numerous multilobated lymphocytes. These same cells are present in histologic sections taken from a biopsy of the mediastinal mass. Based on these clinical findings the diagnosis of adult T-cell leukemia/lymphoma (ATLL) is made. Which of the following statements is an important predisposing factor involved in the pathogenesis of this malignancy?

a. Exposure to beta-naphthylamine
b. Exposure to ionizing gamma radiation
c. Infection with a mutated hepadnavirus
d. Infection with a retrovirus
e. Mutations of the ras oncogene

93. A 19-year-old man is being evaluated for the development of numerous small skin tumors. Physical examination reveals multiple polypoid skin tumors measuring up to 5 mm in diameter along with several cafe-au-lait spots on his back and a pigmented growth on his right iris. A biopsy from one of the skin tumors is diagnosed as being a plexiform neurofibroma. The development of multiple skin tumors in an individual with this man's disease is related to abnormalities involving a particular gene that normally codes for which protein?

a. A protein that downregulates the ras oncoprotein product
b. A glycoprotein that is the patched receptor ligand for smo receptor signaling
c. A lipoprotein that inhibits the binding of the c-sis oncoprotein to its receptor
d. An enzyme that stimulates the conversion of Gs-GDP to Gs-GTP
e. A protein that upregulates membrane receptors for tyrosine kinase

94. A 4-year-old African boy develops a rapidly enlarging mass that involves the right side of his face. Biopsies of this lesion reveal a prominent "starry sky" pattern produced by proliferating small, noncleaved malignant lymphocytes. Based on this microscopic appearance, the diagnosis of Burkitt's lymphoma is made. This neoplasm is associated with chromosomal translocations that involve which one of the following oncogenes?

a. bcl-2
b. c-abl
c. c-myc
d. erb-B
e. N-myc

95. The product of the p53 antioncogene is a nuclear protein that regulates DNA replication and prevents the proliferation of cells with damaged DNA. It does this by stopping the cell cycle at which point?

a. Between G1 and S
b. Between G2 and M
c. Between M and G1
d. Between S and G2
e. During G3

96. A 76-year-old man farmer presents with a 2-cm mass on the left side of his forehead. A biopsy reveals squamous cell carcinoma. Which one of the following causes the formation of pyrimidine dimers in DNA and is associated with the formation of squamous cell carcinoma?

a. Aflatoxin B1
b. Vinyl chloride
c. UVC
d. UVB
e. Epstein-Barr virus

97. A 17-year-old man presents with a lesion on his face that measures approximately 1.5 cm in its greatest dimension. He has a history of numerous similar skin lesions that have occurred mainly in sun-exposed areas. The present lesion is biopsied and reveals an invasive squamous cell carcinoma. This patient most probably has one type of a group of inherited diseases associated with unstable DNA and increased incidence of carcinoma. Which of the following is the most likely diagnosis?

a. Xeroderma pigmentosa
b. Wiskott-Aldrich syndrome
c. Familial polyposis
d. Sturge-Weber syndrome
e. Multiple endocrine neoplasia type I

98. A 56-year-old man presents with a 25-pound weight loss over the past 6 months. He says that he has no appetite for food and over the past several weeks has also developed an "ache" in his stomach region. Gastroscopy finds a fungating mass involving the distal portion of the lesser curvature of his stomach. Biopsies from this mass reveal infiltrating groups of highly atypical cells forming glandular structures. The malignant cells extend through the muscularis mucosa into the submucosa, but they do not extend into the muscularis externa. This type of malignancy is most frequent in which one of the following geographic locations?

a. Canada
b. France
c. Japan
d. United Kingdom
e. United States

99. A 57-year-old man presents with signs of fatigue that are the result of anemia. Workup reveals that his anemia is the result of bleeding from a colon cancer located in the sigmoid colon. The lesion is resected and at the time of surgery no metastatic disease is found. Which of the following markers would be most useful for future follow-up of this patient for the evaluation of possible metastatic disease from his colon cancer?

a. α fetoprotein (AFP)
b. Carcinoembryonic antigen (CEA)
c. Chloroacetate esterase (CAE)
d. Human chorionic gonadotropin (hCG)
e. Prostate-specific antigen (PSA)

100. A 23-year-old woman presents with the recent onset of vaginal discharge. Physical examination reveals multiple clear vesicles on her vulva and vagina. A smear of material obtained from one of these vesicles reveals several multinucleated giant cells with intranuclear inclusions and ground-glass nuclei. These vesicles are most likely the result of infection with which one of the following organisms?

a. Cytomegalovirus (CMV)
b. Herpes simplex virus (HSV)
c. Human papillomavirus (HPV)
d. *Candida albicans*
e. *Trichomonas vaginalis*

101. Five days after returning from a trip to mainland China a 25-year-old previously healthy woman acutely develops a cough, shortness of breath, and fever with chills, headaches, diarrhea, nausea, and vomiting. She is found to have a peripheral lymphopenia. After appropriate laboratory tests are performed the diagnosis of severe acute respiratory syndrome (SARS) is made. What type of virus is the cause of this disorder?

a. Alphavirus
b. Coronavirus
c. Filovirus
d. Flavivirus
e. Hantavirus

102. A 6-year-old boy develops a facial rash that has the appearance of a slap to the face ("slapped cheek" appearance). The rash, which is composed of small red spots, subsequently involves the upper and lower extremities. This boy also has arthralgia and suddenly develops a life-threatening aplastic crisis of the bone marrow. What is the most likely diagnosis?

a. Rubeola (first disease)
b. Scarlet fever (second disease)
c. Rubella (third disease)
d. Atypical scarlet fever (fourth disease)
e. Erythema infectiosum (fifth disease)

103. A 32-year-old man presents to the emergency room with the acute onset of shaking chills and fever, blood-tinged mucoid sputum, and pleuritic chest pain. Physical examination finds fever and an increased respiratory rate, while there is dullness to percussion over the right lower lobe. Examination of his peripheral blood reveals increased numbers of neutrophils and bands. A chest x-ray reveals consolidation of the entire lower lobe of his right lung. Which of the following organisms is the most common cause of this type of pneumonia?

a. *Haemophilus influenzae*
b. *Klebsiella pneumoniae*
c. *Legionella pneumophila*
d. *Staphylococcus pyogenes*
e. *Streptococcus pneumoniae*

104. A 33-year-old man in an underdeveloped country presents with a markedly edematous right foot that has multiple draining sinuses. A Gram stain from one of these draining sinuses reveals gram-positive filamentous bacteria that are partially acid-fast. What is this organism?

a. *Actinomyces israelii*
b. *Corynebacterium diphtheriae*
c. *Listeria monocytogenes*
d. *Nocardia asteroides*
e. *Pneumocystis carinii*

105. A 39-year-old man presents with an enlarging lesion on his right hand. He said that the lesion started out 3 days prior as a small bump. Physical examination finds a 1-cm vesicle with a black center of dead tissue. Cultures from this lesion grow colonies of bacteria that grossly are tangled having a "medusae head" appearance. Gram stains reveal parallel chains of boxcar-shaped gram-positive organisms. What is the best diagnosis?

a. Anthrax
b. Leprosy
c. Plague
d. Scrofula
e. Syphilis

106. A 22-year-old woman presents with the new onset of a watery, foul-smelling vaginal discharge. A gram stain of this discharge reveals squamous epithelial cells that are covered by small gram variable rods. Pap smears show the presence of "clue cells." This abnormality is most closely associated with which one of the listed organisms?

a. *Calymmatobacterium donovani*
b. *Gardnerella vaginalis*
c. *Haemophilus ducreyi*
d. *Neisseria gonorrhoeae*
e. *Treponema pallidum*

107. A 34-year-old woman living on Martha's Vineyard, a small island off the New England coast, develops the sudden onset of chills and fever. Microscopic examination of a peripheral blood smear reveal inclusions within the red blood cells, some of which form distinctive Maltese cross forms. What is the best diagnosis?

a. Babesiosis
b. Leishmaniasis
c. Lyme disease
d. Atypical malaria
e. Toxoplasmosis

108. A 32-year-old man presents with arthritis and conjunctivitis. No rheumatoid factor is found in his serum (i.e., seronegative spondylo-arthropathy). A detailed history reveals that he also has severe pain with urination (nongonococcal urethritis). The combination in this patient of arthritis, urethritis, and conjunctivitis is consistent with a diagnosis of Reiter syndrome, a disorder that is associated with HLA-B27. Which of the following organisms is most closely associated with Reiter syndrome?

a. *Shigella*
b. *Salmonella*
c. *Yersinia*
d. *Campylobacter*
e. *Chlamydia*

109. A 35-year-old woman who lives in the southeastern portion of the United States and likes to hike in the Great Smoky Mountains presents with a spotted rash that started on her extremities and spread to her trunk and face. A biopsy of one of these lesions reveals necrosis and reactive hyperplasia of blood vessels. Which of the following is the most likely causative agent of her disease?

a. *Bartonella henselae*
b. *Bartonella quintana*
c. *Coxiella burnetii*
d. *Rickettsia prowazekii*
e. *Rickettsia rickettsii*

110. A 22-year-old hiker living in western North Carolina develops fever, chills, headaches, and myalgia after being bitten by a tick. Examination of his peripheral blood reveals rare "asterisk-shaped" inclusion bodies in his neutrophils. What is the most likely cause of his illness?

a. Chlamydia psittaci
b. Ehrlichia chaffeensis
c. Francisella tularensis
d. Nocardia asteroides
e. Trypanosoma brucei

111. A 21-year-old college athlete presents with a nagging cough and a 20-lb weight loss. In addition to the chronic cough and weight loss, his main symptoms consist of fever, night sweats, and chest pains. Examination of his sputum reveals the presence of rare acid-fast organisms. His symptoms are most likely due to an infection with which one of the following organisms?

a. K. pneumoniae
b. L. pneumophila
c. Mycobacterium avium-intracellulare
d. Mycobacterium tuberculosis
e. Mycoplasma pneumoniae

112. A 21-year-old HIV-positive man presents with malaise, fever, weight loss, diarrhea, and increasing size of lymph nodes in his right cervical region. Physical examination finds tender hepatosplenomegaly along with the enlarged lymph nodes. A microscopic section from one of the enlarged lymph nodes, which has a yellow color grossly, that is stained with an acid-fast stain reveals aggregates of foamy macrophages with numerous ("too many to count") intracellular acid-fast organisms. Granulomas are not found. Which of the following organisms is the most likely cause of this patient's acute illness?

a. M. avium-intracellulare
b. M. marinum
c. M. leprae
d. M. tuberculosis
e. M. fortuitum

I 13. An adult migrant farm worker in the San Joaquin Valley of California has been hospitalized for 2 weeks with progressive lassitude, fever of unknown origin, and skin nodules on the lower extremities. A biopsy of one of the deep dermal nodules shown in the photomicrograph below reveals the presence of which abnormality?

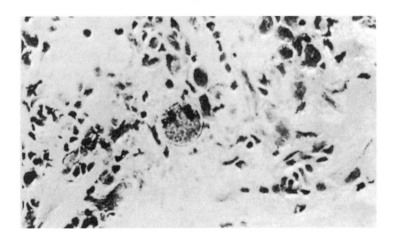

a. Russell bodies
b. Malignant lymphoma
c. Coccidioides spherule
d. Lymphomatoid granulomatosis
e. Erythema nodosum

I 14. A 31-year-old woman living in southern Ohio presents with a low-grade fever and a nonproductive cough. She says that over the last few days she has had some left-sided chest pain along with shortness of breath. A chest x-ray reveals a diffuse infiltrate in the lower lobe of her left lung. Histologic sections of lung from this area reveal organisms morphologically consistent with Blastomyces dermatitidis. Which one of the following abnormalities was most likely seen in these histologic sections?

a. Acute angle-branching, septate hyphae
b. Broad-based budding of yeast
c. Large spheres with external budding
d. Nonbranching pseudohyphae and blastocysts
e. Wide angle–branching, nonseptate hyphae

115. A 38-year-old man with AIDS presents with decreasing mental status. The workup at this time includes a spinal tap. Cerebrospinal fluid (CSF) is stained with a mucicarmine stain and India ink. The mucicarmine stain reveals numerous yeasts that stain bright red. The India ink prep reveals through negative staining that these yeasts have a capsule. Which of the following is the most likely diagnosis?

a. Chromomycosis
b. Coccidioidomycosis
c. Cryptococcosis
d. Cryptosporidiosis
e. Paracoccidioidomycosis

116. A patient who presents to the hospital with severe headaches develops convulsions and dies. At autopsy the brain grossly has a "Swiss cheese" appearance due to the presence of numerous small cysts containing milky fluid. Microscopically, a scolex with hooklets is found within one of these cysts. Which of the following is the causative agent for this disease?

a. *Taenia saginata*
b. *Taenia solium*
c. *Diphyllobothrium latum*
d. *Echinococcus granulosa*
e. *Toxocara canis*

117. A 27-year-old man develops acute diarrhea consisting of foul-smelling, watery stools, along with severe abdominal cramps and flatulence, after returning from a trip to the Caribbean. The associated photomicrograph is from a duodenal aspiration smear. These signs and symptoms are caused by infection with which one of the following organisms?

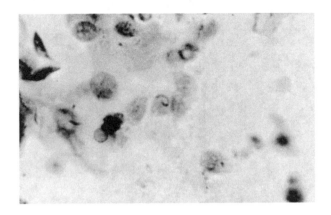

a. Acanthamoeba
b. *Entamoeba histolytica*
c. *E. vermicularis*
d. *Giardia lamblia*
e. Sporothrix

118. A 7-year-old girl presents with signs of acute appendicitis including fever and right lower quadrant abdominal pain. A section from the resected appendix is seen in the associated picture. Which one of the listed laboratory tests is most commonly used to diagnose infection with this organism?

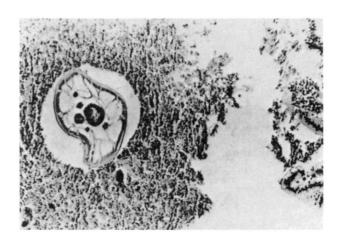

a. Examine the stool with an acid-fast stain
b. Measure vitamin B_{12} levels in the serum
c. Perform an anal "Scotch-tape" test
d. Quantitate the amount of fecal fat in a 24-h stool specimen
e. Test the absorption of D-xylose in the colon

119. Soon after returning from a trip to Costa Rica, a 41-year-old woman develops recurrent chills and high fever that recur every 48 h. Examination of her peripheral blood reveals red granules (*Schüffner's dots*) in enlarged, young erythrocytes. Which of the following organisms is most likely to have produced her signs and symptoms?

a. *Afipia felis*
b. *Ancyclostoma duodenale*
c. *B. microti*
d. *P. ovale*
e. *Toxoplasma gondii*

120. An apathetic male infant in an underdeveloped country is found to have peripheral edema, a "moon" face, and an enlarged, fatty liver. Which of the following is the basic defect causing this change in the liver?

a. Decreased protein intake leads to decreased lipoproteins
b. Decreased caloric intake leads to hypoalbuminemia
c. Decreased carbohydrate intake leads to hypoglycemia
d. Decreased fluid intake leads to hypernatremia
e. Decreased fat absorption leads to hypovitaminosis

121. A 32-year-old man presents with dry skin and symptoms of malabsorption including diarrhea and steatorrhea. The increased loss of fat in his stool caused a deficiency of fat-soluble vitamins. Which of the following abnormalities is most likely to develop in this individual without appropriate therapy?

a. Alopecia due to a deficiency of vitamin B_{12}
b. Megaloblastic anemia due to a deficiency of vitamin K
c. Night blindness due to a deficiency of vitamin A
d. Perifollicular hemorrhages due to a deficiency of vitamin D
e. Soft bones due to a deficiency of vitamin E

122. A 7-year-old girl is being evaluated for growth retardation and soft bones. A bone biopsy reveals a relative excess of woven bone with wide osteoid seams. Increased dietary cholecalciferol has no effect on her signs and symptoms. Which of the following enzymes is most likely to be deficient in this girl?

a. 1-α-hydroxylase
b. 5-α-reductase
c. 7-α-hydroxylase
d. 11-hydroxylase
e. 21-hydroxylase

123. A 22-year-old man presents with increasing fatigue and is being evaluated for anemia. Examination of a peripheral blood smear reveals a dimorphic population of red blood cells. That is, some of the red cells are normal in appearance, while others are hypochromic and microcytic. A bone marrow biopsy reveals an increase in the number of ring sideroblasts along with the presence of a few abnormal-appearing erythroid precursors. No chromosomal abnormalities are identified, but a deficiency of 5-aminolevulinic acid synthetase is found in the red blood cells. This individual should first be treated with a trial therapy using which one of the following substances?

a. Biotin
b. Cyanocobalamin
c. Pyridoxine
d. Riboflavin
e. Selenium

124. A 62-year-old male alcoholic is brought into the emergency room acting very confused. Physical examination reveals a thin, emaciated man who has problems with memory, ataxia, and paralysis of his extraocular muscles. These signs and symptoms, which are caused by a dietary deficiency of vitamin B_1, are most closely associated with hemorrhages into which one of the following areas of the central nervous system?

a. Cerebellar vermis
b. Mammillary bodies
c. Medial pons
d. Precentral gyrus
e. Substantia nigra

125. A 41-year-old man presents with slowly progressive diarrhea along with a dark discoloration of the skin of his neck ("necklace" dermatitis). Mental status evaluation finds changes suggestive of early dementia. Laboratory evaluation finds increased urinary 5-hydroxyindole acetic acid, and further workup finds a 4-cm tumor in the distal small intestines. Sections of this tumor were interpreted by the pathologist as being consistent with a carcinoid tumor. In this individual, the tumor produced serotonin from tryptophan and subsequently caused a deficiency of tryptophan. This in turn led to a deficiency of niacin, which produced the clinical signs of dermatitis, diarrhea, and dementia. Which of the following is the most likely diagnosis?

a. Beriberi
b. Marasmus
c. Pellagra
d. Rickets
e. Scurvy

126. A 70-year-old woman is brought to the emergency room by her granddaughter because she has developed ecchymosis covering many areas of her body. Her granddaughter states that her grandmother lives alone at home and has not been eating well. Her diet has consisted of mainly tea and toast, as she does not drink milk or eat fruits or vegetables. Your physical examination reveals small hemorrhages around hair follicles, some of these follicles having an unusual "corkscrew" appearance. You also notice swelling and hemorrhages of the gingiva. The signs and symptoms in this individual are most likely caused by a deficiency of which one of the following substances?

a. Thiamine
b. Pyridoxine
c. Niacin
d. Vitamin D
e. Vitamin C

127. A 67-year-old woman is brought to the emergency room by paramedics after she was involved in a motor vehicle accident. Among her many injuries is a linear tear of her scalp measuring approximately 3.5 cm in length. Small thin strands of tissue are seen crossing this wound. Which of the following is the best term that classifies this lesion?

a. Abrasion
b. Avulsion
c. Contusion
d. Incision
e. Laceration

128. A 7-year-old boy living in an old, run-down house is being evaluated for behavior problems in school. Pertinent medical history includes several recent episodes of abdominal colic. Examination of his peripheral blood reveals basophilic stippling of some of the erythrocytes. His white cell count and differential are within normal limits. Further laboratory evaluation finds increased free erythrocyte protoporphyrin in the serum. Which of the following substances is most likely to be increased in the urine of this boy?

a. Delta-aminolevulinic acid
b. Formic acid
c. Hydroxy-indoleacetic acid
d. N-formiminoglutamate
e. Vanillylmandelic acid

129. A 19-year-old woman is brought to the emergency room by her friends who say that she has been acting strangely for the past 6 h. They say that she had seemed depressed lately after breaking up with her boyfriend. Physical examination finds that she is quite drowsy and does not respond appropriately to questions. Her respiratory rate is increased and her optic disks are hyperemic. Laboratory examination finds a metabolic acidosis with a high-anion gap. These findings are most consistent with this woman having ingested which one of the following substances?

a. Cadmium
b. Cobalt
c. Laetrile
d. Mercury
e. Methanol

130. A 65-year-old woman presents to the hospital with increasing confusion. Pertinent clinical history is that she had been taking large amounts of laetrile as part of a metabolic therapy program consisting of a special diet and high-dose vitamin supplementation. Physical examination finds weakness of her arms and legs along with bilateral ptosis. Her skin has a cherry-red color, and the strong odor of bitter almonds is present. Which of the following is the most likely diagnosis?

a. Arsenic ingestion
b. Carbon monoxide toxicity
c. Carbon tetrachloride exposure
d. Cyanide poisoning
e. Ethylene glycol ingestion

131. Which of the following sets of serum levels is most likely to be seen in a young woman with exercise-induced amenorrhea?

	Follicle-Stimulating Hormone (FSH)	Luteinizing Hormone (LH)	Estrogen
a.	Increased	Increased	Increased
b.	Increased	Increased	Decreased
c.	Increased	Decreased	Increased
d.	Decreased	Increased	Decreased
e.	Decreased	Decreased	Decreased

132. A 22-year-old woman presents for a routine ultrasound examination during her first pregnancy. She has not taken any drugs or medications during this pregnancy. The ultrasound finds a male fetus with duplication of the first digit on his right hand. No other physical abnormalities are seen. Chromosomal studies on chorionic villi are within normal limits. In the absence of an identifiable familial syndrome, extra digits are most likely associated with mutations involving which one of the following genes?

a. Cdx-1 gene
b. HOX D13 gene
c. PATCHED gene
d. PAX-2 gene
e. Sonic Hedgehog gene

133. An 8-year-old boy is found to have progressive corneal vasculariza-tion, deafness, notched incisors, and a flattened nose. The most likely cause of these changes is congenital infection with which one of the fol-lowing organisms?

a. Toxoplasma
b. Rubella
c. Cytomegalovirus
d. Herpes simplex virus
e. *T. pallidum*

134. A newborn female infant develops edema, jaundice, and trouble breathing. The blood type of the mother is AB negative, while the baby and the father are both B positive. The mother's only other pregnancy was unre-markable, and she has never received any blood or blood products. Labo-ratory examination reveals a positive Coombs' (DAT) test. Which of the following is the most likely diagnosis?

a. ABO hemolytic disease of the newborn
b. Hemoglobin H disease
c. Hyaline membrane disease of the newborn
d. Hydrops fetalis
e. Rh hemolytic disease of the newborn

135. A premature male infant born at 29 weeks' gestation to a 22-year-old woman with gestational diabetes develops problems breathing about 14 h after delivery. Physical examination finds cyanosis, tachypnea, and nasal flaring. A chest x-ray reveals a bilateral diffuse reticular ("ground glass") appearance. His respiratory problems worsen and he is put on a ventilator. Which one of the following therapies should also be given at this time?

a. Dietary vitamin C
b. Intramuscular insulin
c. Intranasal vasopressin
d. Intratracheal surfactant
e. Intravascular epinephrine

136. A male infant is born markedly prematurely at 25 weeks' gestation. Due to the immaturity of his lungs, therapy with oxygen is used. Because of extensive medical intervention, this premature infant survives, but unfortunately he is found to be blind resulting from the use of oxygen. Which one of the following pathologic abnormalities correctly describes the pathology that caused this infant's blindness?

a. Accumulation of abnormal material in the ganglion cells of the retina
b. Fibrous obliteration of the canal of Schlemm
c. Formation of a fibrovascular mass behind the lens
d. Lipid accumulation at the periphery of the cornea
e. Severe degeneration of the macula

137. Physical examination of a newborn infant reveals underdeveloped forming short stumps without fingers or toes (phocomelia). This developmental abnormality is most consistent with intrauterine exposure to which substance?

a. 13-cis-retinoic acid
b. Diethylstilbestrol
c. Hydantoin
d. Alcohol
e. Thalidomide

138. A 14-month-old male infant presents with an enlarging abdominal mass. Laboratory examination reveals increased urinary levels of metanephrine and vanillylmandelic acid (VMA). A histologic section from the mass reveals a tumor composed of small, primitive-appearing cells with hyperchromatic nuclei and little to no cytoplasm. Occasional focal groups of tumor cells are arranged in a ring around a central space. Which of the following is the most likely diagnosis?

a. Adrenal cortical carcinoma
b. Ganglioneuroma
c. Nephroblastoma
d. Neuroblastoma
e. Pheochromocytoma

139. An elevated serum level of C-reactive protein (CRP) is now used as a clinical marker for determining an increased risk for developing which one of the listed disorders?

a. encephalopathy in patients with liver failure
b. myocardial infarction in patients with coronary artery disease
c. osteoporosis in patients with the nephrotic syndrome
d. pulmonary emboli in patients with peripheral vascular disease
e. thrombocytopenia in patients receiving heparin therapy

140. Which one of the listed substances is a fairly specific serum marker for ventricular dilatation and is used clinically to monitor a patient with congestive heart failure?

a. 5'-nucleotidase (5'-NT)
b. B-type natriuretic peptide (BNP)
c. Lactate dehydrogenase (LDH)
d. Mannan-binding protein (MBP)
e. Serum amyloid A (SAA)

141. Specificity of a test is defined by which one of the following expressions?

a. True negatives/(true negatives + false negatives)
b. True negatives/(true negatives + false positives)
c. True positives/(true positives + false negatives)
d. True positives/(true positives + false positives)
e. (True positives + false negatives)/(true negatives + false positives)

General Pathology

Answers

1. The answer is e. (*Kumar, pp 35–37, 41–42. Chandrasoma, 3/e, pp 8–10.*) Substances that can form clear spaces in the cytoplasm of cells as seen with a routine H&E stain include glycogen, lipid, and water. In the liver, clear spaces within hepatocytes are most likely to be lipid, this change being called fatty change or steatosis. In the normal metabolism of lipid by the liver, free fatty acids are either esterified to triglyceride, converted to cholesterol, oxidized into ketone bodies, or incorporated into phospholipids that can be excreted from the liver as very-low-density lipoproteins (VLDLs). Abnormalities involving any of these normal metabolic pathways may lead to the accumulation of triglycerides (not cholesterol) within the hepatocytes. For example, increased formation of triglycerides can result from alcohol use, as alcohol causes excess NADH formation (high NADH/NAD ratio), increases fatty acid synthesis, and decreases fatty acid oxidation.

In contrast to lipid, calcium appears as a dark blue-purple color with routine H&E stains, while hemosiderin, which is formed from the breakdown of ferritin, appears as yellow-brown granules. Lipofuscin also appears as fine, granular, golden-brown intracytoplasmic pigment. It is an insoluble "wear and tear" (aging) pigment found in residual bodies in the cytoplasm of aging cells, typically neurons, cardiac myocytes, or hepatocytes. Lipofuscin is composed of polymers of lipids and phospholipids derived from lipid peroxidation by free radicals of polyunsaturated lipids of subcellular membranes.

2. The answer is b. (*Alberts, pp 853–858, 878–880. Kumar, pp 9–100, 335–336.*) Many extracellular substances cause intracellular actions via second-messenger systems. These second messengers may bind to receptors that are located either on the surface of the cell or within the cell itself. Substances that react with intracellular receptors are lipid-soluble (lipophilic) molecules that can pass through the lipid plasma membrane. Examples of these lipophilic substances include thyroid hormones, steroid hormones, and the fat-soluble vitamins A and D. Once inside the cell these substances generally travel to the nucleus and bind to the hormone response element (HRE) of DNA.

Some substances that react with cell surface receptors bind to guanine-nucleotide regulatory proteins. These proteins, called G proteins, may be classified into four categories, namely, Gs, Gi, Gt, and Gq. Two of these receptors, Gs and Gi, regulate the intracellular concentration of adenosine 3', 5'-cyclic monophosphate (cAMP). In contrast, Gt regulates the intracytoplasmic levels of cyclic guanosine 3', 5'-monophosphate (cGMP), and Gq regulates the intracytoplasmic levels of calcium ions. Gs and Gi regulate intracellular cAMP levels by their actions on adenyl cyclase, an enzyme located on the inner surface of the plasma membrane that catalyzes the formation of cAMP from ATP. The adenylate cyclase G protein complex is composed of the following components: the receptor, the catalytic enzyme (i.e., adenyl cyclase), and a coupling unit. The coupling unit consists of GTP-dependent regulatory proteins (G proteins), which may either be stimulatory (Gs) or inhibitory (Gi). When bound to GTP and active, Gs stimulates adenyl cyclase and increases cAMP levels. (Gs can be thought of as the "on switch.") In contrast, when bound to GTP and active, Gi inhibits adenyl cyclase and decreases cAMP levels. (Gi can be thought of as the "off switch.") It is important to note that cholera toxin and pertussis toxin both act by altering this adenyl cyclase pathway. Cholera toxin inhibits the conversion of Gs-GTP to Gs-GDP. In contrast, pertussis toxin inhibits the activation of Gi-GDP to Gi-GTP. Therefore, both cholera toxin and pertussis toxin prolong the functioning of adenyl cyclase and therefore increase intracellular cAMP, but their mechanisms are different. Cholera toxin keeps the "on switch" in the "on" position, while pertussis toxin keeps the "off switch" in the "off" position.

3. The answer is a. *(Kumar, pp 61–62, 243–244. Rubin, pp 67, 1088.)* Patients with chronic granulomatous disease have defective functioning of phagocytic neutrophils and monocytes due to an inability to produce hydrogen peroxide. That is, their phagocytic cells have a decreased oxidative or respiratory burst. The most common cause of chronic granulomatous disease is defective NADPH oxidase, which is an enzyme on the membrane of lysosomes that converts O_2 to superoxide and stimulates oxygen burst. This deficiency results in recurrent infections with catalase-positive organisms, such as *S. aureus*. The classic form of chronic granulomatous disease usually affects boys and causes death before the age of 10. Key findings in chronic granulomatous disease include lymphadenitis, hepatosplenomegaly, eczematoid dermatitis, pulmonary infiltrates that are associated with hypergammaglobulinemia, and defective ability of neutrophils to kill bacteria.

A defect in the enzyme adenosine deaminase (ADA) is seen in the autosomal recessive (Swiss) form of severe combined immunodeficiency disease (SCID), while a defect in the IL-2 receptor is seen in the X-linked recessive form of SCID. A developmental defect at the pre-B stage is seen in X-linked agammaglobulinemia of Bruton, while developmental failure of pharyngeal pouches 3 and 4 is characteristic of DiGeorge's syndrome.

4. The answer is e. (*Kumar, pp 68–69.*) Certain drugs are important in the control of acute inflammation because they inhibit portions of the metabolic pathways involving arachidonic acid. For example, corticosteroids induce the synthesis of lipocortins, a family of proteins that are inhibitors of phospholipase A_2. They decrease the formation of arachidonic acid and its metabolites, prostaglandins, and leukotrienes. Aspirin, indomethacin, and other nonsteroidal anti-inflammatory drugs (NSAIDs), in contrast, inhibit cyclooxygenase and therefore inhibit the synthesis of prostaglandins and thromboxanes. The prostaglandins have several important functions. For example, prostaglandin E_2 (PGE$_2$), produced within the anterior hypothalamus in response to IL-1 secretion from leukocytes, results in fever. Therefore aspirin can be used to treat fever by inhibiting PGE$_2$ production. PGE$_2$ is also a vasodilator that can keep a ductus arteriosus open. At birth, breathing decreases pulmonary resistance and reverses the flow of blood through the ductus arteriosus. The oxygenated blood flowing from the aorta into the ductus inhibits prostaglandin production and closes the ductus arteriosus. Therefore, PGE$_2$ can be given clinically to keep the ductus arteriosus open, while indomethacin can be used to close a patent ductus. Prostaglandin F_2 (PGF$_2$) causes uterine contractions, which can result in dysmenorrhea. Indomethacin can be used to treat dysmenorrhea by inhibiting the production of PGF$_2$. Bradykinin is a nonapeptide that increases vascular permeability, contracts smooth muscle, dilates blood vessels, and causes pain. It is part of the kinin system and is formed from high-molecular-weight kininogen (HMWK). Histamine, a vasoactive amine that is stored in mast cells, basophils, and platelets, acts on H_1 receptors to cause dilation of arterioles and increased vascular permeability of venules.

5. The answer is c. (*Kumar, pp 91–95.*) Stem cells are unique cells that are characterized by their ability for asymmetric replication, which refers to the fact that one of the products of cell division is capable of self-renewal. Embryonic stem cells are pluripotential, that is, they are capable of forming all the tissues of the body, while adult stem cells are usually only able to differentiate into a particular tissue. Stem cells, which have been identified in many different tissues, are located in special sites called niches. For example, cells located in the canals of Hering of the liver can give rise to precursor cells called oval cells, which are capable of forming hepatocytes and biliary cells. Satellite cells, located in the basal lamina of myotubules, can differentiate into myocytes after injury, while limbus cells located in the canals of Schlemm are stem cells for the cornea. Other sites for stem cells are the base of the crypts of the colon and the dentate gyrus of the hippocampus. In contrast to stem cells, Ito cells, which are located in the subendothelial space of Disse, store vitamin A, and Paneth cells, located near the bottom of crypts, provide host defense against microorganisms.

6. The answer is b. (*Henry, pp 643–646, 656–657. Kumar, pp 129–130. Ayala, p 196.*) Two important control points of the coagulation cascade are the fibrinolytic system and certain plasma protease inhibitors. The main component of the fibrinolytic system is plasmin, which is converted from plasminogen by either factor XII or a plasminogen activator (PA). Examples of PAs include tissue plasminogen activator (tPA), urokinase plasminogen activator, and streptokinase. Once formed, plasmin splits fibrin and also degrades both fibrinogen and coagulation factors VIII and V. Plasma protease inhibitors include antithrombin III and protein C. Antithrombin III in the presence of heparin inhibits thrombin, XIIa, XIa, Xa, and IXa, while protein C inhibits Va and VIIIa. The significance of these control mechanisms is illustrated by the fact that abnormalities of these systems, such as deficiencies of antithrombin III, protein C, or protein S, are associated with hypercoagulable states and increased risk of thrombosis, as the main factors leading to thrombosis include injury to endothelium, alterations in blood flow, and hypercoagulability of the blood. Hypercoagulability may be a primary (genetic) or secondary abnormality. Primary hypercoagulable states include the previously mentioned deficiencies of antithrombin III, protein C, or protein S. These deficiencies are associated with recurrent thromboembolism in early adult life and recurrent spontaneous abortions in women. The causes of secondary hypercoagulable states are numerous and include severe trauma, burns, disseminated cancer, and pregnancy. Lower risk factors for the development of secondary hypercoagulable states include age, smoking, and obesity. Some patients with high titers of autoantibodies against anionic phospholipids such as cardiolipin (the antibody being called a lupus anticoagulant) have a high frequency of arterial and venous thrombosis. To summarize, it is important to remember that the differential diagnosis of recurrent spontaneous abortions in women includes deficiencies of protein C and protein S, and the presence of the lupus anticoagulant, which is part of the antiphospholipid syndrome.

7. The answer is e. (*Kumar, pp 151–152.*) Inheritance of single abnormal genes generally follows one of the following patterns of inheritance: autosomal dominant (AD), autosomal recessive (AR), or X-linked. The key point about X-linked disorders is that there is no male-to-male transmission. [Note that in males the terms dominant and recessive do not apply (since they have only one X chromosome). Also note that X-linked inheritance is different from sex-influenced AD inheritance, an example of which is baldness.] Examples of X-linked recessive (XR) disorders include a few hematology diseases, such as glucose-6-phosphate dehydrogenase deficiency, factor VIII deficiency (hemophilia A), and factor IX deficiency (hemophilia B). Characteristics of XR disorders include: an affected male does not transmit the disease to his sons (e.g., individual III-5 in the pedigree), but all daughters are carriers (individual III-3); sons of carrier females have a one in two chances of the disorder (individual III-8), but all daughters are asymptomatic (individual II-3); and the trait occurs in maternal uncles and in male cousins descended from the mother's sisters (oblique transmission). Affected females are rare and may be homozygous for the disease or may have an unfavorable lyonization. Evaluating the pedigree with this question finds that individual I-1 is a carrier for hemophilia A and individual II-6 could also be a carrier and transmit the disease to a male offspring.

In contrast to XR disorders, characteristics of X-linked dominant (XD) disorders, which are quite rare, include no skipped generations (dominant inheritance) and no male-to-male transmission (X-linked inheritance). A key point is to note that females are affected twice as often as males. Affected females transmit the disease to 50% of their daughters and 50% of their sons. Affected males transmit the disease to all of their daughters and none of their sons. A subtype of X-linked dominant disease is seen when the condition is lethal in utero in hemizygous males. Therefore the condition is seen clinically in heterozygous females, who also have an increase in the number of abortions.

Finally, characteristics of AD inheritance include symptoms manifested in the heterozygous state, males and females affected equally, and vertical transmission. Characteristics of AR inheritance include manifestations in the homozygous state, horizontal transmission, males and females affected equally, and common occurrence of complete penetrance and consanguineous relations.

8. The answer is e. (*Kumar, pp 33, 185, 1341–1342. Damjanov, pp 298–299.*) Almost all genes occur on chromosomes within the nucleus. There are a few genes, however, that are located within the mitochondria. These mitochondrial genes are found on mitochondrial DNA (mtDNA). These genes are all of maternal origin, possibly because ova have mitochondria within the large amount of cytoplasm while sperm do not. This maternal origin means that mothers transmit all of the mtDNA to both male and female offspring, but only the daughters transmit it further. No transmission occurs through males. This mtDNA contains genes that mainly code for oxidative phosphorylation enzymes, such as NADH dehydrogenase, cytochrome c oxidase, and ATP synthase. Symptoms of deficiencies of these enzymes occur in organs that require large amounts of ATP, such as the brain, muscle, liver, and kidneys. The mtDNA of these patients may be composed of either a mixture of mutant and normal DNA (heteroplasm) or of mutant DNA entirely (homoplasmy). The severity of these diseases correlates with the amount of mutant mtDNA that is present. One disease associated with mitochondrial inheritance is Leber hereditary optic neuropathy (LHON), which is characterized by progressive bilateral loss of central vision and usually occurs between 15 and 35 years of age. Other examples of mitochondrial inheritance include mitochondrial myopathies, which are characterized by the presence in muscle of mitochondria having abnormal sizes and shapes. These abnormal mitochondria may result in the histologic appearance of the muscle as ragged red fibers. Electron microscopy reveals the presence within large mitochondria of rectangular crystals that have a "parking lot" appearance.

9. The answer is c. (*Kumar, pp 158–165.*) One group of lysosomal storage diseases is characterized by the abnormal accumulation of sphingolipids (SLs). Some types of sphingolipids are typically found within the central nervous system, and therefore abnormal accumulation of these substances produces neurologic signs and symptoms. For example, ganglion cells within the retina, particularly at the periphery of the macula, may become swollen with excess sphingolipids. The affected area of the retina appears pale when viewed through an ophthalmoscope. In contrast, the normal color of the macula, which does not have accumulated substances, appears more red than normal. This is referred to as a cherry-red spot or a cherry-red macula. Substances that may produce this cherry-red spot include sphingomyelin, which is increased in individuals with Niemann-Pick disease, and gangliosides, which may be increased in individuals with Tay-Sachs disease, Sandhoff disease, or G_{M1} gangliosidosis.

Autosomal recessive disorders tend to be more common in areas in which inbreeding is more common. An example of this is the increased frequency of several autosomal recessive genes in Ashkenazi Jews. Ashkenazi denotes an ethnic group, mostly of the Jewish faith, from Eastern Europe. People of this faith tend to marry other members of the faith. Two storage diseases that have a higher incidence in Ashkenazi Jews are Tay-Sachs disease and type I Gaucher disease. Tay-Sachs disease is due to a deficiency of hexosaminidase A. This same enzyme is decreased in patients with Sandhoff disease. Hexosaminidase A is composed of an α subunit and a β subunit. In contrast, hexosaminidase B is composed of two β subunits. Patients with Tay-Sachs disease have a deficiency of the α subunit. Therefore, they have a deficiency of hexosaminidase A, but not hexosaminidase B. In contrast, patients with Sandhoff disease have a deficiency of the β subunit, and thus they have a deficiency of both hexosaminidase A and hexosaminidase B. In patients with Tay-Sachs disease, accumulation of G_{M2} ganglioside occurs within many tissues, including the heart, liver, spleen, and brain. Electron microscopy reveals cytoplasmic whorled lamellar bodies within lysosomes. There are several clinical forms of Tay-Sachs disease, but the most severe is the infantile type. Patients develop mental retardation, seizures, motor incoordination, and blindness (amaurosis), and usually die by the age of 3 years.

Type I Gaucher disease is due to a deficiency of β-glucocerebrosidase. Patients may have increased serum levels of acid phosphatase (an enzyme that is typically found in the prostate), erythrocytes, and platelets. Patients with Gaucher disease have accumulation of excess glucocerebrosides within phagocytic cells, not ganglion cells. Sphingomyelinase is decreased in patients with Niemann-Pick disease, while arylsulfatase is decreased in patients with MLD.

10. The answer is d. (*Kumar, pp 153, 1311. Champe, pp 348–349.*) Purine synthesis involves adding carbons and nitrogens to ribose 5-phosphate (R5P), which is a product of the hexose monophosphate (HMP) shunt. R5P is then converted to ribose phosphate pyrophosphate (RPPP), which is subsequently converted to 5'-phosphoribosylamine, the latter step being the committed step in purine nucleotide biosynthesis. Through a series of steps RPPP is converted to inosine 5'-monophosphate (IMP). Several of these biochemical steps involve transferring methyl groups from folate. This is important because folate analogues, such as methotrexate, inhibit DNA synthesis, especially in rapidly growing tumor cells, by inhibiting purine synthesis. Finally IMP is converted into either adenosine monophosphate (AMP) or guanosine monophosphate (GMP). These last biochemical steps are also connected to biochemical reactions that involve adenosine deaminase, an enzyme that is deficient in individuals with the autosomal recessive form of SCID, and hypoxanthine-guanine phosphoribosyltransferase (HGPRT), an enzyme of the purine salvage pathway for recycling guanine and hypoxanthine that is deficient in individuals with the X-linked recessive disorder Lesch-Nyhan syndrome. This disorder is characterized by excess uric acid production, which may produce symptoms of gout, mental retardation, spasticity, self-mutilation, and aggressive behavior. In contrast, a deficiency of homogentistic oxidase, which is involved in the conversion of homogentisic acid to methylacetoacetate, is associated with alkaptonuria. Abnormal degradation of galactocerebroside is seen in Krabbe's disease, while abnormal breakdown of branched-chain amino acids is seen in maple syrup urine disease.

11. The answer is d. (*Damjanov, p 252. Kumar, p 179.*) A 47,XXY karyotype is the classic karyotype for Klinefelter syndrome, a disorder that is associated with the presence of two or more X chromosomes and one or more Y chromosomes. In most cases the extra X chromosome is inherited from the mother, and therefore this disorder is associated with increased maternal age. Klinefelter syndrome is an important cause of hypogonadism in men. Patients have small, firm, atrophic testes, often associated with a micropenis. Histologic sections of the testes reveal atrophy of the tubules, Leydig cell hyperplasia, and lack of sperm production. Therefore, individuals with Klinefelter syndrome are infertile (Klinefelter syndrome is the principle cause of male infertility). Because of the testicular atrophy, patients have decreased levels of testosterone, which leads to increased blood levels of FSH and LH. Estradiol levels are also increased, but the cause of this increase is unknown. The combination of decreased testosterone and increased estradiol leads to eunuchoidism, lack of secondary male characteristics, and a female distribution of hair. Patients tend to be tall due to delayed fusion of the epiphysis that results from a lack of testosterone.

Patients also develop a high voice and gynecomastia, and they have an increased incidence of breast cancer. Patients have a slight decrease in IQ, but they are not severely mentally retarded.

12. The answer is a. (*Kumar, pp 149, 181–183. Rubin, pp 263–264.*) Fragile X syndrome is one of four diseases that are characterized by long repeating sequences of three nucleotides. The other diseases are Huntington's disease, myotonic dystrophy, and spinal and bulbar muscular atrophy. The fragile X syndrome, which is more common in males than females, is one of the most common causes of familial mental retardation. Additional clinical features of this disorder include developmental delay, a long face with a large mandible, large everted ears, and large testicles (macroorchidism). Examination of the DNA from patients with fragile X syndrome reveals multiple tandem repeats of the nucleotide sequence CGG on the X chromosome. Normally these repeats average up to 50 in number, but in patients with fragile X syndrome there are more than 230 repeats. This number of repeats is called a full mutation. Normal transmitting males (NTMs) and carrier females have between 50 and 230 CGG repeats. This number of repeats is called a premutation. During oogenesis, but not spermatogenesis, premutations can be converted to mutations by amplification of the triplet repeats. This explains the much higher incidence of mental retardation in grandsons rather than brothers of NTMs (Sherman's paradox), as the premutation is amplified in females but not in males. Since the premutation is not amplified in males, no daughters of NTMs are affected. An additional finding associated with these repeat units is anticipation, which refers to the fact that the disease is worse in subsequent generations.

13. The answer is d. (*Kumar, pp 235–236.*) The combination of dry eyes (keratoconjunctivitis) and dry mouth (xerostomia) in an adult woman is suggestive of Sjögren's syndrome, an autoimmune disorder characterized by immunologic destruction of the lacrimal and salivary glands. This disorder is characterized by the presence of SS-A and SS-B autoantibodies, but the diagnosis of Sjögren syndrome is confirmed by finding a lymphocytic infiltrate within minor salivary glands from a biopsy of the lip. Lymphocytic infiltrates are characteristic of organs affected by autoimmune diseases. In addition to enlargement of the salivary glands, the lymph nodes of patients with Sjögren's syndrome may be enlarged due to a pleomorphic infiltrate of B lymphocytes. Indeed patients have an approximately 40-fold increased risk for developing non-Hodgkin's lymphoma, especially marginal zone lymphoma. The majority of individuals with Sjögren syndrome have manifestations of other autoimmune disorders, such as systemic lupus erythematosus (SLE), rheumatoid arthritis, or systemic sclerosis, and involvement of the lungs and kidneys does occur. Glomerular lesions are very rare, but a mild tubulointerstitial nephritis is quite common and may result in renal tubular acidosis.

14. The answer is a. (*Kumar, pp 240–245. Rubin, pp 129–133.*) In X-linked agammaglobulinemia (XLA) of Bruton, B cells are absent but numbers and function of T cells are normal. This abnormality results from defective maturation of B lymphocytes beyond the pre-B stage. This block results from a mutation in the gene coding for a particular tyrosine kinase called Bruton tyrosine kinase (Btk). This maturation defect leads to decreased or absent numbers of plasma cells, and therefore immunoglobulin levels are markedly decreased. Male infants with Bruton disease begin having trouble with recurrent bacterial infections at about the age of 9 months, which is when maternal antibodies are no longer present in the affected infant. Therapy for Bruton disease consists primarily of IV gamma globulin.

Common variable immunodeficiency (CVI; adult-onset agammaglobulinemia) has a variable clinical presentation but it is characterized by decreased immunoglobulin (especially IgG) levels with hyperplastic B cell areas and no plasma cells. In contrast to patients with XLA, patients with CVI have normal numbers of B cells in the peripheral blood. Patients develop recurrent infections, especially bacteria and *Giardia* infections, and have an increased incidence of autoimmune diseases and lymphoid malignancies.

DiGeorge's syndrome is a T cell-deficiency disorder that results from hypoplasia of the thymus due to abnormal development of the third and fourth pharyngeal pouches. The parathyroid glands are also abnormal, and these individuals develop hypocalcemia and tetany. Congenital heart defects are also present.

Isolated deficiency of IgA is probably the most common form of immunodeficiency. It is due to a block in the terminal differentiation of B lymphocytes. Most patients are asymptomatic, but some develop chronic sinopulmonary infections. Patients are prone to developing diarrhea (Giardia infection) and also have an increased incidence of autoimmune disease, such as Hashimoto's thyroiditis.

Finally, Omenn's syndrome is a rare autosomal recessive form of SCID caused by mutations in the RAG-1 and RAG-2 genes. This results in the inability to rearrange the VDJ regions in the T-cell and B-cell receptors. Clinically newborns with Omenn's syndrome develop dermatitis and diarrhea in the first weeks of life and then develop severe infections with viruses, bacteria, and fungi.

15. The answer is d. (*Kumar, pp 335, 1043. Chandrasoma, pp 307–308.*) An embryonal carcinoma is a testicular malignancy that secretes alpha-fetoprotein (α-AFP) and is composed of undifferentiated cells along with primitive glandular differentiation. Once the diagnosis of malignancy is established, clinicians estimate the prognosis for the patient through the process of grading and staging the malignancy. It is important to understand the difference between these two terms. First of all, note that these terms are applied only to malignant neoplasms. Basically, grading is done histologically, while staging is done clinically. Grading of a malignant tumor is based on the histologic degree of differentiation of the tumor cells and on the number of mitoses that are present. These histologic features are thought to be indicators of the aggressiveness of the malignant neoplasm. Cancers are generally classified into grades I through IV. Lower grades, such as grades I and II, are more differentiated, less aggressive and have a better prognosis, while higher grades, such as grades III and IV, are less differentiated, more aggressive and have a worse prognosis. Tumors composed of malignant cells that appear primitive or undifferentiated are classified as high grade tumors.

In contrast to grading, the staging of cancers is based on the size of the primary lesion, the presence of lymph node metastases, and the presence of blood-borne metastases. These characteristics are determined by clinical means. The two main staging systems were developed by the Union Internationale Contre le Cancer (UICC) and the American Joint Committee (AJC) on Cancer Staging. The UICC classification is called the TNM classification where the T refers to the tumor size, the N refers to the presence of lymph node metastases, and the M refers to the presence of non-lymph node metastases. The location of the tumor is also important, as the TNM classification uses different staging systems depending on the location of the primary tumor. In contrast, the AJC staging system generally divides cancers into stages 0 through IV. Lower stage tumors are smaller, localized, and have a better prognosis, while higher stage tumors are larger, widespread, and have a worse prognosis. Staging has proved to be of greater clinical value than grading.

16. The answer is a. (*Kumar, pp 319–323, 924.*) Many chemicals are associated with an increased incidence of malignancy. These substances are called chemical carcinogens. Although there are direct-acting chemical carcinogens, such as the direct-acting alkylating agents that are used in chemotherapy, most organic carcinogens first require conversion to a more reactive compound. Polycyclic aromatic hydrocarbons, aromatic amines, and azo dyes must be metabolized by cytochrome P450–dependent mixed-function oxidases to active metabolites. Vinyl chloride is metabolized to an epoxide and is associated with angiosarcoma of the liver, not hepatocellular carcinoma. Azo dyes, such as butter yellow and scarlet red, are metabolized to active compounds that have induced hepatocellular cancer in rats, but no human cases have been reported. β-naphthylamine is an exception to the general rule involving cytochrome P450, as the hydrolysis of the nontoxic conjugate occurs in the urinary bladder by the urinary enzyme glucuronidase. In the past there has been an increase in bladder cancer in workers in the aniline dye and rubber industries who have been exposed to these compounds. Aflatoxin B1, a natural product of the fungus *Aspergillus flavus*, is metabolized to an epoxide. The fungus can grow on improperly stored peanuts and grains and is associated with the high incidence of hepatocellular carcinoma in some areas of Africa and the Far East. Hepatitis B virus is also highly associated with liver cancer in these regions.

17. The answer is b. (*Kumar, pp 333–335. Chandrasoma, p 858.*) Symptoms not caused by either local or metastatic effects of tumors are called paraneoplastic syndromes. Bronchogenic carcinomas are associated with the development of many different types of paraneoplastic syndromes. These syndromes are usually associated with the secretion of certain substances by the tumor cells. For example, ectopic secretion of ACTH may produce Cushing's syndrome, while ectopic secretion of antidiuretic hormone (syndrome of inappropriate ADH secretion) may produce hyponatremia. Hypocalcemia may result from the production of calcitonin, while hypercalcemia may result from the production of parathyroid hormone–related peptide (PTHrP), which is a normal substance produced locally by many different types of tissue. PTHrP is distinct from parathyroid hormone (PTH). Therefore, patients with this type of paraneoplastic syndrome have increased calcium levels and decreased PTH levels. As a result of decreased PTH production, all of the parathyroid glands in these patients are atrophic. Other tumors associated with the production of

PTHrP include clear cell carcinomas of the kidney, endometrial adenocarcinomas, and transitional carcinomas of the urinary bladder. Lung cancers are also associated with multiple, migratory venous thromboses. This migratory thrombophlebitis is called Trousseau's sign and is more classically associated with carcinoma of the pancreas. Hypertrophic osteoarthropathy is a syndrome consisting of periosteal new bone formation with or without digital clubbing and joint effusion. It is most commonly found in association with lung carcinoma, but it also occurs with other types of pulmonary disease. Erythrocytosis is associated with increased erythropoietin levels and some tumors, particularly renal cell carcinomas, hepatocellular carcinomas, and cerebellar hemangioblastomas. It is not particularly associated with bronchogenic carcinomas.

18. The answer is e. *(Kumar, pp 359, 372–374. Ayala, pp 136, 294.)* Toxic shock syndrome (TSS) is caused mainly by infection with certain types of *S. aureus* that secrete the toxin toxic shock syndrome toxin 1 (TSST-1). TSS can also be caused by *Streptococcus pyogenes* that secretes exotoxins A and B. All of these toxins are types of superantigens that bind to both the class II major histocompatibility complex (MHC) and T-cell receptor (TCR) outside of the normal antigen-binding groove. As such, these toxins can react with up to 10% of peripheral T cells, which leads to massive T-cell activation and shock. Clinically, TSS caused by *S. aureus* is most often seen in women who use certain tampons that have been colonized with Staphylococcus. Either sex can be affected by TSS caused by *Streptococcus*. In either case, symptoms include fever, chills, watery diarrhea, myalgias, hypotension, and a diffuse rash that begins on the trunk and spreads to the arms and legs. The rash typically involves the palms and soles.

In contrast, erysipelas is caused by a dermal streptococci (*S. pyogenes*) infection of the face or scalp. It is characterized by a rapidly spreading, erythematous swelling that usually begins on face in a "butterfly" distribution. There is a sharp demarcation between the affected and unaffected skin, this being due to degradation of hyaluronic acid in ground substance of the skin. In contrast to erysipelas, cellulitis refers to a deeper infection of the skin that involves the dermis and subcutaneous tissue. The most common organisms are group A streptococci (*S. pyogenes*) and *Staphylococcus aureus*. Impetigo is caused by a superficial epidermal infection with either *Staphylococcus aureus* or *Streptococcus pyogenes* (group A strep). Characteristically pustules (blisters filled with pus) are found on the face of children. They can rupture to form a thick yellow (honey-colored) crust. Neonatal impetigo is caused by Staph that produces epidermolytic toxin, which leads to bullae formation and denuded skin ("scalded skin syndrome"). Finally, the skin lesions seen with secondary syphilis are typically maculopapular, scaly, or pustular, and secondary syphilis is not associated with high fever, nausea, or diarrhea.

19. The answer is d. (*Kumar, pp 397–401, 754–755. Rubin, pp 432–440.*) *H. capsulatum*, a dimorphic fungus, causes one of the three major fungal infections in the United States that may result in systemic infection (*Blastomyces* and *Coccidioides* are the other two). Although *H. capsulatum* commonly produces asymptomatic primary disease, it can result in granulomatous inflammation, especially granulomatous lung disease. Multiple small yeasts surrounded by clear zones may be found within the cytoplasm of macrophages. The source for *Histoplasma* is soil contaminated by the excreta of birds (starlings and chickens) and bats. The typical location for individuals to develop histoplasmosis is the Ohio and Mississippi Valley areas. *Aspergillus* species produce several clinical disease states, including allergic aspergillosis, systemic aspergillosis, and aspergilloma. Typically *Aspergillus* species are seen in tissue as acute angle-branching septate hyphae; however, they may form fruiting bodies in cavities, such as within cystic cavities of the lungs. There they may form a large mass called a fungus ball or aspergilloma. Blastomycosis is a chronic granulomatosis disease caused by a dimorphic fungus, *B. dermatitidis*. In tissues this fungus is seen as a thick-walled yeast having broad-based budding. Without the budding, Blastomyces may be mistaken for *Cryptococcus*. The infection, also known as Gilchrist's disease, is seen in individuals living in the Ohio and Mississippi Valley areas and is usually confined to the lungs. Candida species, which frequently cause human infections, grow as yeasts, elongated chains of yeast without hyphae (pseudohyphae), or septate hyphae. Mucocutaneous candidal infections can produce white plaques called thrush. Mucormycosis (zygomycosis) is a disease caused by "bread mold fungi" such as *Rhizopus, Mucor,* and *Absidia* species. These infections typically occur in neutropenic patients or diabetics. One form of the disease, typically found in diabetics, is called rhinocerebral mucormycosis and is characterized by facial pain, headache, changing mental status, and a blood-tinged nasal discharge. Tissue sections reveal characteristic broad, nonseptate, right angle–branching hyphae.

20. The answer is e. (*Kumar, p 456. Schneider, p 192.*) Vitamin K compounds include phylloquinone (K_1), which is the major form of vitamin K in plants, and menaquinone (K_2), which is produced by bacteria. Up to 50% of the vitamin K needed by the body is provided by the normal bacteria of the GI tract. Therefore a deficiency of vitamin K can result from a decrease in the normal number of vitamin K-producing bacteria in the gut, which in adults can result from the use of broad-spectrum antibiotics. In neonates vitamin K deficiency can result from inadequate colonization of the gut by bacteria or rarely from breast milk, which is low in vitamin K. This deficiency in neonates can result in hemorrhagic disease of the newborn, which typically occurs prior to day 7 of life. In adults, a deficiency of vitamin K can also result from a dietary deficiency or decreased absorption, which can result from fat malabsorption, pancreatitis, or diffuse liver disease.

Vitamin K is required for the posttranslational conversion of glutamyl residues in some proteins into gamma-carboxylates. It participates in the hepatic carboxylation of four procoagulants (factors II, VII, IX, and X) and plasma proteins C and S. For these four proclotting factors, this gamma-carboxylation provides the calcium-binding sites necessary for the calcium-dependent interaction with a phospholipid surface. Because of this, a deficiency of vitamin K produces a bleeding diathesis characterized by hematomas, ecchymoses, hematuria, melena, and bleeding from the gums. Laboratory tests reveal an increased bleeding with prolonged PT and PTT and normal bleeding time.

In contrast, a deficiency of vitamin A is associated with night blindness, dry eyes, dry skin, and recurrent infections; a deficiency of vitamin B_1 (thiamine) with beriberi; a deficiency of vitamin B_6 (pyridoxine) with sideroblastic anemia, and vitamin C (ascorbic acid) with scurvy.

21. The answer is c. (*Kumar, pp 14–15, 23–24.*) Damage to cells may result in reversible or irreversible injury. Common mediators of cell injury include chemicals, toxins, free radicals, and decreased oxygen delivery by the blood. Decreased blood flow (ischemia) decreases ATP production by aerobic cellular processes because of the deficiency of oxygen. This results in decreased oxidative phosphorylation by mitochondria, which decreases the functioning of the ATP-dependent sodium pump of the plasma membrane. This decreases the efflux of sodium ions outside the cell and decreases the influx of potassium out of the cell, which increases the sodium ions inside the cell and increases the potassium ions outside the cell. The resultant net gain of intracellular ions causes isosmotic water accumulation and hydropic swelling (cloudy swelling) of the cell and the organelles of the cell. Decreased aerobic respiration by mitochondria also increases anaerobic glycolysis, which decreases intracellular pH by increasing lactic acid production (lactic acidosis). The decreased pH causes chromatin clumping and may activate lysosomal enzymes. Additionally, ribosomes can dissociate from the endoplasmic reticulum (RER), which decreases protein production by cell. All of these changes that result from hypoxia are characteristic of reversible cellular injury, as they are reversible if blood flow and oxygen supply are restored.

22. The answer is b. (*Kumar, pp 15–16, 37–38.*) With prolonged ischemia, certain cellular events occur that are not reversible, even with restoration of oxygen supply. These cellular changes are referred to as irreversible cellular injury. This type of injury is characterized by severe damage to mitochondria (vacuole formation), extensive damage to plasma membranes and nuclei, and rupture of lysosomes. Severe damage to mitochondria is characterized by the influx of calcium ions into the mitochondria and the subsequent formation of large, flocculent densities within the mitochondria. These flocculent densities are characteristically seen in irreversibly injured myocardial cells that undergo reperfusion soon after injury. Less severe changes in mitochondria, such as mitochondrial swelling, are seen with reversible injury. Cytochrome c released from damaged mitochondria can induce apoptosis, a process through which irreversibly injured cells can shrink and increase the eosinophilia of their cytoplasm. These shrunken apoptotic cells (apoptotic bodies) may be engulfed by adjacent cells or macrophages. Myelin figures are derived from plasma membranes and organelle membranes and can be seen with either reversible or irreversible injury. Psammoma bodies are small, laminated calcifications, while Russell bodies are round, eosinophilic aggregates of immunoglobulin.

23. The answer is c. (*Kumar, pp 39–42. Carson, pp 119–123, 142–144, 159–162, 214–215.*) The differential for brown (or yellow-brown) granules in hepatocytes as seen with routine hematoxylin and eosin (H&E) stain includes hemosiderin, bile, and lipofuscin. The special histologic stain for hemosiderin, which contains iron, is the Prussian blue stain. Hemosiderin stains blue with a Prussian blue stain. Causes of excess iron deposition in the liver include hemosiderosis, which can result from excessive blood transfusions, and familial hemochromatosis, which results from excessive iron absorption from the gut. In contrast, excess bile in the liver can be seen with jaundice, while lipofuscin deposition is seen with aging, cachexia, and severe malnutrition.

In contrast to the Prussian blue stain, the oil red O stain and the Sudan black B stain are both used to demonstrate neutral lipids in tissue sections, while the PAS (periodic acid–Schiff) stain is used to demonstrate carbohydrates. For example, glycogen is PAS-positive, and this staining characteristically is diastase-sensitive. Finally the trichrome stain is used to demonstrate collagen or smooth muscle in tissue. With this stain collagen appears blue, while smooth muscle appears red.

24. The answer is c. (*Kumar, pp 34, 37–41, 423, 905.*) Hyalin is a nonspecific term that is used to describe any material, inside or outside the cell, that stains a red homogenous color with the routine H&E stain. There are many different substances that have the appearance of hyalin. Alcoholic hyaline inclusions (Mallory bodies) are irregular eosinophilic hyaline inclusions that are found within the cytoplasm of hepatocytes. Mallory bodies are composed of prekeratin intermediate filaments. They are a nonspecific finding and can be found in patients with several diseases other than alcoholic hepatitis, such as Wilson's disease, and in patients who have undergone bypass operations for morbid obesity. Immunoglobulins may form intracytoplasmic or extracellular oval hyaline bodies called Russell bodies. Excess plasma proteins may form hyaline droplets in proximal renal tubular epithelial cells or hyaline membranes in the alveoli of the lungs (hyaline membrane disease). The hyalin found in the walls of arterioles of kidneys in patients with benign nephrosclerosis is composed of basement membranes and precipitated plasma proteins. Lipofuscin is an intracytoplasmic aging pigment that has a yellow-brown, finely granular appearance with H&E stains. Its appearance does not resemble that of hyaline material.

25. The answer is b. (*Kumar, pp 41–42. Henry, pp 195–196.*) Calcification within tissue can be classified as being dystrophic or metastatic. Dystrophic calcification is characterized by calcification in abnormal (dystrophic) tissue, while metastatic calcification is characterized by calcification in normal tissue. Examples of dystrophic calcification include calcification within severe atherosclerosis, calcification of damaged or abnormal heart valves, and calcification within tumors. Small (microscopic) laminated calcifications within tumors are called psammoma bodies and are due to single-cell necrosis. Psammoma bodies are characteristically found in papillary tumors, such as papillary carcinomas of the thyroid and papillary tumors of the ovary (especially papillary serous cystadenocarcinomas), but they can also be found in meningiomas or mesotheliomas. Dystrophic calcification within tumors of the central nervous system (CNS), which can be seen with x-rays, is useful in the differential diagnosis of these CNS tumors. For example, calcification of a tumor of the cortex in an adult is suggestive of an oligodendroglioma, while calcification of a hypothalamus tumor is suggestive of a craniopharyngioma. Additional periventricular calcification in children is most commonly caused by infection with cytomegalovirus (CMV) or toxoplasmosis. With dystrophic calcification the serum calcium levels are normal, while with metastatic calcification the serum calcium levels are elevated (hypercalcemia). Causes of hypercalcemia include certain paraneoplastic syndromes, such as secretion of parathyroid hormone–related peptide, hyperparathyroidism, iatrogenic causes (drugs), immobilization, multiple myeloma, increased milk consumption (milk-alkali syndrome), and sarcoidosis.

26. The answer is a. (*Kumar, pp 26–32. Rubin, pp 25–27.*) Apoptosis is a distinctive pattern of cell death that is described as a "programmed suicide" process of cells through which stimulation of endogenous endonucleases causes cleavage of nuclear chromatin. Apoptosis as originally defined is a purely morphologic process that differs from necrosis in several respects. Apoptosis involves single cells, not large groups of cells, and with apoptosis the cells shrink and there is increased eosinophilia of cytoplasm. The shrunken apoptotic cells form apoptotic bodies, which may be engulfed by adjacent cells or macrophages. With apoptosis there is no inflammatory response, the cell membranes do not rupture, and there is no release of macromolecules. Importantly, apoptosis is an active process in which activation of endonucleases causes peripheral condensation of chromatin (the most characteristic feature) and formation of multiples of DNA base pair fragments (called a DNA "ladder").

In contrast to apoptosis, necrosis, which is usually due to hypoxia or toxins, involves the death of many cells or clusters of cells. With necrosis the cells swell, and inflammation is present (cell membrane ruptures). Autophagy and heterophagy are two processes through which lysosomes degrade macromolecules derived from either intracellular organelles (autophagy) or extracellular products (heterophagy). Finally metaplasia is a term that describes the conversion of one cell type to another histologic type that is otherwise normal in appearance.

27. The answer is e. (*Kumar, pp 21–22.*) The cause of cell injury and death may sometimes be inferred from the type of necrosis present. Liquefactive necrosis is the type of necrosis produced by acute bacterial infections. With liquefactive necrosis the dead cells are completely dissolved by hydrolytic enzymes from acute inflammatory cells and all that remains is a liquid mass. Liquefactive necrosis can also be seen with fungal infections, and it is the type of necrosis that is produced by ischemic necrosis of the brain. More commonly, however, ischemia produces coagulative necrosis, which is characterized by loss of the cell nucleus, acidophilic change of the cytoplasm, and preservation of the outline of the cell. Sudden, severe ischemia produces coagulative necrosis in practically every tissue except the brain. Myocardial infarction, which results from the sudden occlusion of the coronary artery, is a classic example of coagulative necrosis.

Caseous necrosis is a combination of coagulative and liquefactive necrosis, but the necrotic cells are not totally dissolved and remain as amorphic, coarsely granular, eosinophilic debris. This type of necrosis grossly has the appearance of clumped cheese. It is classically seen in tuberculous infections. Gangrenous necrosis of extremities is also a combination of coagulative and liquefactive necrosis. In dry gangrene the coagulative pattern is predominate, while in wet gangrene the liquefactive pattern is predominate. Fat necrosis, seen with acute pancreatic necrosis, is fat cell death caused by lipases. Fibrinoid necrosis is an abnormality seen sometimes in injured blood vessels where plasma proteins abnormally accumulate within the vessel walls.

28. The answer is c. (*Kumar, pp 26–32. Schneider, pp 6–7. Rubin, pp 25–27.*) Apoptosis is the type of cell death in which activation of a cell's own enzymes eventually leads to its death. The process of apoptosis has two basic phases: an initiation phase, during which caspases are activated, and an execution phase, during which cell death occurs. The initiation phase has two distinct pathways: the extrinsic (receptor mediated) pathway and the intrinsic (or mitochondrial) pathway. The extrinsic pathway is mediated by cell surface death receptors, which are members of the tumor necrosis factor receptor family. These receptors contain a cytoplasmic death domain (DD). Two examples of death receptors are type 1 TNF receptor (TNFR1) and Fas (CD95). Fas ligand (FasL), which is produced by immune cells, stimulates apoptosis by binding to Fas, which activates the cytoplasmic Fas-associated death domain protein (FADD), which in turn activates the caspase cascade via the activation of caspase 8. Similarly tumor necrosis factor (TNF) binds to TNFR1 and the complex activates the cytoplasmic TNF-receptor-adaptor protein with a death domain (TRADD), which in turn activates FADD. Another function of TNF, however, is to activate the transcription factor nuclear factor κB (NF-κB) by degrading an inhibitor of NF-κB called IκB.

In contrast to the extrinsic pathway, the intrinsic pathway does not involve death receptors and instead results from increased permeability of mitochondria. For example, cytochrome c can be released into the cytoplasm from mitochondria via bax channels, these channels being upregulated by p53. Cytochrome c then binds to and activates apoptosis activating factor 1 (Apaf-1), which then in turn stimulates the caspase cascade. Note that the product of the *bcl-2* oncogene, which is normally located on the outer mitochondrial membrane, endoplasmic reticulum, and nuclear envelope, inhibits apoptosis by blocking bax channels and by binding to and sequestering Apaf-1.

29. The answer is c. (*Kumar, pp 4–7, 665–666.*) There are many adaptive mechanisms of cells to persistent stimuli. Hypertrophy is an increase in the size of cells. Examples of hypertrophy include enlarged skeletal muscle in response to repeated exercise or anabolic steroid use and enlarged cardiac muscle in response to volume overload or hypertension. In contrast to hypertrophy, hyperplasia is an increase in the number of cells. Hyperplasia may be the result of a physiologic response or a pathologic process. Examples of physiologic hyperplasia include the increased size of the female breast or uterus in response to hormones. Pathologic hyperplasia may be compensatory to some abnormal process, or it may be a purely abnormal process. Examples of compensatory pathologic hyperplasia include the regenerating liver, increased numbers of erythrocytes in response to chronic hypoxia, and increased numbers of lymphocytes within lymph nodes in response to bacterial infections [follicular (nodular) hyperplasia]. Examples of purely pathologic hyperplasia include abnormal enlargement of the endometrium (endometrial hyperplasia) and the prostate (benign prostatic hyperplasia). Atrophy is a decrease in the size and function of cells. Examples of atrophy include decreased size of limbs immobilized by a plaster cast or paralysis, or decreased size of organs affected by endocrine insufficiencies or decreased blood flow. Metaplasia is a term that describes the conversion of one histologic cell type to another. Examples of metaplasia include respiratory epithelium changing to stratified squamous epithelium (squamous metaplasia) in response to prolonged smoking, the normal glandular epithelium of the endocervix changing to stratified squamous epithelium (squamous metaplasia) in response to chronic inflammation, or the normal stratified squamous epithelium of the lower esophagus changing to gastric-type mucosa in response to chronic reflux. In contrast to metaplasia, dysplasia refers to disorganized growth and is characterized by the presence of atypical or dysplastic cells. Dysplasia can be seen in many organs, such as within the epidermis in response to sun damage (actinic keratosis), the respiratory tract, or the cervix (cervical dysplasia).

30. The answer is e. (*Kumar, pp 95–97, 107–109.*) Angiogenesis (blood vessel formation in adults) is a complex process that involves many different cells and substances. It may be initiated from endothelial precursor cells in the bone marrow or from pre-existing blood vessels. In either event, perhaps the most important growth factor is vascular endothelial growth factor (VEGF). It together with nitric oxide cause vasodilation and increased vascular permeability, which are the first steps in angiogenesis from pre-existing vessels. VEGF, which is secreted by many mesenchymal and stromal cells, also stimulates endothelial cell migration and proliferation.

Other growth factors are also involved in angiogenesis. For example, once new blood vessels are formed they are fragile and must become "stabilized," a process that involves platelet derived growth factor (PDGF) and transforming growth factor-beta (TGF-β). PDGF, which is found in platelets, activated macrophages, endothelial cells, and smooth muscle cells, can also cause migration and proliferation of fibroblasts, smooth muscle cells, and monocytes. TGF-β, produced by platelets, endothelial cells, T cells, and macrophages, stabilizes new blood vessels by increasing the production of extracellular matrix proteins. It is also associated with fibrosis. In low concentrations it causes the synthesis and secretion of PDGF, but in high concentrations it inhibits growth due to inhibition of the expression of PDGF receptors.

Finally, the epidermal growth factor family includes epidermal growth factor (EGF) and transforming growth factor alpha (TGF-alpha). These substances can cause proliferation of many types of epithelial cells and fibroblasts. The EGF receptor is c-erb B1.

31. The answer is e. (*Kumar, pp 57–60, 194–196.*) Leukocytes are a type of inflammatory cell that are important in the process of inflammation, a process that can be defined as the reaction of vascularized living tissue to local injury. During this process leukocytes are activated through several mechanisms that involve substances binding to different receptors on their surface. Toll-like receptors (TLRs), which stimulate one of the immune responses directed against microbes, are an example of one of these leukocyte activation receptors. TLRs bind to pathogen-associated molecular patterns (PAMPs), which are small molecular sequences found commonly on pathogens. Examples of PAMPs include bacterial lipopolysaccharide (LPS), lipoteichoic acid, and peptidoglycan. LPS is probably the prototypical PAMP. TLRs, in conjunction with CD14, bind to LPS (endotoxin), and activate leukocytes to produce cytokines and reactive oxygen intermediates (ROIs).

Other examples of leukocyte receptors involved in their activation include G-protein-coupled receptors (GPCRs), cytokine receptors, the mannose receptor, and receptors for opsonins. Activation of the GPCRs, which have seven transmembrane portions, increases intracytoplasmic calcium which in turn stimulates leukocyte migration. These G-protein receptors bind to multiple substances such as N-formylmethionyl residues of bacteria, lipid mediators of inflammation such as prostaglandin E and leukotriene B_4, and complement chemotactic factors such as C5a. Other leukocyte receptors for cytokines include the receptor for gamma-interferon, which is secreted by activated T lymphocytes and natural killer cells. Finally the mannose receptor recognizes terminal mannose and fucose residues of glycoproteins and glycolipids on microbial cell walls.

32. The answer is e. (*Kumar, pp 64–67.*) The complement system is a cascade of plasma proteins whose basic function is the direct lysis of cells, attraction of leukocytes to sites of inflammation (chemotaxis), and activation of leukocytes. The complement system can be activated by one of two basic pathways. The classic pathway is initiated by antigen-antibody (immune) complexes binding to C1. The antibodies that are involved in forming these complement-activating immune complexes are IgM and IgG (subtypes 1, 2, and 3). There are also some non-immunologic activators of the classic complement pathway, such as urate crystals, which may be part of the pathophysiologic process of gout. In contrast, with the alternate complement pathway the early complement components (C1, C4, and C2) are bypassed and C3 is activated directly by such things as bacterial endotoxins, cobra venom factor, lipopolysaccharide, and aggregated immunoglobulin (mainly IgA, but also IgE). C3 nephritic factor is an unusual substance capable of activating the alternate complement system within the glomerulus, producing glomerular injury.

Finally, the mechanism through which organisms with increased amounts of sialic acid can inhibit the activation of the alternate complement system is as follows: first note that normally low levels of C3 in the blood are converted into C3a and C3b by a slow process called "C3 tick-over." The C3b may combine with factor B to form C3bB, which subsequently will react with factor D and properdin, both of which are part of the alternate complement pathway. Some of the C3b formed by "C3 tick-over" may instead attach to factor H. This will cause C3b to be inactivated by being converted to C3bi by factor I. This attachment to factor H is increased by sialic acid.

33. The answer is e. *(Kumar, pp 42–43. Lekstrom-Himes, pp 1703–1714.)* Progeria (or Hutchinson-Gilford syndrome) is a disease characterized by symptoms of premature aging, which include baldness, stiffness of joints, cardiovascular problems, wrinkled skin, and dwarfism. Symptoms begin around the age of 6–12 months of age. Werner's syndrome is a similar appearing disease that first causes symptoms in affected individuals in their late teens. Werner's syndrome is typically first identified when an adolescent fails to have a normal growth spurt. In contrast to progeria, the cause of which is unknown, Werner's syndrome is caused by a mutation in the WS gene which results in the production of a defective DNA helicase.

In contrast, DiGeorge's syndrome results from abnormal developmental of pharyngeal pouches 3 and 4 due to a deletion involving chromosome 22: Signs of DiGeorge's syndrome include abnormal face (hypertelorism with low set ears), abnormal thymus with decreased cell-mediated immunity, and hypocalcemia due to the absence of the parathyroid glands.

Leukocyte adhesion deficiency type 1 is an autosomal recessive disorder that results from a deficiency of the beta chain of the beta-2-integrins. This beta-2 chain is also called CD18. A deficiency of this beta-2 chain will affect the three main beta-2-integrins, namely LFA-1, CR3 (complement receptor 3), and CR4 (complement receptor 4). Symptoms caused by decreased functioning of these integrins include recurrent severe bacterial infections and decreased wound healing, which leads to delayed separation of the umbilical cord. Additionally, since neutrophils cannot bind to endothelial cells and migrate into the interstitial tissues, they are not found at sites of infection, which heal very slowly. Instead there are increased numbers of neutrophils in the peripheral blood, even when no infection is present.

Finally, decreased numbers of neutrophils in the peripheral blood, neutropenia, are seen with congenital neutropenias, two examples of which are cyclic neutropenia and the Shwachman-Diamond syndrome. Both of these disorders are associated with recurrent severe bacterial infections. In addition, the Shwachman-Diamond syndrome is characterized by insufficiency of the exocrine pancreas, skeletal abnormalities, and dysfunction of the bone marrow.

34. The answer is b. (*Kumar, pp 61–62, 155–156. Rubin, pp 1089, 1106.*) Chédiak-Higashi syndrome is an autosomal recessive disorder characterized by the abnormal fusion of phagosomes with lysosomes, which results in ineffective bactericidal capabilities of neutrophils and monocytes. These abnormal leukocytes develop giant intracytoplasmic lysosomes. Abnormal formation of melanosomes in these individuals results in oculocutaneous albinism. Most of these patients eventually develop an "accelerated phase" in which an aggressive lymphoproliferative disease, possibly the result of an Epstein-Barr viral infection, results in pancytopenia and death.

Ataxia-telangiectasia is a chromosome instability syndrome that is characterized by increased sensitivity to x-rays (causing a markedly increased risk of lymphoid malignancies), recurrent infections, oculocutaneous telangiectasias (dilated blood vessels), and cerebellar ataxia. Chronic granulomatous disease is an X-linked recessive disorder characterized by recurrent bacterial infections due to deficient NADPH oxidase. Ehlers-Danlos syndrome results from many different defects in formation of collagen and is generally characterized by fragile skin and hypermobile joints. Sturge-Weber syndrome is characterized by capillary-venous malformation of leptomeninges and superficial cortex of one cerebral hemisphere with ipsilateral port-wine stains (nevus flammeus) in the trigeminal region of the face.

35. The answer is b. (*Kumar, pp 64–67.*) Complement assays can be used clinically to help determine the causes and pathomechanisms of certain diseases. For example, activation of the complement cascade can produce local deposition of C3, which can be seen with special histologic techniques. If a patient has widespread activation of the complement system, then serum assays of C3 levels might be decreased. In particular, activation of the classic complement pathway decreases levels of the early complement components, namely, C1, C4, and C2. In contrast, activation of the alternate complement pathway, which bypasses these early complement components, decreases levels of C3, but the levels of the early factors (C2 and C4) are normal. An example of a disorder associated with the activation of the alternate complement system is IgA nephropathy (Berger's disease), which is characterized by the deposition of IgA in the mesangium of the glomeruli.

36. The answer is b. (*Kumar, pp 66–67.*) Deficiencies of components of the complement system are associated with specific abnormalities. Patients with congenital deficiencies in the early components of the complement cascade have recurrent symptoms resembling those of systemic lupus erythematosus (SLE) due to the deposition of immune complexes. Patients with deficiencies of the middle complement components (C3 and C5) are at risk for recurrent pyogenic infections, while those lacking terminal complement components (C6, C7, or C8, but not C9) are prone to developing recurrent infections with *Neisseria* species. A deficiency of decay accelerating factor (DAF), which breaks down the C3 convertase complex, is seen in paroxysmal nocturnal hemoglobinuria (PNH), a disorder that is characterized by recurrent episodes of hemolysis of red cells because of the excessive intravascular activation of complement. Deficiencies of C1 esterase inhibitor result in recurrent angioedema, which refers to episodic nonpitting edema of soft tissue, such as the face. Severe abdominal pain and cramps, occasionally accompanied by vomiting, may be caused by edema of the gastrointestinal tract (GI). To understand how a deficiency of C1 inhibitor can cause vascular-produced edema (angioedema), note that not only does C1 inhibitor inactivate C1, but it also inhibits other pathways, such as the conversion of prekallikrein to kallikrein and kininogen to bradykinin. A deficiency of C1 inhibitor also leads to excess production of C2, a product of C2 called C2 kinin, and bradykinin. It is the uncontrolled activation of bradykinin that produces the angioedema, as bradykinin increases vascular permeability, stimulates smooth muscle contraction, dilates blood vessels, and causes pain. In contrast, a defect involving β_2-integrins is seen with leukocyte adhesion deficiency, while defects involving NADPH of leukocytes are characteristic of chronic granulomatous disease.

37. The answer is e. (*Kumar, pp 68–70.*) Products of arachidonic acid (AA) metabolism are involved extensively in inflammation. In this pathway, AA is broken down into leukotrienes (vasoconstrictors) and prostaglandins (vasodilators). AA is a polyunsaturated fatty acid that is normally found esterified in plasma membrane phospholipids. It is released by the activation of phospholipases, such as phospholipase A_2. Cyclooxygenase transforms AA into the prostaglandin endoperoxide PGG_2, which is then converted into PGH_2 and subsequently into three products: thromboxane A_2 (TxA_2), prostacyclin (PGI_2), and the more stable prostaglandins PGE_2, PGF_2, and PGD_2. Thromboxane, found in platelets, is a potent platelet aggregator and blood vessel constrictor.

In contrast, prostacyclin, which is found in the walls of blood vessels, is a potent inhibitor of platelet aggregation and is also a vasodilator. Prostaglandin E and prostacyclin probably account for most of the vasodilation that is seen in inflammation. The prostaglandins are also involved in producing pain and fever in inflammation. In contrast to cyclooxygenase, lipoxygenase converts AA into hydroperoxyl derivatives, namely 12-HPETE in platelets and 15-HPETE in leukocytes. 5-HPETE gives rise to HETE and the leukotrienes (Lts). While many substances can be chemotactic, few are known to be as potent as several of the leukotrienes. Leukotriene B_4 is a potent chemotactic agent that also causes aggregation and adhesion of leukocytes. Additionally, leukotrienes C_4, D_4, and E_4 cause increased vascular permeability, bronchoconstriction, and vasoconstriction. Other chemotactic factors for neutrophils include C5a and IL-8, but these substances are not formed from AA.

38. The answer is d. (*Kumar, pp 50–53, 79–82.*) Vasoactive amines are important mediators of the early signs and symptoms of acute inflammation. Two important vasoactive amines are histamine and serotonin. Histamine is found in mast cells, basophils, and platelets and is primarily responsible for the initial swelling found in acute inflammation. This swelling results from histamine binding to H_1 receptors and increasing the permeability of venules. Histamine release is induced by temperature changes (both hot and cold), antibodies (a type I hypersensitivity reaction), anaphylatoxins, IL-1, and IL-8. Neuropeptides, such as substance P, can cause vasodilation and increased vascular permeability directly and by stimulating histamine release by mast cells. Serotonin (5-hydroxytryptamine) is found in platelets and enterochromaffin cells and has actions similar to those of histamine, although these may not be physiologically significant in humans.

39. The answer is d. (*Kumar, pp 79–82, 122, 562. Henry, p 522.*) Most tissue macrophages originate from a committed bone marrow stem cell that differentiates into a monoblast and then a promonocyte, and then finally matures into a monocyte in the circulating peripheral blood. When called upon, the circulating monocyte can enter into an organ or tissue bed as a tissue macrophage (sometimes called a histiocyte). Examples of tissue macrophages are Kupffer cells (liver), alveolar macrophages (lung), osteoclasts (bone), Langerhans cells (skin), microglial cells (central nervous system), and possibly the dendritic immunocytes of the dermis, spleen, and lymph nodes. The entire system, including the peripheral blood monocytes, constitutes the mononuclear phagocyte system. In the lung, alveolar macrophages can phagocytize the red blood cells that accumulate in alveoli in individuals with congestive heart failure. These cells contain hemosiderin and are referred to as "heart failure cells."

40. The answer is a. *(Kumar, pp 56–57, 79–82.)* There are several types of leukocytes; all have specific structures that enable them to participate in specific types of inflammatory reactions. Acute inflammatory processes, such as pyogenic bacterial infections and tissue necrosis, are associated with infiltrates of neutrophils into tissue and increased numbers of neutrophils in the blood; hence neutrophils are thought of as acute inflammatory cells. Neutrophils are also called polymorphonuclear leukocytes (PMNs or "polys") because they characteristically have nuclei with three to five lobes. Myeloperoxidase is an enzyme within the primary (azurophilic) granules of neutrophils, while alkaline phosphatase is an enzyme in their secondary (specific) granules. Neutrophils have a short life span and do not divide. IL-1 causes an increased number of neutrophils to be released from the bone marrow. In contrast, chronic inflammatory processes are associated with increased numbers of monocytes and lymphocytes. Monocytes are mononuclear leukocytes with a "bean-shaped" or "horseshoe-shaped" nucleus. Their tissue form is called a macrophage or histiocyte. The activated form of macrophages have abundant eosinophilic cytoplasm and are called epithelioid cells. They secrete many different types of products and may fuse to form giant cells. Lymphocytes are smaller mononuclear leukocytes that have a round to oval nucleus and little cytoplasm. There are two types of lymphocytes, B and T lymphocytes. These types of lymphocytes look histologically identical. B lymphocytes (B cells) mature into plasma cells, which have an eccentric nucleus with a "clock-face" appearance of their chromatin. Plasma cells secrete immunoglobulin, while certain T lymphocytes (T cells) secrete lymphokines. Numbers of lymphocytes are increased in acute viral infections or chronic disease.

Eosinophils are bilobed leukocytes that contain abundant eosinophilic granules within their cytoplasm. These granules contain many different types of substances, such as major basic protein (which is toxic to helminthic parasites), arylsulfatase (which neutralizes leukotrienes), and histaminase (which neutralizes histamine). They participate in specific types of inflammatory processes, such as allergic disorders, parasitic infections, and some diseases of the skin. Basophils are a type of leukocyte that have numerous deeply basophilic granules within their cytoplasm that completely hide the nucleus. Basophils participate in certain specific types of immune reactions because they have surface receptors for IgE. When activated they release vasoactive substances, such as histamine. Mast cells, although not exactly the same as basophils, are found in tissue and are very similar to basophils.

41. The answer is d. (*Kumar, pp 79–83, 381–386.*) Granulomatous inflammation is characterized by the presence of granulomas, which by definition are aggregates of activated macrophages (epithelioid cells, not epithelial cells). These cells may be surrounded by mononuclear cells, mainly lymphocytes, and multinucleated giant cells. These cells result from the fusion of several epithelioid cells together. The source of macrophages (histiocytes) are monocytes from the peripheral blood.

Granulomatous inflammation is a type of chronic inflammation initiated by a variety of infectious and noninfectious agents. Indigestible organisms or particles, or T cell–mediated immunity to the inciting agent, or both, appear essential for formation of granulomas. Tuberculosis is the classic infectious granulomatous disease and is characterized by finding rare acid-fast bacilli within areas of caseous necrosis. In addition to tuberculosis, several other infectious disorders are characterized by formation of granulomas, including deep fungal infections (coccidioidomycosis and histoplasmosis), schistosomiasis, syphilis, brucellosis, lymphogranuloma venereum, and cat-scratch disease. In sarcoidosis, a disease of unknown cause, the granulomas are noncaseating, which may assist in histologic differentiation from tuberculosis. No organisms are found in the noncaseating granulomas of sarcoidosis.

42. The answer is c. (*Kumar, pp 107, 110, 112–113.*) Tissue repair occurs through the regeneration of damaged cells and the replacement of tissue by connective tissue. Tissue repair involves the formation of granulation tissue, which histologically is characterized by a combination of proliferating fibroblasts and proliferating blood vessels. Proliferating cells are cells that are rapidly dividing and usually have prominent nucleoli. This histologic feature should not be taken as a sign of dysplasia or malignancy. It is important not to confuse the term granulation tissue with the similar-sounding term granuloma. The latter refers to a special type of inflammation that is characterized by the presence of activated macrophages (epithelioid cells).

43. The answer is b. (*Kumar, pp 103–105. Rubin, pp 78–84.*) The extracellular matrix (ECM) is composed of fibrous structural proteins and interstitial matrix, the latter being composed of adhesive glycoproteins embedded within a ground substance. The structural proteins of the ECM include collagen fibers, reticular fibers, and elastic fibers. Collagen is a triple helix of three polypeptide α-chains that is secreted by fibroblasts and has a high content of glycine and hydroxyproline. Collagens may be either fibrillar or nonfibrillar. The fibrillar (interstitial) types of collagen (types I, III, and V) are found within the ECM (interstitial tissue), while the nonfibrillar type IV collagen is found within the basement membranes, which are special organizations of the interstitial matrix found around epithelial, endothelial, and smooth-muscle cells. Type I collagen is found in skin, tendon, bone, dentin, and fascia; type II collagen is found only in cartilage; and type III collagen (reticulin) appears in the skin, blood vessels, uterus, and embryonic dermis.

The adhesive glycoproteins include fibronectin and laminin. Laminin, the most abundant glycoprotein in basement membranes, is a cross-shaped glycoprotein that is capable of binding multiple matrix components, such as type IV collagen and heparan sulfate. It also binds to specific receptors on the surface of some cells. Fibronectin, secreted by fibroblasts, monocytes, and endothelial cells, is also capable of binding many substances, such as collagen, fibrin, proteoglycans, and integrins. Basically, fibronectin links the ECM component and macromolecules to integrins and is chemotactic for fibroblasts and endothelial cells. Instead of being cross-shaped like laminin, fibronectin is a large glycoprotein composed of two chains held together by disulfide bonds. Albumin is secreted by hepatocytes and is mainly responsible for intravascular oncotic pressure, while immunoglobulins are secreted by plasma cells and are important in mediating humoral immunity.

44. The answer is d. (*Kumar, pp 104, 154–155. Ayala, p 179.*) Several diseases result from abnormalities involving defects in structural proteins. Marfan's syndrome is an autosomal dominant disorder that results from defective synthesis of fibrillin causing connective tissue abnormalities. It is characterized by specific changes involving the skeleton, the eyes, and the cardiovascular system. Skeletal changes seen in individuals with Marfan's syndrome include arachnodactyly (spider fingers) and a large skeleton causing increase in height. Eyes in patients with Marfan's syndrome typically have a subluxed lens (ectopia lentis) in which the lens is found in the anterior chamber. The lens dislocation in Marfan's syndrome is usually upward, in contrast to the downward dislocation seen with homocystinuria. Cardiovascular lesions associated with Marfan's syndrome include MV prolapse and cystic medial necrosis of the aorta.

Abnormalities of copper metabolism is seen with Wilson's disease, which is characterized by varying liver disease and neurologic symptoms due to excess copper deposition within the liver and basal ganglia of the brain. Decreased levels of vitamin D can produce rickets in children or osteomalacia in adults. Type VI Ehlers-Danlos syndrome is characterized by decreased lysyl hydroxylation of collagen, which causes decreased crosslinking of collagen. These individuals have eye problems along with hyperextensible skin and joint hypermobility. Finally, osteogenesis imperfecta (OI) results from defective synthesis of type I collagen. These patients have "brittle bones" and also typically develop blue scleras and hearing loss.

45. The answer is c. (*Kumar, pp 120–122, 714–715.*) Edema is the accumulation of excess fluid in the interstitial tissue or body cavities. It may be caused by inflammation (inflammatory edema) or it may be due to abnormalities involving the Starling forces acting at the capillary level (noninflammatory edema or hemodynamic edema). Inflammatory edema is caused by increased capillary permeability, which is the result of vasoactive mediators of acute inflammation. An exudate is inflammatory edema fluid resulting from increased capillary permeability. It is characterized by a high protein content, much cellular debris, and a specific gravity greater than 1.020. Pus is an inflammatory exudate containing numerous leukocytes and cellular debris. In contrast, transudates result either from increased intravascular hydrostatic pressure or from decreased osmotic pressure. They are characterized by a low protein content and a specific gravity of <1.012. Noninflammatory edema is the result of abnormalities of the hemodynamic (Starling) forces acting at the level of the capillaries. Increased hydrostatic pressure may be caused by arteriolar dilation, hypervolemia, or increased venous pressure. Hypervolemia may be caused by sodium retention seen in renal disease, and increased venous hydrostatic pressure can be seen in venous thrombosis, congestive heart failure, or cirrhosis. Decreased plasma oncotic pressure is caused by decreased plasma protein, the majority of which is albumin. Decreased albumin levels may be caused by loss of albumin in the urine, which occurs in the nephrotic syndrome, or by reduced synthesis, which occurs in chronic liver disease. Lymphatic obstruction may be caused by tumors, surgical resection, or infections (for example, infection with filarial worms and consequent elephantiasis).

46. The answer is a. (*Kumar, pp 122–124.*) Hyperemia refers to excess amounts of blood within an organ. It may be caused by increased arterial supply (active hyperemia) or impaired venous drainage (passive hyperemia). Examples of active hyperemia include increased blood flow during exercise, blushing (such as embarrassment associated with being asked a question during a lecture), or inflammation. Examples of passive hyperemia, or congestion, include the changes produced by chronic heart failure. These changes include chronic passive congestion of the lung or the liver. The lung changes are characterized by intraalveolar, hemosiderin-laden macrophages, called "heart failure cells." Congestion in the liver is characterized by centrilobular congestion, which is seen grossly as a "nutmeg" appearance of the liver. In contrast to hyperemia, hemorrhage refers to the leakage of blood from a blood vessel. Blood may escape into the tissue, producing a hematoma, or it may escape into spaces, producing a hemothorax, hemopericardium, or hemarthrosis. Superficial hemorrhages into the skin or mucosa are classified as petechiae (small, pinpoint capillary hemorrhages), purpura (diffuse, multiple superficial hemorrhages), or ecchymoses (larger, confluent areas of hemorrhages).

47. The answer is e. (*Kumar, pp 68–69, 126–127.*) The contrasting actions of the arachidonic acid metabolites prostacyclin and thromboxane produce a fine-tuned balance for the regulation of clotting. Thromboxane, a product of the cyclooxygenase pathway of arachidonic acid metabolism, is synthesized in platelets and is a powerful platelet aggregator and vasoconstrictor. The prostaglandin prostacyclin, also a product of the cyclooxygenase pathway but produced by endothelial cells, inhibits platelet aggregation and causes vasodilation. Aspirin is a cyclooxygenase inhibitor that blocks the synthesis of both thromboxane and prostacyclin. The inhibition of prostacyclin production within endothelial cells, however, can be somewhat overcome, but not the production of thromboxane within platelets. That is, aspirin will selectively inhibit the production of thromboxane more than prostacyclin, which is the reason why it can be used to prevent thrombosis in patients with coronary artery disease.

In addition to producing prostacyclin, endothelial cells produce other substances with anticoagulant activities, such as thrombomodulin and plasminogen activator. Endothelial cells, however, produce both procoagulant and anticoagulant substances. Examples of procoagulant substances produced by endothelial cells include tissue factor (thromboplastin), which can activate the extrinsic coagulation cascade, von Willebrand factor, and platelet-activating factor, both of which stimulate platelet aggregation. Finally fibrinogen, which is cleaved by thrombin to form fibrin, is produced by the liver and not endothelial cells or platelets.

48. The answer is a. (*Kumar, pp 127–130, 649. Henry, pp 642–646.*) The coagulation cascade involves the formation of fibrin through the intrinsic, extrinsic, and common pathways. The intrinsic pathway is initiated by contact of factor XII with several types of biologic surfaces. Activated XII (XIIa) initiates the formation of XIa and IXa. The extrinsic pathway is initiated by contact of tissue factor with factor VII. Activated factor VII acts together with IXa, VIIIa, and platelet factor 3 (PF-3), which is a phospholipid complex located on the surface of platelets, to produce activated factor X. This begins the common pathway, which continues with the interaction of Xa, Va, PF-3, and Ca^{2+} to cleave prothrombin, forming thrombin, which in turn cleaves fibrinogen to form fibrin.

Two laboratory tests that are used to evaluate the functioning of the coagulation cascade are prothrombin time (PT) and partial thromboplastin time (PTT). Abnormalities of the extrinsic pathway prolong (not shorten) the PT, while abnormalities of the intrinsic pathway prolong (not shorten) the PTT. Note that abnormalities of the common pathway prolong both the PT and the PTT. To illustrate, deficiencies of factor VII produce an abnormal (prolonged) PT with a normal PTT. Compare these results to each of the following: a normal PT with an abnormal PTT can be seen with deficiencies of factors XII, XI, IX, or VIII, while abnormal PT and PTT are seen with deficiencies of X, V, prothrombin, or fibrinogen.

49. The answer is a. (*Kumar, pp 130–135.*) A thrombus is a blood clot that is formed within a blood vessel and remains at the site of its origin. In contrast, a hematoma is formed outside of blood vessels and emboli do not remain at their site of origin. Thrombi may form within the venous system (venous thrombi) or within the arterial system (arterial thrombi). Venous thrombi, which are almost invariably occlusive, are found most often in the legs, in superficial varicose veins, or deep veins. Those of the larger outflow veins of the leg may embolize. It is important to be able to tell postmortem clots from venous thrombi. The postmortem clot is usually rubbery, gelatinous, and lacks fibrin strands and attachments to the vessel wall. Large postmortem clots may have a "chicken fat" appearance overlying a dark "currant jelly" base.

In contrast, arterial thrombi, which can form within the heart or the arteries, may have laminations, called the lines of Zahn, formed by alternating layers of platelets admixed with fibrin, separated by layers with more cells. Mural thrombi within the heart are associated with myocardial infarcts and arrhythmias, while thrombi in the aorta are associated with atherosclerosis or aneurysmal dilatations. Arterial thrombi are usually occlusive; however, in the larger vessels they are not.

50. The answer is c. (*Kumar, pp 135–137.*) An embolus is a detached intravascular mass that has been carried by the blood to a site other than where it was formed. Most emboli originate from thrombi (thrombotic emboli), but they can also originate from material other than thrombi (nonthrombotic emboli). Types of nonthrombotic emboli include fat emboli, air emboli, and amniotic fluid emboli. Fat emboli, which result from severe trauma and fractures of long bones, will stain positively with an oil red O stain or Sudan black stain. They can be fatal as they can damage the endothelial cells and pneumocytes within the lungs. Air emboli are seen in decompression sickness, called caisson disease or the bends, while amniotic fluid emboli are related to the rupture of uterine venous sinuses as a complication of childbirth. Amniotic fluid emboli can also lead to a fatal disease, disseminated intravascular coagulopathy (DIC), which is marked by the combination of intravascular coagulation and hemorrhages. In this setting DIC results from the high thromboplastin activity of amniotic fluid.

It is important to remember, however, that most emboli arise from thrombi (thromboemboli) that are formed in the deep veins of the lower extremities. These thrombi may embolize to the lungs and form thrombotic pulmonary emboli (venous emboli). The majority of small pulmonary emboli do no harm, but, if they are large enough, they may occlude the bifurcation of the pulmonary arteries (saddle embolus), causing sudden death. In contrast, arterial emboli most commonly originate within the heart on abnormal valves (vegetations) or mural thrombi following myocardial infarctions. If there is a patent foramen ovale, a venous embolus may cross over through the heart to the arterial circulation, producing an arterial (paradoxical) embolus.

51. The answer is e. (*Kumar, pp 137–139, 1040.*) Infarcts are localized areas of ischemic coagulative necrosis. They can be classified on the basis of their color into either red or white infarcts, or by the presence or absence of bacterial contamination into either septic or bland infarcts. White infarcts, also referred to as pale or anemic infarcts, are usually the result of arterial occlusion. They are found in solid organs such as the heart, spleen, and kidneys. Red or hemorrhagic infarcts, in contrast, may result from either arterial or venous occlusion. They occur in organs with a dual blood supply, such as the lung, or in organs with extensive collateral circulation, such as the small intestine and brain. These infarcts are hemorrhagic because there is bleeding into the necrotic area from the adjacent arteries and veins that remain patent. Hemorrhagic infarcts also occur in organs in which the venous outflow is obstructed (venous occlusion). Examples of this include torsion of the ovary or testis. In the latter, twisting of the spermatic cord occludes the venous outflow, but the arterial inflow remains patent because these arterial blood vessels have much thicker walls. This results in venous infarction. Testicular torsion is usually the result of physical trauma in an individual with a predisposing abnormality, such as abnormal development of the gubernaculum testis.

52. The answer is c. (*Champe, pp 352–353.*) The synthesis of pyrimidines begins with the conversion of glutamine to carbamoyl phosphate. This step, which is the committed step in pyrimidine synthesis, is catalyzed by the enzyme carbamoyl phosphate synthetase II (CPSII) and requires 2ATP and CO_2. After several biochemical steps orotate is formed; orotate is then converted to orotidine 5′-monophosphate (OMP) by the enzyme orotate phosphoribosyl transferase. Subsequently OMP is converted to uridine 5′-monophosphate (UMP) by the enzyme OMP decarboxylase. A deficiency of either of these two enzymes leads to a disorder called orotic aciduria, which is characterized by orotate in the urine, abnormal growth, and megaloblastic anemia. Next UMP is converted to CTP, while dUMP is converted by thymidylate synthase to dTMP. This latter step also involves folate and is inhibited by the folate analogue methotrexate, while thymidylate synthase is inhibited by the thymine analogue 5-flurouracil (5-FU). Finally, the ribonucleoside diphosphates (ADP, GDP, CDP, and UDP) are converted to deoxyribonucleoside diphosphates by ribonucleotide reductase, an enzyme that is inhibited by increased levels of dATP, as seen in individuals with the autosomal recessive (Swiss type) form of SCID, which is due to a deficiency of adenosine deaminase (ADA).

53. The answer is e. (*Jorde, pp 339–351. Kumar, pp 149–151, 470–472.*) There are several similar clinical terms that are used to describe various types of abnormal physical development. A sequence is a recognized pattern that results from a single preexisting abnormality; that is, a sequence refers to the combination of a primary defect along with its secondary structural changes. Examples of this include the Pierre Robin sequence and the oligohydramnios sequence. The Robin sequence is characterized by the triad of micrognathia, cleft palate, and glossoptosis. In this disorder the primary defect is the micrognathia and this leads to the secondary structural changes. In the oligohydramnios (Potter) sequence the primary defect is the oligohydramnios (which may have several causes, such as renal agenesis) and this leads to the secondary structural changes seen as the classic facial appearance (flattened facies).

The term "syndrome" is often confused with the term "sequence." Syndrome refers to multiple anomalies having a recognizable pattern and known pathogenesis (e.g., Down syndrome). Other confusing terms include "disruption," "association," and "deformation." A disruption is a defect that results from interference in a normally developing process. A classic example of a disruption is rupture of the amnion in utero forming amniotic bands that can wrap around, compress, and possibly amputate arms or legs. An association is a pattern of nonrandom anomalies with an unknown mechanism, an example being the VATER association. VATER is an acronym that refers to the body part that can be affected: vertebrae, anus, trachea, esophagus, and radius. The cause of the VATER association is unknown. Finally a deformation is an alteration of a normally formed body part by mechanical forces. For example, a prolonged breech presentation can dislocate the hip and produce a flattened, elongated "breech head."

54. The answer is a. (*Kumar, pp 150–151, 155–156.*) There are several general clinical differences between autosomal dominant (AD) disorders and autosomal recessive (AR) disorders. In general, AD mutations usually involve complex structural proteins or regulatory proteins, while AR disorders are more likely to result from abnormalities of proteins that function as enzymes. Examples of AD disorders involving abnormalities of structural proteins include Marfan's syndrome (fibrillin), osteogenesis imperfecta (collagen), hereditary spherocytosis (spectrin), and several types of Ehlers-Danlos syndrome (EDS; collagen). This later syndrome refers to a group of related disorders characterized by defects in collagen synthesis or structure. These defects produce abnormalities of the skin and joints. The skin in these patients is fragile and hyperextensible, while the joints are hypermobile. There are at least 10 variants or subtypes of EDS, encompassing three types of Mendelian inheritance. EDS types I, II, III, IV, and VIII have abnormalities involving the structural protein collagen, either collagen types I, III, or V, and all of these have AD modes of inheritance. In particular, type IV EDS is related to abnormal type III collagen and as such is associated with ruptured intestinal organs and blood vessels.

Examples of AD disorders involving abnormalities of regulatory proteins include familial hyperlipidemia (LDL receptor), von Willebrand's disease (von Willebrand factor), and hereditary angioedema (C1 esterase inhibitor). Enzyme deficiencies are usually not associated with AD inheritance, because decreased levels of enzymes can usually be compensated for. Examples of AR disorders involving enzyme deficiencies include storage diseases and several amino acid diseases. Also note that, when compared with AD diseases, AR disorders tend to be more uniform in expression and the age of onset is frequently early in life. Examples of this latter fact include diseases of the blood (sickle cell anemia and thalassemia) and the infantile form of polycystic renal disease, which has an AR inheritance. In contrast, the adult form of polycystic renal disease has an AD pattern of inheritance.

55. The answer is d. (*Kumar, pp 152, 655–656.*) X-linked patterns of inheritance are seen with disorders involving genes located on the X chromosome. X-linked inheritance can be either X-linked recessive (XR) or X-linked dominant (XD). Examples of XR disorders include a few hematology diseases, such as glucose-6-phosphate dehydrogenase deficiency, factor VIII deficiency (hemophilia A), and factor IX deficiency (hemophilia B). To reiterate, since hemophilia is an X-linked recessive disorder, the gene that codes for coagulation factor VIII must be on the X chromosome. Other XR disorders include a few immunodeficiency diseases (Bruton's agammaglobulinemia, one form of severe combine immune deficiency disease, chronic granulomatous disease, and Wiskott-Aldrich syndrome); a few, rare storage diseases (Fabry's disease and Hunter's syndrome); a few muscle diseases (Duchenne and Becker's muscular dystrophy); rare metabolic diseases (diabetes insipidus and Lesch-Nyhan); and a few other diseases (red-green color blindness and Menkes "kinky hair" syndrome). Finally, examples of XD disorders include hypophosphatemic rickets, pseudohypoparathyroidism, some forms of Alport's syndrome, and ornithine-transcarbamylase deficiency (hyperammonemia).

56. The answer is c. (*Kumar, pp 489–490. Jorde, pp 57–59.*) Cystic fibrosis is an autosomal recessive disorder that results from mutations in the cystic fibrosis transmembrane conductance regulator (CFTR) gene located on chromosome 7. It is the most common lethal genetic disease that affects Caucasian populations in the United States (1 in 3200 live births), but is rare in African-Americans (1 in 15,000 live births) and Asians (1 in 31,000 live births). The probability that a child will inherit a particular gene found on only one chromosome of a chromosome pair from one parent is 1 in 2 (e.g., 50%). Therefore, the probability that a child will inherit the cystic fibrosis (CF) gene from a parent is 50% and the probability that they will inherit an abnormal gene from both parents and be homozygous for cystic fibrosis is 25% (e.g., 1/2 * 1/2). This is the same probability (25%) that a child will inherit a normal gene from both parents, that is, the child is homozygous normal. The remaining possibility, which is 50%, is the chance that a child will be a heterozygous carrier of the disease. This can be seen in the following Punnett Square where "C" is the normal gene and "c" is the abnormal gene. Also note that with autosomal recessive disorders one-third of normal appearing offsprings are homozygous normal noncarriers and two-thirds are heterozygous carriers.

Mother's gametes

	C	C
C	CC	Cc
c	cC	Cc

Father's gametes

57. The answer is d. (*Jorde, pp 59, 62.*) The Hardy-Weinberg principle predicts population genotype frequencies based on gene frequencies. The principle, which assumes random mating, states that given gene frequencies p (for an allele A) and q (for another allele a), then the aa genotype (homozygous) is q * q and the Aa genotype (heterozygous carriers) is 2pq. The latter can also be written as (p * q) + (p * q).

58. The answer is e. (*Kumar, pp 165–167. Rubin, pp 255–257.*) The glycogen storage diseases are due to defective metabolism of glycogen, and at least 11 syndromes stemming from genetic defects in the responsible enzymes have been described. Most of these glycogenoses are inherited as autosomal recessive disorders. von Gierke's disease (type I) results from deficiency of glucose-6-phosphatase, the hepatic enzyme needed for conversion of G6P to glucose, with glycogen accumulation particularly in the enlarged liver and kidney and hypoglycemia. Diagnosis requires biopsy demonstration of excess liver glycogen plus either absent or low liver glucose-6-phosphatase activity, or a diabetic glucose tolerance curve, or hyperuricemia. von Gierke's disease is the major hepatic or hepatorenal type of glycogenosis. Lysosomal glucosidase deficiency causes Pompe's disease (type II). Glycogen storage is widespread but most prominent in the heart (cardiomegaly). In brancher glycogenosis (type IV) there is accumulation of amylopectin or abnormal glycogen in the liver, heart, skeletal muscle, and brain. The major myopathic form, McArdle's disease (type V), is due to lack of muscle phosphorylase.

59. The answer is d. (*Kumar, pp 158–165.*) Sphingomyelin, a lipid composed of phosphocholine and a ceramide, is characteristically found in abnormally high concentrations throughout the body tissues of patients who have one of the two forms of Niemann-Pick disease: type A and type B. Type A, the acute neuronopathic form, is the more common type. The lack of sphingomyelinase in type A is the metabolic defect that prevents the hydrolytic cleavage of sphingomyelin, which then accumulates in the phagocytic cells of the liver (causing hepatomegaly), spleen (causing splenomegaly), lymph nodes (causing lymphadenopathy), and bone marrow. In the brain ballooning degeneration of neurons is diffuse, and a "cherry-red spot" of the retina may be present. Patients who have the type A form usually show hepatosplenomegaly at 6 months of age, progressively lose motor functions and mental capabilities, and die during the third year of life. Type B is characterized by organomegaly, but lacks the involvement of the central nervous system seen in type A.

In contrast, patients with Fabry's disease, an X-linked recessive disorder, is characterized by the accumulation of ceramide trihexose, while Gaucher disease has the accumulation of excess glucocerebrosides within phagocytic cells. Hurler's and Hunter's syndrome, two types of mucopolysaccharidoses, have accumulations of heparan sulfate, while metachromatic leukodystrophy, an autosomal recessive disorder, has the accumulation of sulfatides in lysosomes. This substance stains metachromatically with cresyl violet.

60. The answer is a. (*Kumar, pp 165, 1397–1398. Damjanov, pp 293–294.*) The mucopolysaccharidoses (MPSs) result from deficiencies of specific enzymes involved in the breakdown of glycosaminoglycans (GAGs), which are also called MPSs. The seven major types of GAGs are hyaluronic acid, chondroitin sulfate, keratin sulfate, dermatan sulfate, heparan sulfate, and heparin. The MPSs are characterized by accumulation of partially degraded GAGs in multiple organs, including the liver, spleen, heart, and blood vessels. Accumulations of GAGs within leukocytes produce Alder-Reilly bodies, while accumulations within neurons can produce zebra bodies. The MPSs are also characterized by the excretion of excess acid mucopolysaccharides in the urine, a finding that helps to differentiate the MPSs from the mucolipidoses. Most of the MPSs are associated with coarse facial features, clouding of corneas, joint stiffness, and mental retardation. The characteristic appearance of patients with type IH MPS (Hurler's syndrome), which results from a deficiency of alpha-1-iduronidase, has been described as "gargoylism." These patients excrete excess dermatan sulfate and heparan sulfate, both of which are mucopolysaccharides, in the urine. Type II MPS (Hunter's syndrome) is the only MPS that has an X-linked recessive type of inheritance. These patients have a much milder disease than Hurler's syndrome patients, but they also secrete dermatan sulfate and heparan sulfate in the urine. Type IV MPS, known as Morquio's syndrome, is characterized by short stature, aortic valvular disease, and normal intelligence. These patients are prone to development of subluxation of the spine, which can produce quadriplegia. They secrete keratan sulfate in the urine.

In contrast to the MPSs, the mucolipidoses (MLs) are characterized by abnormalities affecting both the MPSs and the sphingolipidoses (SLs). Similar to the MPSs, the MLs involve abnormal bone development (dysostosis), while similar to some of the SLs, cherry-red maculae and peripheral demyelination are also seen. The MLs, however, unlike the MPSs, do not involve excessive urinary excretion of acid MPSs. The metabolism of the carbohydrates in glycoproteins and glycolipids is abnormal in the MLs and results in excess accumulation of oligosaccharides. There are three main types of MLs: type I is sialidosis, type II is inclusion cell (I cell) disease, and type III is pseudo-Hurler's disease. Patients with type II ML lack the enzyme N-acetylglucosamine phosphotransferase, which catalyzes the first step in the formation of mannose-6-phosphate. Many lysosomal enzymes in these patients, such as acid hydrolases (which includes glycoprotein and ganglioside sialidases), do not reach the cellular lysosomes and are instead secreted into the plasma. The name I cell originated from the finding of cytoplasmic granular inclusions in affected patients' fibroblasts when cultured in vitro and observed under a phase-contrast microscope. These cytoplasmic inclusions are lysosomes that are swollen with many different types of contents. I cell disease is a slowly progressive disease that starts at birth and is fatal in childhood. Treatment is symptomatic only.

61. The answer is d. (*Rubin, pp 257–260. Kumar, pp 167–168.*) Several autosomal recessive disorders involve inborn errors of amino acid metabolism. Alkaptonuria (ochronosis) is caused by the excess accumulation of homogentisic acid. This results from a block in the metabolism of the phenylalanine-tyrosine pathway, which is caused by a deficiency of homogentisic oxidase. Excess homogentisic acid causes the urine to turn dark upon standing after a period of time. It also causes a dark coloration of the scleras, tendons, and cartilage. After years, many patients develop a degenerative arthritis. Phenylketonuria (PKU), also called hyperphenylalaninemia, results from a deficiency of phenylalanine hydroxylase, an enzyme that oxidizes phenylalanine to tyrosine in the liver. Infants are normal at birth, but rising phenylalanine levels (hyperphenylalaninemia) result in irreversible brain damage. The excess phenylacetic acid in the urine results in a "mousy" odor. A lack of the enzyme fumarylacetoacetate hydrolase results in increased levels of tyrosine (tyrosinemia). Chronic forms of the disease are associated with cirrhosis of the liver, kidney dysfunction, and a high risk of developing hepatocellular carcinoma. Maple syrup urine disease is associated with an enzyme defect that causes the accumulation of branched-chain α-keto acid derivatives of isoleucine, leucine, and valine. Albinism refers to a group of disorders characterized by an abnormality of the synthesis of melanin. Two forms of oculocutaneous albinism are classified by the presence or absence of tyrosinase, which is the first enzyme in the conversion of tyrosine to melanin. Albinos are at a greatly increased risk for the development of squamous cell carcinomas in sun-exposed skin.

62. The answer is d. (*Kumar, pp 173–175, 1110–1112.*) The normal human karyotype consists of 23 pairs of chromosomes, of which 22 are homologous pairs of autosomes and one pair is the sex chromosome. The number of chromosomes found in germ cells (23) is called the haploid number (n), while the number of chromosomes found in all of the remaining cells in the body (46) is called the diploid number (2n). Any exact multiple of the haploid number (n) is called euploid. Note that both haploid and diploid cells are euploid. Chromosome numbers such as 3n and 4n are called polypoid. 3n is called triploid, while 4n is called tetraploid. Triploid karyotypes (69 chromosomes) are found in about 7% of miscarriages. Interestingly, they are also associated with abnormalities of the placenta, including cystic villi and partial hydatidiform moles. Both abnormalities can produce large placentas. Triploid karyotypes are usually due to double fertilization of a haploid ovum by two haploid sperm, that is, there is a total of 69 chromosomes, 46 of which are from the father.

Do not confuse triploid with trisomy; the latter refers to the presence of three copies of one chromosome, which results in 47 chromosomes. Note that any number that is not an exact multiple of n is called aneuploid. Aneuploidy can result from nondisjunction (more commonly) or anaphase lag. Nondisjunction is the failure of paired chromosomes or chromatids to separate at anaphase, either during mitosis or meiosis. Nondisjunction during the first meiotic division is the mechanism responsible for the majority of cases of trisomy 21.

63. The answer is e. (*Kumar, pp 173–175, 1041, 1043.*) An isochromosome of the short arm of chromosome 12, i(12p) is found in virtually all testicular germ cell tumors, regardless of their histologic type. An isochromosome results from abnormal division of the centromere along a transverse plane. That is, one arm of a chromosome is lost and the remaining arm is duplicated. Turner's syndrome can result from an isochromosome of the X chromosome. In contrast, deletion of both ends of a chromosome with fusion of the damaged ends produces a ring chromosome, while two breaks occurring within a single chromosome with the reincorporation of the inverted segment produces an inversion. Finally, a reciprocal translocation between two acrocentric chromosomes is characteristic of the Robertsonian translocation (centric fusion), which results in the formation of one large metacentric chromosome and a small chromosomal fragment, which is usually lost.

64. The answer is e. (*Kumar, pp 175–176. Rubin, pp 228–233.*) Nondisjunction during the first meiotic division is responsible for trisomy 21 in about 93% of patients with Down syndrome. Nondisjunction during mitosis of a somatic cell early during embryogenesis results in mosaicism in about 2% of patients with Down syndrome. Translocation of an extra long arm of chromosome 21 causes about 5% of Down syndrome cases. An important type of translocation, the Robertsonian translocation (centric fusion), involves two nonhomologous acrocentric chromosomes with the resultant formation of one large metacentric chromosome. Carriers of this type of translocation may also produce children with Down syndrome.

It is important to understand these different causes of Down syndrome in order to estimate the chance of recurrence if parents already have one child with Down syndrome. Overall, the risk of recurrence of trisomy 21 after one such child has been born to a family is about 1%. If the karyotypes of the parents are normal, then the recurrence rate is dependent on the age of the mother. For mothers under the age of 30, the risk is about 1.4%. For mothers over the age of 30, the risk is the same as the age-related maternal risk, which at age 30 is 1/900, at age 35 is 1/350, at age 40 is 1/100, and at age 40 and over is 1/25. The recurrence risk is different for a translocation Down syndrome, which may be either a 14q21q Robertsonian translocation or a 21q21q translocation. A carrier of a Robertsonian translocation involving chromosomes 14 and 21 has only 45 chromosomes and can theoretically produce six possible types of gametes. Of these, only three are potentially viable: one that is normal, one that is balanced, and one that is unbalanced, having both the translocated chromosome and a normal chromosome 21. The latter, when combined with a normal gamete, could produce a child with Down syndrome. Therefore, theoretically, the risk of a carrier of this type of Robertsonian translocation producing a child with Down syndrome would be 1 in 3. In practice, about 15% of the progeny of mothers with this type of translocation, and very few of the progeny of fathers with this type of translocation, develop Down syndrome. In contrast, carriers of a 21q21q translocation produce gametes that either have the translocated chromosome or lack any 21 chromosome. Progeny then can have either trisomy 21 or monosomy 21, but, since the latter is rarely viable, approximately 100% of progeny will have Down syndrome.

65. The answer is c. (*Kumar, pp 175–178.*) The three most common trisomies causing human disease are trisomies 13, 18, and 21. Trisomy 13 (Patau's syndrome) is characterized by forebrain and midline facial abnormalities. Patients can develop holoprosencephaly, which is characterized by fused frontal lobes and a single ventricle. Olfactory bulbs are also absent. The midline facial abnormalities that are seen with trisomy 13 include cleft lip, cleft palate, nasal defects, and a single central eye ("cyclops"). Other defects associated with Patau's syndrome include polydactyly, rocker-bottom feet, and congenital heart diseases. Trisomy 18 (Edwards' syndrome) is characterized by mental retardation, micrognathia (tiny jaw), low-set ears, rocker-bottom feet, and congenital heart diseases. Perhaps most characteristic is a clenched fist with overlapping fingers: the index finger overlying the third and fourth fingers, while the fifth finger overlaps the fourth. Edwards' syndrome is also associated with polyhydramnios and a single umbilical artery.

Trisomy 21 (Down syndrome) is the most common chromosomal abnormality and is an important cause of mental retardation. Children with Down syndrome invariably have severe mental retardation, which progressively declines with advancing age. Patients have characteristic facial features that include a flat facial profile, oblique palpebral fissures, and epicanthal folds; a horizontal palmar crease; and a decreased muscle tone at birth that leads to a "floppy baby." About one-third of these children also have congenital heart defects, most commonly ventricular septal defects and AV canal defects. There is also a marked increase in the incidence of acute leukemia, usually acute lymphoblastic leukemia, in children with Down syndrome who are younger than 3 years of age. There is almost a 100% incidence of Alzheimer's disease in patients with Down syndrome by the age of 35. Changes in the brains of patients with Down syndrome similar to those seen in the brains of patients with Alzheimer's disease include senile plaques and neurofibrillary tangles. Patients with Down syndrome also have an increased incidence of infections, GI obstruction, and duodenal ulcers.

Deletions involving chromosome 22 (e.g., 22q11) are associated with both DiGeorge's syndrome and the velocardiofacial (VCF) syndrome. DiGeorge's syndrome is associated with absence of the thymus, which leads to cell-mediated immune deficiencies, and absence of the parathyroids, which leads to hypocalcemia. VCF syndrome is associated with palate (velum) abnormalities and dysfunction of the T cells. DiGeorge's syndrome and VCF syndrome may represent spectrums of the same abnormality. In fact, the acronym CATCH-22 refers to the signs of the 22q11 deletion syndrome: cardiac abnormality, abnormal face, T-cell defect secondary to thymic hypoplasia, cleft palate, and hypocalcemia secondary to hypoparathyroidism.

66. The answer is b. (*Rubin, pp 227, 234. Kumar, pp 176–178.*) Several genetic diseases are characterized by a deletion of part of an autosomal chromosome. The 5p⁻ syndrome is also called the cri-du-chat syndrome, as affected infants characteristically have a high-pitched cry similar to that of a kitten. Additional findings in this disorder include severe mental retardation, microcephaly, and congenital heart disease. 4p⁻, also called Wolf-Hirschhorn syndrome, is characterized by pre- and postnatal growth retardation and severe hypotonia. Affected infants have many defects including micrognathia and a prominent forehead. The 11p⁻ syndrome is characterized by the congenital absence of the iris (aniridia) and is often accompanied by Wilms' tumor of the kidney. The 13q⁻ syndrome is associated with the loss of the Rb suppressor gene and the development of retinoblastoma. Deletions involving chromosome 15 (15q⁻) may result in either Prader-Willi syndrome or Angelman's syndrome depending on whether the defect involves the paternal or the maternal chromosome (genetic imprinting). 17p⁻, also known as Smith-Magenis syndrome, is associated with self-destructive behavior.

67. The answer is a. (*Kumar, pp 10, 185–187, 289, 505.*) Genetic imprinting refers to the fact that different diseases may result from the same chromosomal deletion depending on whether that deletion specifically involves either the maternal chromosome or the paternal chromosome. This finding is in sharp contrast to the classic concept of Mendelian inheritance, which states that the phenotype of a certain allele is independent of whether the chromosome is the maternal or the paternal chromosome. The cause of genetic imprinting is not known, but it may relate to the degree of methylation of genes. Genes that are more highly methylated are less likely to be transcribed into messenger RNA. The best example of genetic imprinting involves deletions involving chromosome 15 (15q⁻). If the deletion involves the maternal chromosome that codes for the gene UBE3A then Angelman's syndrome results. This gene codes for the ubiquitin protein ligase E3A, an enzyme that attaches ubiquitin to proteins destined to be degraded within proteasomes of the cell. Both maternal and paternal copies of the UBE3A gene are active in most organs, but in the brain only the maternal gene is active as the paternal gene is normally imprinted (inactivated). Deletion of the normally active UBE3A gene on maternal chromosome 15 produces Angelman's syndrome, which is characterized by severe mental retardation, seizures, a stiff ataxic gait with jerky movements, inappropriate laughter, and occasional oculocutaneous albinism. Because of the combination of ataxic gait and inappropriate laughter, these patients are sometimes inappropriately referred to as "happy puppets."

In contrast, deletions involving the paternal chromosome 15 result in Prader-Willi syndrome, which is characterized by short stature, obesity, mild to moderate mental retardation, and small hands and feet. Patients also develop hypogonadism, which is characterized in males by cryptorchidism and micropenis and in females by hypoplastic labia. Note that a loss of chromosome 15 can also occur if two parental chromosomes of the same type are derived from the same parent. This condition is called uniparental disomy, whereas the normal condition is called biparental disomy. Inheritance of the same (duplicated) chromosome is called isodisomy, while inheritance of homologues from the same parent is called heterodisomy. To illustrate this concept, consider paternal uniparental disomy of chromosome 15. This refers to inheriting two copies of paternal chromosome 15 and no maternal chromosome 15. Therefore, this is essentially the same as a deletion of maternal chromosome 15, which produces Angelman's syndrome.

Inheriting two copies of paternal chromosome 11 results in Beckwith-Wiedemann syndrome. This is not a trisomy, as the maternal chromosome is lost, and therefore this would be a paternal uniparental disomy for chromosome 11. This syndrome is characterized by exomphalos, macroglossia, and gigantism (EMG). Patients also develop hypoglycemia because the genes for insulin and insulinlike growth factors are located in this region. Smith-Magenis syndrome ($17p^-$) is associated with self-destructive behavior along with short stature, brachydactyly and sleep disturbances, while Wolf-Hirschhorn syndrome ($4p^-$) is characterized by growth retardation, severe hypotonia, and micrognathia.

68. The answer is a. (*Kumar, pp 178–181.*) Turner's syndrome (hypogonadism in phenotypic females) is an important cause of primary amenorrhea. Characteristics of this syndrome include short stature, a webbed neck, and multiple skeletal abnormalities that include a wide carrying angle of the arms where the elbow is out (cubitus valgus), a "shield-shaped" chest, and a high-arched palate. Most cases of Turner's syndrome are associated with a 45,XO karyotype, which has no Barr body, but other causes of Turner's syndrome include isochromosome X and mosaicism. The 45,XO karyotype is associated with the loss of some genes that normally remain active on both X chromosomes. The haploinsufficiency of the short stature homeobox (SHOX) gene may lead to the short stature characteristic of Turner's syndrome.

Individuals with Turner's syndrome are phenotypic females, but they fail to develop secondary characteristics at puberty. Patients have streak gonads, histologic sections of which reveal atrophic, fibrous strands and are devoid of ova and follicles. These hypermaturing ovaries produce decreased estrogen levels, resulting in primary amenorrhea with no menarche. About one-half of patients develop hypothyroidism due to autoantibodies against thyroid hormone. Mental retardation is not associated with Turner's syndrome.

Deletion of chromosome 13, such as with a 45,XX,del(13) karyotype, is seen with Patau's syndrome, while a 47,XX,+21 karyotype is seen with trisomy 21. An XYY karyotype, which most often results from nondisjunction at the second meiosis during spermatogenesis, produces individuals who are phenotypically normal except that they may be tall and have severe acne (cystic acne). The relationship of the extra Y to behavior is controversial, but these individuals do have problems with motor and language development. Multi-X females, such as with a 48,XXXX karyotype, are phenotypically normal, but there is an increased tendency toward mental retardation that is proportional to the number of X chromosomes that are present.

69. The answer is a. (*Kumar, pp 178–181.*) Sexual ambiguity arises when there is disagreement between the various ways of determining sex. Genetic sex is determined by the presence or absence of a Y chromosome. Gonadal sex is based upon the histologic appearance of the gonads. Ductal sex depends on the presence of derivatives of the Müllerian or Wolffian ducts. Phenotypic or genital sex is based on the appearance of the external genitalia. True hermaphroditism refers to the presence of both ovarian and testicular tissue. Pseudohermaphroditism is a disagreement between the phenotypic and gonadal sex. A female pseudohermaphrodite has ovaries but external male genitalia, while a male pseudohermaphrodite has testicular tissue, resulting from an XY genital sex karyotype, but female external genitalia. Female pseudohermaphroditism results from excessive exposure to androgens during early gestation; most often this is the result of congenital adrenal hyperplasia. Male pseudohermaphroditism results from defective virilization of the male embryo, most commonly caused by complete androgen insensitivity syndrome, also called testicular feminization.

Kallmann's syndrome results from a lack of embryonic migration of cells from the olfactory bulb to the hypothalamus and is characterized by primary amenorrhea, lack of secondary sex characteristics, and decreased sense of smell (hyposmia). Laboratory findings include decreased GnRH, LH, and FSH. Mixed gonadal dysgenesis consists of one well-defined testis and a contralateral streak ovary. It is a cause of ambiguous genitalia in the

newborn. Turner's syndrome, which has a 45,XO karyotype, is characterized by a female phenotype and bilateral streak ovaries.

70. The answer is c. (*Kumar, pp 198–199, 672. Braunwald, p 274. Goldman,
pp 954–956.*) The immunologic classification of acute lymphoblastic
leukemia is based on the normal developmental sequence of maturation of
B and T lymphocytes, which is characterized by gene rearrangement and the
acquisition of surface markers. Both B and T lymphocytes originate from a
common lymphoid stem cell that is characterized by the intranuclear
enzyme terminal deoxynucleotidyl transferase (TdT) and the surface antigens CD34 and CD38. The first definable stage of B cell maturation occurs
as the cell begins the process of producing immunoglobulin (Ig). The heavy-
chain genes, which are located on chromosome 14, are first rearranged, but
because this occurs before the rearrangement of the light-chain genes, complete immunoglobulin is not yet expressed on the cell surface. Instead mu
heavy-chain genes are rearranged first and are found within the cytoplasm.
This defines these developing cells as being pre-B cells. These cells also
demonstrate surface CD10 (CALLA) and the pan–B cell markers CD19,
CD20, and CD22. Next these developing B cells begin to synthesize light
chains. Kappa light-chain genes are found on chromosome 2 and are
rearranged first. If something goes wrong in this process, then the lambda
light-chain genes on chromosome 22 are rearranged; otherwise they stay in
their germline configuration. The synthesized light chains then combine
with the intracytoplasmic mu heavy chains to form complete IgM, which is
then transported to the surface, forming surface IgM (sIgM). These cells,
which have also acquired CD21 but have lost TdT and CD10, are called
immature B cells. Next these developing B cells produce IgD, which is also
expressed on the cell surface (sIgD). These cells with surface IgM and IgD
are called mature B cells. They are also called "virgin" B cells because these
cells have not encountered any foreign antigen. (Note that all of the preced-
ing steps occur in the bone marrow of the developing fetus.)

71. The answer is c. (*Henry, pp 878–886, 915–916, 922. Chandrasoma, pp
59–63.*) Follicular hyperplasia is a reactive process involving lymph nodes in
which reactive proliferating B lymphocytes produce hyperplasia of the lymphoid follicles and germinal centers. These B lymphocytes are stimulated to
proliferate by binding of foreign antigen to membrane-bound surface
immunoglobulin (Ig) on the B cells. Upon activation these B cells will then

become either memory cells or plasma cells, the product of which is Ig. Igs are composed of light chains and heavy chains, each of which are composed of a variable region and a constant region. The variable regions of both of these chains form the antigen-binding region of Ig, which is called the Fab portion. The portion of Ig that binds complement is called the Fc portion. There are two types of light chains and five types of heavy chains. The two light chains are the kappa chain, the genes of which are located on chromosome 2, and the gamma chain, the genes of which are located on chromosome 22. The heavy chains are M, D, A, E, and G, the genes of all of these being on chromosome 14. The combination of one type of light chain with a particular heavy-chain forms each of the five types of Ig.

In contrast to Ig, erythropoietin is secreted by the peritubular interstitial cells of the kidney, while interleukin-2 and interleukin-3 are secreted by activated T cells. NK cells and T cells are the only known sources of gamma-interferon.

72. The answer is b. (*Henry, pp 878–886. Chandrasoma, pp 59–63. Ravel, pp 284–285.*) IgM, which constitutes about 5 to 10% of the Ig in the serum, is secreted during the first exposure to antigen (primary immune response). The monomeric form of IgM is found on the surface of some B cells, while the pentameric form is found in the serum and cannot cross the placenta. Because of this, elevated titers of toxoplasma-specific IgM antibodies, which generally persist for less than a year, are an indication, but not confirmation, of current or recent infection. In contrast to IgM, IgG, which is the most abundant Ig in the serum (80%), is secreted in the second response to certain antigens and does not predominate early during the first response. Therefore, toxoplasma-specific IgG titers, which may persist for life, are only diagnostic if the titer is rising or they are particularly high (greater than 1:1024). Additionally, unlike IgM, IgG can cross the placenta, and it is the major protective immunoglobulin in the neonate. IgG can also activate complement, participate in antibody-dependent cell-mediated cytotoxicity (ADCC), neutralize toxins or viruses, and function as an opsonin.

The remaining types of immunoglobulins are IgD, IgE, and IgA. IgD, which forms less than 1% of serum Ig, is found on the cell surface of some B cells and functions in the activation of these B cells. IgE, also known as reaginic antibody, is found on the plasma membrane of mast cells and basophils and participates in type I hypersensitivity reactions, such as allergies, asthma, and anaphylaxis. IgE is used to fight parasitic infections. IgA, which constitutes about 10 to 15% of serum Ig, exists as a monomer in the serum and a dimer in glandular secretions. IgA is synthesized by mucosal plasma cells of the GI tract, lung, and urinary tract—thus making it the immunoglobulin of "secretory immunity"—and is found in saliva, sweat, nasal secretion, and tears. It is secreted as a dimer bound to a secretory piece that stabilizes the molecule against proteolysis.

73. The answer is a. (*Kumar, pp 51–52, 71. Damjanov, pp 400–401.*) The interleukins are a group of cytokines with diverse functions primarily involved in inflammatory reactions and immunity. Two interleukins that are primarily involved in stimulating acute phase reactions, which include fever production, peripheral leukocytosis, and decreased appetite, are interleukin-1 (IL-1) and interleukin-6 (IL-6), both of which are secreted by macrophages. IL-1 is also produced by many other types of cells, including antigen-presenting cells (APCs) and other somatic cells. Other effects of IL-1 important in acute inflammation include increasing vascular permeability and stimulating neutrophils, B cells, and fibroblasts. The functions of IL-1 also include autocrine effects on the APCs and paracrine effects on T cells. The effects of IL-1 on T cells include increased interleukin-2 (IL-2) secretion and increased expression of receptors for IL-2 and gamma-interferon (γ-IFN). IL-6 is the most potent stimulator for acute-phase reactant production by the liver. Additionally, it stimulates B cells and, synergistically with IL-1, T cells. Tumor necrosis factor (TNF) acts with IL-1 and IL-6 to induce systemic acute phase reactions.

In contrast, IL-2 is produced by T-helper cells and stimulates the T-cell response by stimulating CD-8 lymphocytes and NK cells and increasing IL-2 receptors of T-helper cells. Interleukin-3 (IL-3), also known as multi-CSF (multicolony stimulating factor), is a cytokine that stimulates pluripotential stem cells. It can be used clinically in patients with aplastic anemia to increase peripheral neutrophil numbers. Finally, interleukin-5 is produced by T_H2 cells and stimulates B cells, secretion of IgA, and production of eosinophils, while interleukin-12 is produced by B cells and macrophages and stimulates T_H1 and inhibits T_H2 cells.

74. The answer is a. (*Kumar, pp 203–204.*) Histocompatibility antigens are important for the recognition of foreign antigens by T lymphocytes. For example, CD8 cytotoxic T lymphocytes can recognize a foreign antigen only if that antigen is complexed to self-class I antigens. In general, these class I molecules bind to proteins synthesized within the cell; one example is the cellular production of viral antigens. The CD8 molecule of the cytotoxic T cell binds to the nonpolymorphic portion of the class I molecule, while the T-cell receptor on the surface of the T lymphocyte binds to a complex formed by the peptide fragment of the antigen and the class I antigen. In contrast, CD4 helper T lymphocytes can recognize a foreign antigen only if that antigen is complexed to self-class II antigens. In general, class II antigens present foreign antigens that have been processed within the cell in endosomes or lysosomes; one example is bacteria. Macrophages and neutrophils are active phagocytes and have receptors for the Fc portion of IgG and C3b; both of these substances are important opsonins. Macrophages also ingest and present antigens to T cells in conjunction with surface class II antigens. Finally, note that class III antigens are not involved in histocompatibility but include proteins of the complement cascade.

75. The answer is b. (*Kumar, pp 205, 1309.*) A variety of different diseases have an association with certain human leukocyte antigen (HLA) types. The exact mechanism of this association is unknown. These diseases can be grouped into three broad categories: inflammatory diseases, inherited errors of metabolism, and autoimmune diseases. The classic example of an inflammatory disease associated with a certain HLA is the association of ankylosing spondylitis with HLA-B27. Ankylosing spondylitis is one type of spondyloarthropathy that lacks the rheumatoid factor found in rheumatoid arthritis. Other seronegative spondyloarthropathies include Reiter syndrome, psoriatic arthritis, and enteropathic arthritis. All of these are associated with an increased incidence of HLA-B27. Ankylosing spondylitis, also known as rheumatoid spondylitis or Marie-Strümpell disease, is a chronic inflammatory disease that primarily affects the sacroiliac joints of adult males. Calcification of the vertebral and paravertebral ligaments produce low back pain and stiffness and are seen radiographically as a "bamboo spine."

HLA types are also associated with inherited errors of metabolism and autoimmune diseases. An example of an inherited error of metabolism being associated with a certain HLA type is the association of hemochromatosis with HLA-A3, while autoimmune diseases can be associated with the DR locus. Two examples of this are the associations of rheumatoid arthritis with DR4 and of insulin-dependent diabetes with DR3/DR4.

76. The answer is d. (*Kumar, pp 205–210.*) Hypersensitivity diseases are caused by immune mechanisms. They are classified into four different categories based on the immune mechanisms involved. Type I hypersensitivity reactions involve IgE (reaginic) antibodies that have been bound to the surface of mast cells and basophils. These IgE antibodies are formed by a T cell–dependent process. An allergen initially binds to antigen-presenting cells, which then stimulate T_H2 cells to secrete interleukin 4 (IL-4), IL-5, and IL-6. IL-5 stimulates the production of eosinophils, while IL-4 stimulates B cells to transform into plasma cells and produce IgE. This IgE then attaches to mast cells and basophils, because these cells have cell surface receptors for the Fc portion of IgE. When these "armed" mast cells or basophils are reexposed to the allergen, the antigen bridges two IgE molecules and causes mast cells to release preformed (primary) mediators. This antigen-to-antibody binding also causes these cells to synthesize secondary mediators.

The reactions that occur as a result of the primary mediators of type I hypersensitivity are rapidly occurring, since the mediators have already been made and are present within the granules of mast cells. These substances include biogenic amines, such as histamine, chemotactic factors, enzymes, and proteoglycans. Histamine causes increased vascular permeability, vasodilation, and bronchial smooth muscle contraction. The chemotactic factors are chemotactic for eosinophils and neutrophils. Mast cells also produce new products (secondary mediators) via a series of reactions within the cell membrane that lead to the generation of lipid mediators and cytokines. The lipid mediators are generated from arachidonic acid. Membrane receptors bound to IgE activate phospholipase A_2, which then cleaves membrane phospholipids into arachidonic acid. Lipoxygenase produces leukotrienes, including LTB_4 and leukotrienes C_4, D_4, and E_4. These last three leukotrienes are the most potent vasoactive and spasmogenic agents known. They used to be called slow reactive substance of anaphylaxis (SRS-A). Prostaglandin D_2, which is produced via the enzyme cyclooxygenase, is abundant in lung mast cells. It causes bronchospasm and increased mucus production.

Type I reactions may be either local or systemic. Local reactions include urticaria (hives), angioedema, allergic rhinitis (hay fever), conjunctivitis, food allergies, and allergic bronchial asthma. Systemic reactions usually follow parenteral administration of antigen, such as with drug reactions (penicillin) or insect stings. The amount of antigen may be very small. Symptoms include vomiting, cramps, diarrhea, itching, wheezing, and shortness of breath, and death may occur within minutes. The main treatment is epinephrine.

77. The answer is d. (*Kumar, p 210.*) A blood transfusion reaction is a type II hypersensitivity reaction that is mediated by antibodies reacting against antigens present on the surface of blood group antigens or irregular antigens present on the donor's red blood cells. Type II hypersensitivity reactions result from attachment of antibodies to changed cell surface antigens or to normal cell surface antigens. Complement-mediated cytotoxicity occurs when IgM or IgG binds to a cell surface antigen with complement activation and consequent cell membrane damage or lysis. Blood transfusion reactions and autoimmune hemolytic anemia are examples of this form. Systemic anaphylaxis is a type I hypersensitivity reaction in which mast cells or basophils that are bound to IgE antibodies are reexposed to an allergen, which leads to a release of vasoactive amines that causes edema and broncho- and vasoconstriction. Sudden death can occur. Systemic immune complex reactions are found in type III reactions and are due to circulating antibodies that form complexes upon reexposure to an antigen (such as foreign serum), which then activates complement. This process is followed by chemotaxis and aggregation of neutrophils, which leads to release of lysosomal enzymes and eventual necrosis of tissue and cells. Serum sickness and Arthus reactions are examples of type III reactions. Delayed type hypersensitivity is type IV and is due to previously sensitized T lymphocytes, which release lymphokines upon reexposure to the antigen. This takes time—perhaps up to several days following exposure. The tuberculin reaction is the best-known example. T cell–mediated cytotoxicity leads to lysis of cells by cytotoxic T cells in response to tumor cells, allogenic tissue, and virus-infected cells. These cells have CD8 antigens on their surfaces.

78. The answer is a. (*Kumar, pp 215–218. Damjanov, pp 400–401.*) Type IV hypersensitivity reactions do not involve antibody formation, but instead are mediated by T cells (cell-mediated hypersensitivity). There are two subtypes of type IV hypersensitivity reactions, one of which involves CD4 cells [delayed-type hypersensitivity (DTH)] and the other of which involves CD8 cells (cell-mediated cytotoxicity). The classic example of a DTH reaction is the tuberculin skin test (Mantoux reaction), in which a local area of erythema and induration peaks at about 48 h following intracutaneous injection of tuberculin. Other examples of DTH reactions include granulomatous inflammation, poison ivy reactions and contact dermatitis (often the result of sensitivity to nickel, which can be found in some watchbands).

The formation of granulomas (with epithelioid cells) is another example of a type IV hypersensitivity reaction. The pathomechanisms involved in the formation of granulomas is as follows. Upon first exposure to the antigen in DTH reactions, macrophages ingest the antigen and process it in association with class II antigens (HLA-D) to helper T cells (CD4), which differentiate into CD4 T_H1 cells based on the actions of interleukin-12 secreted by macrophages and dendritic cells. Upon reexposure to the antigen, these CD4 T_H1 cells are activated and secrete biologically active factors (the lymphokines). Specifically, T_H1 cells secrete gamma-interferon, interleukin 2, and TNF-alpha. Gamma-interferon is the main cytokine that is responsible for DTH reactions. It activates macrophages (epithelioid cells) and forms granulomas (caseating or noncaseating). Interleukin 2 activates other CD4 cells, while TNF-alpha causes endothelial cells to increase production of prostacyclin and ELAM-1.

Note that type I hypersensitivity reactions involve IgE antibodies, secreted from plasma cells, that attach to the surface of mast cells and basophils. Initially an allergen binds to antigen-presenting cells, which then stimulate T_H2 cells to secrete IL-4, IL-5, and IL-6. IL-5 stimulates the production of eosinophils, while IL-4 stimulates B cells to transform into plasma cells and produce IgE. The activation of mast cells and basophils causes them to secrete many substances, such as histamine. Finally, leukotrienes C4, D4, and E4 increase vascular permeability and cause vasoconstriction and bronchospasm.

79. The answer is c. (*Damjanov, pp 655–658.*) An allograft is also called a homograft and refers to a graft between members of the same species. An autograft is a tissue graft taken from one site and placed in a different site in the same individual. Isografts are grafts between individuals from an inbred strain of animals. A graft between individuals of two different species is a xenograft or heterograft.

80. The answer is e. (*Kumar, pp 218–222.*) The rejection of organ transplants involves both humoral and cell-mediated immunologic reactions. Hyperacute rejection, due to preformed host antibodies that are directed against antigens of the graft, occurs within minutes after transplantation. Histologically, neutrophils are found within the glomerulus and peritubular capillaries. These changes illustrate an antigen-antibody reaction at the vascular endothelium, similar to the Arthus reaction. Acute rejection may occur within days or much longer after transplantation. It is called acute because once it begins, the changes progress rapidly. Acute rejection can result from vasculitis or interstitial lymphocytic infiltration. The vasculitis is the result of humoral rejection (acute rejection vasculitis), while the interstitial mononuclear infiltrate is the result of cellular rejection (acute cellular rejection). Acute cellular rejection is responsive to immunosuppressive therapy, but acute rejection vasculitis is not. Subacute rejection vasculitis occurs during the first few months after transplantation and is characterized by the proliferation of fibroblasts and macrophages in the tunica intima of arteries. In chronic rejection, tubular atrophy, mononuclear interstitial infiltration, and vascular changes are found. The vascular changes are probably the result of the proliferative arteritis seen in acute and subacute stages. The vascular obliteration leads to interstitial fibrosis and tubular atrophy, resulting in loss of renal function.

In contrast, graft-versus-host (GVH) disease occurs when immunocompetent lymphocytes from the donor, usually from bone marrow or liver, attack the recipient's tissue. GVH may be acute or chronic. Acute GVH is manifested by changes in the skin (dermatitis), the intestines (diarrhea, malabsorption), and the liver (jaundice). Chronic GVH produces changes in the skin (fibrosis) that are similar to the skin changes seen in patients with progressive systemic sclerosis.

81. The answer is b. (*Kumar, pp 227–230, 913–915. Goldman, pp 807–809.*) Autoantibodies can be directed against antigens in the nucleus or cytoplasm of cells, or they can be directed against certain cells, proteins, structural antigens, or receptors. Examples of autoantibodies to components of the cytoplasm of cells include antimitochondrial antibodies, anti-smooth-muscle antibodies and antineutrophil cytoplasmic antibodies. Antimitochondrial antibodies are found in the majority of patients with primary biliary cirrhosis, while anti-smooth-muscle antibodies are characteristic of lupoid autoimmune hepatitis. Antineutrophil cytoplasmic antibodies (ANCAs) may be directed against myeloperoxidase or proteinase 3. The former produces a perinuclear pattern (P-ANCAs) and is seen in some patients with Wegener's granulomatosis, but more often is associated with microscopic polyarteritis nodosa. The latter type of ANCA produces a cytoplasmic pattern (C-ANCAs) and is seen mainly in patients with Wegener's granulomatosis.

Autoantibodies against nuclear antigens (antinuclear antibodies or ANAs) can be grouped into several categories. Antibodies may be directed against DNA, histones, nonhistone proteins bound to RNA, or nucleolar antigens. Antibodies to double-stranded DNA are specific for patients with SLE.

Non-DNA nuclear components, called extractable nuclear antigens, include Sm antigen, ribonucleoprotein, SS-A and SS-B reactive antigens, and Scl-70. Autoantibodies to Smith antigen are specific for patients with SLE, antibodies to Scl-70 are specific for patients with progressive systemic sclerosis, and antibodies to either SS-A or SS-B are specific for patients with Sjögren's syndrome. Anticentromere antibodies are found in patients with systemic sclerosis, especially in a subset of patients with the CREST syndrome. Finally note that autoantibodies to IgG (called rheumatoid factor) are present in patients with rheumatoid arthritis. This type of antibody may also be seen in patients with other types of autoimmune diseases.

82. The answer is e. (*Kumar, pp 227–239.*) Systemic lupus erythematosus (SLE) is a chronic, remitting and relapsing, often febrile multisystem disorder that predominantly affects the skin, kidneys, serosal membranes, and joints. SLE has a strong female predominance (10:1), and the disease usually arises in the second and third decades. The classic lesion involving the skin is an erythematous lesion over the bridge of the nose producing a "butterfly" pattern. Sunlight makes the rash worse. Histologically there is liquefactive degeneration of the basal layer of the epidermis with a perivascular lymphoid infiltrate. Deposits of immunoglobulin and complement can be demonstrated at the dermoepidermal junction. Finding immunoglobulin deposits in uninvolved skin is considered highly specific for SLE; this is called the lupus band test.

The most common symptom with SLE is caused by involvement of the joints (arthritis), which produces a nonerosive synovitis. The heart may also be involved in patients with SLE. Small vegetations may develop on the heart valves and are called Libman-Sacks endocarditis. The major cause of death in patients with SLE is involvement of the kidneys leading to renal failure. There are deposits of DNA–anti-DNA complexes within the glomeruli. These deposits are found within the mesangium as well as in subendothelial and subepithelial locations. The subendothelial deposits produce wire-loop lesions and are particularly important. Other sites of involvement include the CNS, which may be life-threatening, and serous membranes, which can produce pleuritis and pleural effusions.

Patients with SLE also have marked B cell hyperactivity. This leads to a polyclonal production of antibodies to self and nonself antigens. Several autoantibodies to both nuclear and cytoplasmic cell components have been found, but antinuclear antibodies (ANAs) are the hallmark of SLE. Damaged cells can lose their nuclei, which then can react with these autoantibodies.

This produces an LE body, or hematoxylin body. These bodies are pathognomonic of lupus. In vitro, these LE bodies can be ingested by phagocytic cells (such as a neutrophil or macrophage), producing an LE cell.

In contrast to the clinical characteristics of SLE, dermatomyositis is characterized by periorbital lilac discoloration with erythema on the dorsal portion of the hands; rheumatoid arthritis is characterized by the combination of arthritis and serum rheumatoid factor; Sjögren's syndrome is characterized by the combination of dry eyes, a dry mouth, and enlarged salivary glands; and amyloidosis is characterized by Congo red–positive extracellular deposits.

83. The answer is c. (*Kumar, pp 238–239.*) The combination of trouble swallowing, hypertension, and sclerosis of the skin should raise the possibility of progressive systemic sclerosis (scleroderma), a multisystem disease that involves the cardiovascular, gastrointestinal, cutaneous, musculoskeletal, pulmonary, and renal systems through progressive interstitial fibrosis. Small arterioles in the aforementioned systems show obliteration caused by intimal hyperplasia accompanied by progressive interstitial fibrosis. In the skin, the changes begin in the fingers and hands and consist of sclerotic atrophy, which is characterized by increased dermal collagen, epidermal atrophy, and loss of skin adnexal structures. Two antinuclear antibodies are unique to systemic sclerosis. One is Scl-70, which is found in diffuse progressive systemic sclerosis, and the other is an anticentromere antibody found in the CREST syndrome, a variant of progressive systemic sclerosis. The CREST syndrome is characterized by calcinosis, Raynaud's syndrome (episodic ischemia of digits), esophageal dysmotility, sclerodactyly, and telangiectasia. Pulmonary hypertension and primary biliary cirrhosis are common in the CREST syndrome, but the kidneys are usually spared.

In contrast to the histologic findings with systemic sclerosis, a conjunctival biopsy that reveals noncaseating granulomas is suggestive of sarcoidosis; a peripheral nerve biopsy that reveals rare acid-fast bacteria is diagnostic of leprosy; and a temporal artery biopsy that reveals fragmentation of the internal elastic lamina is characteristic of temporal arteritis.

84. The answer is a. (*Kumar, pp 258–264, 680.*) Amyloid is a generic term that describes special properties of any protein having a tertiary structure that produces a β-pleated sheet. Amyloid stains brown with iodine ("starch-like"). Histologically, the deposits always begin between or outside of cells. Eventually the amyloid deposits may strangle the cells, leading to atrophy or cell death. The histologic diagnosis of amyloid is based solely on its special staining characteristics. It stains pink with the routine hematoxylin and eosin stain, but, with Congo red stain, amyloid stains dark red and has an apple-green birefringence when viewed under polarized light. There are many different types of proteins that stain as amyloid, and these are associated with a wide variety of diseases. These diseases may be either systemic, such as with immune dyscrasias, reactive diseases, or hemodialysis, or they may be localized, such as with senile or endocrine disorders. Immune dyscrasias, such as multiple myeloma or B cell lymphomas, can secrete amyloid light (AL) chains. Increased serum protein with hypercalcemia is consistent with a diagnosis of multiple myeloma. Bone pain can result from the lytic bone lesions that are characteristic of myeloma. Deposition of AL chains in the kidneys is the most common cause of renal amyloidosis in the United States. Patients can develop the nephrotic syndrome with marked proteinuria.

Systemic deposits of amyloid-associated (AA) protein complicate various chronic infections and inflammatory processes, most commonly rheumatoid arthritis, other connective tissue diseases, bronchiectasis, and inflammatory bowel disease. Reactive systemic diseases may be associated with the deposition of amyloid-associated (AA) protein, which is a polypeptide derived from serum AA protein produced in the liver. Patients on chronic hemodialysis may develop amyloid deposits consisting of β_2-microglobulin. Patients with senile cardiac disease may develop amyloid deposits in the heart consisting of amyloid transthyretin (ATTR), while patients with senile cerebral disease, such as Alzheimer's disease, may develop amyloid deposits in the brain consisting of β_2-amyloid protein. Do not confuse β_2-amyloid protein with β_2-microglobulin, a component of the MHC class I molecule. Patients with medullary carcinoma of the thyroid, a malignancy of the calcitonin-secreting parafollicular C cells of the thyroid, characteristically have amyloid deposits of pro-calcitonin within the tumor. Patients with type II diabetes mellitus may have amyloid deposits within pancreatic islets consisting of islet amyloid peptide.

85. The answer is c. (*Kumar, pp 240–245. Flake, pp 1806–1810, 1996.*) Patients with severe combined immunodeficiency disease (SCID) have defects of lymphoid stem cells involving both T and B cells. These patients have severe abnormalities of immunologic function with lymphopenia. They are at risk for infection with all types of infectious agents, including bacteria, mycobacteria, fungi, viruses, and parasites. Patients have a skin rash at birth, possibly due to a graft-versus-host reaction from maternal lymphocytes. Patients are particularly prone to chronic diarrhea, due to rotavirus and bacteria, and to oral candidiasis. The most common form of SCIDs is X-linked and related to a mutation in the common gamma chain subunit of cytokine receptors. In particular, the cytokine receptor that is mainly responsible for this defect is the receptor for interleukin-7. The remaining cases of SCIDs have an autosomal recessive inheritance (Swiss type of SCIDs) and lack the enzyme adenosine deaminase (ADA) in their red cells and leukocytes. This leads to accumulation of adenosine triphosphate and deoxyadenosine triphosphate, both of which are toxic to lymphocytes.

The Wiskott-Aldrich syndrome (WAS) is also an X-linked recessive disorder, but it is characterized by the combination of recurrent pyogenic infections, eczema, and thrombocytopenia. WAS is associated with a mutation in a gene on the X chromosome that codes for the Wiskott-Aldrich syndrome protein (WASP). The immune abnormalities associated with WAS are characterized by progressive loss of T-cell function and decreased IgM. The other immunoglobulin levels are normal or increased. There are decreased numbers of lymphocytes in the peripheral blood and paracortical (T cell) areas of lymph nodes. Both cellular and humoral immunity are affected, and, because patients fail to produce antibodies to polysaccharides, they are vulnerable to infections with encapsulated organisms.

In patients with chronic granulomatous disease (CGD), another X-linked recessive disorder, the neutrophils and macrophages have deficient H_2O_2 production due to abnormalities involving the enzyme NADPH oxidase. These individuals have frequent infections that are caused by catalase-positive organisms, such as S. aureus, because the catalase produced by these organisms destroys the little hydrogen peroxide that is produced.

Finally, hyper-IgM immunodeficiency is paradoxically a T-cell disorder as a defect in CD40L prevents T lymphocytes from inducing isotype switching in B lymphocytes. Therefore, there is decreased levels of IgG, IgE, and IgA but increased levels of IgM. The most common form of this disease is X-linked (XLM).

86. The answer is b. (*Kumar, pp 246–255. Ravel, 272–273. Ayala, pp 239–241.*) Acquired immunodeficiency syndrome (AIDS) is caused by infection with the human immunodeficiency virus (HIV), which is an RNA retrovirus. The first laboratory test used in the diagnosis of HIV infection is the enzyme-linked immunoassay (ELISA) test, which detects the presence of HIV antibodies. If the ELISA test is positive, the Western blot test is usually done to confirm the diagnosis. The Western blot assay detects the presence of gp24, gp41, and gp120/160. These are HIV proteins that are produced by the major genes of HIV, which are the *gag*, *pol*, and *env* genes. The *gag* gene encodes for precursor protein p55, which is processed by viral protease into other components that include p24 (the major core protein) and p7 (nucleocapsid). The *pol* gene encodes viral enzymes including protease, reverse transcriptase, and integrase. Reverse transcriptase is an RNA-dependent DNA polymerase that converts viral RNA to DNA so it can be integrated into the host DNA. Finally, the *env* gene encodes for envelope proteins, including gp120 and gp41.

87. The answer is d. (*Kumar, pp 270–273. Chandrasoma, pp 264–268.*) The names given to tumors are based on the parenchymal component of the tumor, which consists of the proliferating neoplastic cells. In general, benign tumors are designated by using the suffix -oma attached to a name describing either the cell of origin of the tumor or the gross or microscopic appearance of the tumor. Examples of benign tumors whose names are based on their microscopic appearance include adenomas, which have a uniform proliferation of glandular epithelial cells; papillomas, which are tumors that form finger-like projections; fibromas, which are composed of a uniform proliferation of fibrous tissue; leiomyomas, which originate from smooth muscle cells and have elongated, spindle-shaped nuclei; hemangiomas, which are formed from a uniform proliferation of endothelial cells; and lipomas, which originate from adipocytes. The suffix -oma is unfortunately still applied to some tumors that are not benign. Examples of this misnaming include melanomas, lymphomas, and seminomas.

88. The answer is e. (*Kumar, pp 270–276.*) Malignant tumors are generally classified as being either carcinomas or sarcomas. Carcinomas are malignant tumors of epithelial origin, while sarcomas are malignant tumors of mesenchymal tissue. Examples of malignant epithelial tumors (carcinomas) include adenocarcinomas, which consist of a disorganized mass of malignant cells that form glandular structures, and squamous cell carcinomas, which consist of a disorganized mass of malignant cells that produce keratin. Examples of malignant mesenchymal tumors include rhabdomyosarcomas, leiomyosarcomas, fibrosarcomas, and liposarcomas. One clue that a tumor has developed from skeletal muscle, such as a rhabdomyosarcoma, is the presence of cross-striations. These individual cells, seen histologically, are called strap cells. The wall of the stomach consists of smooth muscle, and a tumor that originates from these smooth-muscle cells will consist of proliferating cells with elongated, spindle-shaped nuclei. If a tumor of this type is benign, it is called a leiomyoma, while if it is malignant, it is called a leiomyosarcoma. This distinction is based on the number of mitoses that are present and the degree of atypia displayed by the neoplastic cells.

89. The answer is b. (*Kumar, pp 272–281, 288. Schneider, p 89. Chandrasoma, pp 260–264.*) Neoplasms are clonal proliferations of cells. This fact can be used to demonstrate the difference between normal tissue (polyclonal) and neoplasms (monoclonal). In the past, clonality of tumors was assessed by looking at the heterozygosity of polymorphic X-linked markers in women, such as the enzyme glucose-6-phosphate dehydrogenase. Currently, however, the most common method to assess clonality of tumors is by analyzing the highly pleomorphic locus for the human androgen receptor (HUMARA).

In addition, several gross and microscopic features help to differentiate benign neoplasms from malignant neoplasms. Benign neoplasms grow slowly with an expansile growth pattern that often forms a fibrous capsule. This histologic feature can also be useful in distinguishing a benign neoplastic lipoma from normal nonneoplastic adipose tissue. Benign neoplasms characteristically remain localized and do not metastasize. Histologically, benign neoplastic cells tend to be uniform and well differentiated; that is, they appear similar to their tissue of origin. This histologic feature may not distinguish between benign neoplasms and normal tissue.

In contrast to benign tumors, malignant neoplasms grow rapidly in a crablike pattern and are capable of metastasizing. Histologically, the malignant cells are pleomorphic because they differ from one another in size and shape. These cells have hyperchromatic nuclei and an increased nuclear-to-cytoplasmic ratio. Malignant cells tend to have nucleoli, and mitoses may be frequent. These two features only indicate rapidly proliferating cells and can also be seen in reactive or reparative processes. The mitoses in malignancies, however, tend to be atypical, such as tripolar mitoses. Malignant tumors are graded by their degree of differentiation as well differentiated, moderately differentiated, or poorly differentiated. Marked pleomorphism is described as anaplasia. This histologic feature is usually seen in poorly differentiated or undifferentiated malignancies.

90. The answer is d. (*Kumar, pp 324, 1073–1079.*) Some epithelial malignancies (carcinomas) are preceded by disordered growth (dysplasia) of the epithelium. One example of this is the development of squamous cell carcinoma of the uterine cervix. The normal cervix is lined by a stratified layer of squamous epithelium, while the endocervix is composed of mucus-secreting columnar epithelial cells. In response to chronic inflammation, the columnar epithelial cells change to stratified squamous epithelial cells. This change—squamous metaplasia—is characterized histologically by normal-appearing stratified squamous epithelium overlying endocervical glands. Next, infection with human papillomavirus (HPV) causes dysplastic changes within the epithelium. These dysplastic changes are characterized by disorganized stratified squamous epithelium with mitoses located above the basal layers of the epithelium. The cells themselves are pleomorphic and have hyperchromatic nuclei. The intraepithelial dysplasia is divided into three types based on the degree of dysplasia present and the location of mitoses. In mild dysplasia there are mitoses in the basal one-third of the epithelium; in moderate dysplasia mitoses occur in the middle one-third of the epithelium; and in severe dysplasia there are mitoses in the upper one-third of the epithelium. When the dysplastic changes involve the full thickness of the epithelium, it is referred to as carcinoma in situ (CIS). Next, the neoplastic cells start to invade the underlying tissue, forming an invasive squamous cell carcinoma.

91. The answer is c. (*Kumar, pp 1016–1018, 1071.*) The most common histologic type of cancer at a given site generally reflects the normal histology of that site. For example, squamous cell carcinomas arise in organs that are normally lined by stratified squamous epithelium. That is, sites associated with the development of squamous cell carcinoma include the skin, lung, esophagus, and cervix. Adenocarcinomas arise from glandular epithelium, and therefore sites associated with the development of adenocarcinoma include the lung, colon, stomach, prostate, and endometrium. Sites for transitional cell carcinoma include the urinary bladder and kidney (renal pelvis). Two types of cancer associated with special sites include clear cell carcinoma and signet cell carcinoma. Sites for clear cell carcinoma include the kidney (renal cortex) and vagina, the latter being associated with previous diethylstilbestrol (DES) exposure, while signet cell carcinoma is seen in the stomach and ovaries. In this malignancy the cells infiltrate individually instead of forming recognizable glandular structures.

Each individual cell is filled with a large drop of mucin, which pushes the nucleus to the side, giving it the appearance of a signet ring.

92. The answer is d. (*Kumar, p 327. Rubin, pp 173–183. Braunwald, p 275.*) Retroviruses are important because they are types of RNA viruses that have been implicated as causing immunodeficiency or malignancy. There are two classes of retroviruses that infect man, namely the lenti-viruses, e.g., HIV-1, and the BLV-HTLV retroviruses, e.g., HTLV-1, which stands for human T cell–lymphotropic virus. This retrovirus is the causative agent of adult T-cell leukemia/lymphoma, which is a type of malignancy that is endemic in southern Japan and the Caribbean. Patients with adult T-cell leukemia/lymphoma have increased serum levels of calcium and numerous malignant cells in their lymph nodes and blood. These cells are multilobated and have a characteristic "4-leaf clover" appearance. HTLV-1 produces two novel proteins called Tax and Rex. These are *trans*-regulatory proteins as they can promote at a distance from their transcription of the activity of other genes involved in cellular proliferation. This is in addition to the three specific genes for retroviruses: *gag* (which codes for core protein), *pol* (which codes for the polymerase reverse transcriptase), and *env* (which codes for the envelope protein). These genes are flanked by long terminal repeat units (LTRs), which can turn on genes that are located near to the LTRs. This is important because these LTRs can turn on nearby cellular proto-oncogenes (p-oncs), which are cellular genes that promote normal growth and differentiation. Abnormal activation of these oncogenes turns them into c-oncs, which are genes associated with the production of tumors.

93. The answer is a. (*Kumar, pp 296–297, 305, 1413. Rubin, pp 173–183.*) Classic neurofibromatosis (NF-1) is characterized by the formation of multiple skin tumors (neurofibromas) along with café-au-lait skin macules, axillary freckling, plexiform neurofibromas, and Lisch nodules (pigmented iris hamartomas). The abnormal gene for the classic form (NF-1) is located on chromosome 17. It encodes for neurofibromin, a protein that regulates the function of p21 ras oncoprotein. There are three members of the ras gene family, namely K-*ras*, N-*ras*, and H-*ras*. These genes code for similar proteins called p21, which are attached to the inner surface of the cell membrane. Mutation of the *ras* gene is the single most common abnormality of dominant oncogenes in human tumors and is found in about one-third of all human tumors. Normal *ras* protein (p21) flips back and forth between an activated, signal-transmitting form and an inactive state. In the inactive state, p21 binds GDP, but when cells are stimulated by growth factors, p21 becomes activated by exchanging GDP for GTP, and it can then stimulate MAP kinases and protein kinase C. In normal cells, the activated signal-transmitting stage of ras protein bound to GTP is transient because its intrinsic GTPase activity hydrolyzes GTP to GDP, which returns it to its inactive state. The GTPase activity of normal ras protein is accelerated by GTPase-activating proteins (GAPs), which function as brakes to prevent uncontrolled ras activity. Neurofibromin is a form of GAP. When it is not functioning normally, such as with type I neurofibromatosis, it cannot downregulate the ras oncoprotein product and multiple tumors develop.

94. The answer is c. (*Kumar, pp 293–298.*) There are several mechanisms through which proto-oncogenes (p-oncs) can become oncogenic (c-oncs). Normal cellular genes (proto-oncogenes) may become oncogenic by being incorporated into the viral genome (forming v-oncs), or they may be activated by other processes to form cellular oncogenes (c-oncs). These other processes include gene mutations, chromosomal translocations, and gene amplifications. Gene mutations, such as point mutations, are associated with the formation of cancers by mutant c-*ras* oncogenes. Chromosomal translocations are associated with the development of many types of cancers, one example of which is Burkitt's lymphoma. The most common translocation associated with Burkitt's lymphoma is t(8;14), in which the c-*myc* oncogene on chromosome 8 is brought in contact with the immunoglobulin heavy-chain gene on chromosome 14. Two other examples of chromosomal translocations are the association of chronic myelocytic leukemia (CML) with t(9;22), which is the Philadelphia chromosome, and the association of follicular lymphoma with the translocation t(18;14). The former involves the proto-oncogene c-*abl*, which is rearranged in proximity to a break point cluster region (bcr) on chromosome 22. The resultant chimeric c-*abl/bcr* gene encodes a protein with tyrosine kinase activity. The t(18;14) translocation involves the *bcl*-2 oncogene on chromosome 18. Expression of the oncogene *bcl*-2 is associated with the prevention of apoptosis in germinal centers. Examples of associations that involve gene amplification include N-*myc* and neuroblastoma, c-*neu* and breast cancer, and *erb*-B and breast and ovarian cancer. Gene amplifications can be demonstrated by finding doublet minutes or homogenous staining regions.

95. The answer is a. (*Kumar, pp 292, 302–303, 339.*) In contrast to proto-oncogenes, which are genes that encode for proteins stimulating cell growth, cancer suppressor genes (antioncogenes) encode for proteins that suppress cell growth. Examples of tumor suppressor genes are Rb (associated with retinoblastoma), p53, APC, NF1, DCC, and WT1. In general, these tumor suppressor genes encode proteins that can function as cell surface molecules, regulators of signal transduction, or regulators of nuclear transcription. The DCC gene codes for a cell surface molecule that can transmit negative signals such as contact inhibition. NF1 is associated with regulating signal transduction. It codes for a GAP that binds to a ras protein and then increases GTPase activity, which inactivates ras product. Loss of normal NF1 functioning causes ras to be trapped in an active state. Genes that regulate nuclear transcription include Rb, p53, and WT1. Products of these genes are found within the nucleus and are involved in regulation of the cell cycle. The product of the Rb gene is a nuclear phosphoprotein that regulates the cell cycle at several points. It exists as an active unphosphorylated form (pRb) and an inactive phosphorylated form (pRb-P). The active unphosphorylated form (pRb) normally stops the cell cycle at G1 going to S. It does this by binding to transcription factors such as the product of c-myc and the E2F protein. When pRb is phosphorylated, the cell can enter S and complete the cell cycle. Inactivation of the pRb stop signal causes the cell to continually cycle and undergo repeated mitosis. The product of the p53 gene is also a nuclear protein that regulates DNA replication. The normal p53 prevents the replication of cells with damaged DNA. It does this by pausing cells during G1 (before S), giving the cells time to repair the damaged DNA. The p53 gene, located on chromosome 17, is the single most common target for genetic alterations in human cancers. It is found in many cases of colon, breast, and lung cancers. Mutations in the adenomatous polyposis coli (APC) gene lead to the development of tumors that may progress to adenocarcinomas of the colon, while deletion of WT1, located on chromosome 11, is associated with the development of Wilms' tumor, a childhood neoplasm of the kidney.

96. The answer is d. (*Kumar, pp 320–324.*) Ultraviolet rays are associated with the formation of skin cancers, including squamous cell carcinoma, basal cell carcinoma, and malignant melanoma. The ultraviolet portion of the spectrum (ultraviolet rays) is divided into three wavelength ranges: UVA (320 to 400 nm), UVB (280 to 320 nm), and UVC (200 to 280 nm).

UVB is the wavelength range that is responsible for the induction of skin cancers. The carcinogenic property of UVB is related to the formation of pyrimidine dimers in DNA. UVC, although a potent mutagen, is not significant because it is filtered out by the ozone layer around the earth. Some DNA viruses and RNA viruses are associated with the development of dysplasia and malignancy. For example, infection with human papillomavirus (HPV), especially types 16 and 18, is associated with cervical dysplasia; Epstein-Barr virus (EBV) is associated with Burkitt's lymphoma and nasopharyngeal carcinoma; hepatitis B virus (HBV) and hepatitis C virus (HCV) are associated with primary hepatocellular carcinoma; and HHV-8 is associated with Kaposi's sarcoma. HTLV-I is an RNA retrovirus that is associated with the formation of a peculiar type of hematologic malignancy called adult T-cell leukemia/lymphoma. These patients have malignant cells in their lymph nodes and blood. This malignancy is endemic in southern Japan and the Caribbean region.

97. The answer is a. (*Kumar, pp 307, 323, 1245.*) Hereditary factors are important in the development of many types of cancers. They are particularly important in several inherited neoplasia syndromes. The autosomal recessive DNA-chromosomal instability syndromes include ataxia-telangiectasia, Bloom's syndrome, Fanconi anemia, and xeroderma pigmentosa. These disorders have in common abnormalities involving the normal repair of DNA. Patients with xeroderma pigmentosa have defective endonuclease activity, which normally repairs the pyrimidine dimers found in DNA damaged by ultraviolet (UV) light. These patients have an increased incidence of skin cancers, including basal cell carcinoma, squamous cell carcinoma, and malignant melanoma. Wiskott-Aldrich syndrome, characterized by thrombocytopenia and eczema, is an immunodeficiency disease associated with an increased incidence of lymphomas and acute leukemias. Familial polyposis is characterized by the formation of numerous neoplastic adenomatous colon polyps. These individuals have a 100% risk of developing colorectal carcinoma unless surgery is performed. Sturge-Weber syndrome is a rare congenital disorder associated with venous angiomatous masses in the leptomeninges and ipsilateral port-wine nevi of the face. Multiple endocrine neoplasia (MEN) syndrome type 1 (Wermer's syndrome) refers to the combination of adenomas of the pituitary, adenomas or hyperplasia of the parathyroid glands, and islet cell tumors of the pancreas.

98. The answer is c. (*Kumar, pp 283–284, 822–826. Rubin, pp 207–210.*) There are marked differences in the incidence of various types of cancer in different parts of the world. The highest rates for gastric carcinoma are found in Japan, Chile, China, and Russia, while it is much less common in the United States, the United Kingdom, Canada, and France. The high rates for gastric cancer in Japan might be related to dietary factors, such as eating smoked and salted foods.

Other examples of geographic variations in the incidence of neoplasms include nasopharyngeal carcinoma, liver cancer, and trophoblastic disease. Nasopharyngeal carcinoma, associated with the Epstein-Barr virus, is rare in most parts of the world, except for parts of the Far East, especially China. Liver cancer is associated with both hepatitis B infection and high levels of aflatoxin B1. It is endemic in large parts of Africa and Asia. Trophoblastic diseases, including choriocarcinoma, have high rates of occurrence in the Pacific rim areas of Asia. In contrast, Asian populations have a very low incidence of prostate cancer.

99. The answer is b. (*Henry, pp 1034–1035, 1038–1041. Kumar, pp 335–339.*) Tumor markers are a diverse group of biochemical substances associated with the presence of some tumors. These tumor markers include hormones, oncofetal antigens, isozymes, proteins, mucins, and glycoproteins. Carcinoembryonic antigen (CEA) is a glycoprotein associated with many cancers including adenocarcinomas of the colon, pancreas, lung, stomach, and breast. It is used clinically to follow up patients with certain malignancies, such as colon cancer, and to evaluate them for recurrence or metastases. Human chorionic gonadotropin (hCG) is a hormone associated with trophoblastic tumors, especially choriocarcinoma. α-fetoprotein (AFP) is a glycoprotein synthesized by the yolk sac and the fetal liver and is associated with yolk sac tumors of the testes and liver cell carcinomas. Prostate-specific antigen (PSA) and prostatic acid phosphatase (PAP) are associated with cancer of the prostate. Chloroacetate esterase (CAE), not to be confused with CEA, is a histochemical stain used in the differentiation of acute leukemias. It is not considered to be a tumor marker.

100. The answer is b. (*Mandell, pp 1685–1691. Joklik, pp 1060–1063. Rubin, pp 361–364. Kumar, pp 365–366.*) The cytopathic effect of viruses is often a clue to the diagnosis of the type of infection that is present. There are several types of herpesviruses, which are relatively large, double-stranded DNA viruses. Infection by herpes simplex virus (HSV) or varicella-zoster virus (VZV) is recognized by nuclear homogenization (ground-glass nuclei), intranuclear inclusions (Cowdry type A bodies), and the formation of multinucleated cells. Herpes simplex type 2, a sexually transmitted viral disease, results in the formation of vesicles that ulcerate and cause burning, itching, and pain. These lesions heal spontaneously, but the virus remains dormant in the lumbar and sacral ganglia. Recurrent infections may occur, and transmission to the newborn during delivery is a feared complication that may be fatal to the infant. Shingles and chickenpox are caused by herpes zoster, which is identical to varicella. Cytomegalovirus (CMV) causes both the nucleus and the cytoplasm of infected cells to become enlarged. Infected cells have large, purple intranuclear inclusions surrounded by a clear halo and smaller, less prominent basophilic intracytoplasmic inclusions. Adenoviruses can produce similar inclusions, but the infected cells are not enlarged. Adenoviruses also produce characteristic smudge cells in infected respiratory epithelial cells. Human papillomavirus (HPV) infection may produce a characteristic effect that is called koilocytosis. Histologic examination reveals enlarged squamous epithelial cells that have shrunken nuclei ("raisinoid") within large cytoplasmic vacuoles. Candidiasis is the most common fungal infection of the vagina and is especially common in patients who have diabetes or take oral contraceptives. Candida infection causes vulvar itching and produces a white discharge. Microscopic examination of the vaginal discharge reveals yeast and pseudohyphae. *T. vaginalis*, a large, pear-shaped, flagellated protozoan, causes severe vaginal itching with dysuria. It produces a thick yellow-gray discharge.

101. The answer is b. (*Kumar, p 752. Damjanov, pp 886–887, 928–930. Duchin, pp 949–955.*) Severe acute respiratory distress syndrome (SARS) is a highly contagious and very severe atypical pneumonia that was first described in the fall of 2002. The illness was particularly prevalent among the young and health care workers. In March of 2003, investigators identified the cause of SARS as a novel coronavirus (SARS-CoV). Note that the two main strains of human coronaviruses, types 229E and OC43, are major causes of the common cold. It appears that the SARS-CoV may be the first coronavirus to cause severe disease in otherwise healthy individuals as it differs from previous coronaviruses because it can infect the lower respiratory tract and spread throughout the body. Patients develop a dry cough with fever, chills, and malaise after an incubation of up to 10 days. In contrast to atypical pneumonia caused by Mycoplasma, SARS is not usually associated with a sore throat. Up to one-third of the patients improve, but the majority of patients progress to severe respiratory distress and almost 10% die from the disease.

The diagnosis of SARS relies on the presence of fever and respiratory symptoms. Interestingly, the most consistent laboratory finding occurring early in the disease is peripheral lymphopenia. Examination of lung tissue from confirmed cases has revealed the presence of hyaline membrane formation, interstitial mononuclear inflammation, and desquamation of pneumocytes into the alveoli. The Center for Disease Control (CDC) has defined several criteria to be used in the diagnosis of SARS. One of the epidemiologic criteria is: "travel (including transit in an airport) within 10 days of symptom onset to an area with current, recently documented, or suspected community transmission of SARS", such as China or Hong Kong.

In contrast to Coronavirus, the Hantavirus genus belongs to the Bunyaviridae family and includes the causative agent of a group of diseases that occur throughout Europe and Asia and are referred to as hemorrhagic fever with renal syndrome. The characteristic features of this syndrome are hematologic abnormalities, renal involvement, and increased vascular permeability. Respiratory involvement is generally minimal in these diseases. Although several species of rodents in the United States are known to be infected with Hantavirus, no human cases were reported until an outbreak of severe, often fatal respiratory illness occurred in the United States in May 1993 in the Four Corners area of New Mexico, Arizona, Colorado, and Utah. This illness resulted from a new member of the genus Hantavirus that caused a severe disease characterized by a prodromal fever, myalgia, pulmonary edema, and hypotension. The main distinguishing feature of this illness, which is called Hantavirus pulmonary syndrome, is noncardiogenic pulmonary edema resulting from increased permeability of the pulmonary capillaries. Laboratory features common to both Hantavirus pulmonary syndrome and hemorrhagic fever with renal syndrome include leukocytosis, atypical lymphocytes, thrombocytopenia, coagulopathy, and decreased serum protein concentrations. Abdominal pain, which can mimic an acute abdomen, may be found in both Hantavirus pulmonary syndrome and hemorrhagic fever with renal syndrome.

Dengue fever virus is a type of flavivirus, and flaviviruses are similar to alphaviruses. Dengue fever (breakbone fever) is initially similar to influenza but then progresses to a rash, muscle pain, joint pain, and bone pain. It can produce a potentially fatal hemorrhagic disorder. Ebola virus is a member of the Filoviridae family, which causes a severe hemorrhagic fever. Outbreaks occur in Africa and typically make the national news.

102. The answer is e. (*Joklik, pp 1060–1063. Goldman, p 2467. Rubin, pp 361–364. Kumar, pp 347, 373–374.*) Human parvovirus may cause a serious aplastic crisis in patients with an underlying chronic hemolytic anemia. In children, infection with parvovirus produces a characteristic rash, called erythema infectiosum or fifth disease, which first appears on the face and is described as a "slapped-cheek" appearance. Human parvovirus infection in adults produces a nonspecific syndrome of fever, malaise, headache, myalgia, vomiting, and a transient rash. Arthralgia is more common in adults than in children.

Erythema infectiosum is called fifth disease because it is one of the six classic childhood exanthems (skin eruptions associated with certain infectious diseases). Rubeola virus, an RNA paramyxovirus, is the cause of measles (first disease). After an incubation period of 10 to 21 days, measles is characterized by fever, rhinorrhea, cough, skin lesions, and mucosal lesions (Koplik spots). Scarlet fever (second disease) is caused by infection of the tonsils with group A beta-hemolytic streptococci (*S. pyogenes*). Rubella virus, another RNA virus, produces German measles (third disease). Rubella is a mild, acute febrile illness, but if the infection occurs in the first trimester of pregnancy it can produce developmental abnormalities such as cardiac lesions, ocular abnormalities, deafness, and mental retardation. Roseola (exanthem subitum or sixth disease) is caused by human herpesvirus 6 (HHV6). Symptoms include the acute onset of high fever which lasts for about 3 days. As the fever quickly subsides there appears a diffuse pink rash with papules or blanchable macular erythema. Finally, note that chickenpox is yet another eruptive skin disorder of children. It is the primary manifestation of infection with varicella-zoster virus (VZV). Varicella is an acute febrile illness that is usually self-limited. Skin lesions include macules, papules, vesicles ("dew drops on a rose petal"), pustules, and scabs. Children develop recurrent crops of skin lesions every 3 to 5 days. VZV remains latent for years in dorsal root ganglia. Reactivation in adults produces shingles, which is characterized by painful eruptions along dermatomes corresponding to the affected dorsal root ganglia.

103. The answer is e. (*Kumar, pp 373–374, 748–751. Mandell, pp 717–735.*) Most cases of lobar pneumonia are caused by *S. pneumoniae* (reclassification of the pneumococcus). Streptococcal or pneumococcal pneumonia involves one or more lobes and is often seen in alcoholics or debilitated persons. Type 3 pneumococcus (*S. pneumoniae*) causes a virulent lobar pneumonia characterized by mucoid sputum, which is also seen with *K. pneumoniae* (Friedländer's bacillus). This bacteria usually produces a bronchopneumonia, rather than lobar pneumonia, but this is clinically indistinguishable from pneumococcal lobar pneumonia. Legionella species cause a fibrinopurulent lobular pneumonia that tends to be confluent, almost appearing lobar.

104. The answer is d. (*Kumar, pp 376–377. Chandrasoma, pp 488, 794, 882–883. Mandell, pp 2646–2647.*) Nocardia (*N. asteroides*) and *Actinomyces* species are classified as filamentous soil bacteria, although they are often described among the fungi. *A. israelii* is a normal inhabitant of the mouth; it can be seen in the crypts of tonsillectomy specimens. *Actinomyces* is a branched, filamentous gram-positive bacteria. Two forms of disease produced by Actinomyces are cervicofacial actinomyces and pelvic actinomyces. The former consists of an indurated (lumpy) jaw with multiple draining fistulas or abscesses. Small yellow colonies called sulfur granules may be seen in the draining material. Histologic section reveals tangled masses of gram-positive filamentous bacteria. Cultures of Actinomyces grow as white masses with a domed surface, which is called a "molar tooth" appearance. Another filamentous gram-positive bacteria is *N. asteroides*. A characteristic that helps to differentiate these two is the fact that *Nocardia* is partially acid-fast. "Partial" means using weak mineral acids in the acid-fast stain. *Nocardiae* are aerobic and acid-fast, in contrast to *Actinomyces* species, which are strict anaerobes and not acid-fast. Inhaled nocardial bacteria produce lung or skin infections. Progressive pneumonia with purulent sputum and abscesses is suggestive of nocardiosis, especially if dissemination to the brain or subcutaneous tissue occurs. *Nocardia* is also one cause of mycetoma, a form of chronic inflammation of the skin that causes indurated abscesses with multiple draining sinuses. Patients who develop nocardiosis are often immunosuppressed, and transplant rejection, steroid therapy, AIDS, or alveolar proteinosis are often antecedent. Organisms in sputum, pus, or bronchial lavage specimens are gram-positive. A modified acid-fast stain should be used for diagnosis.

 C. diphtheriae is a small, pleomorphic gram-positive bacillus that may have club-shaped swellings at either pole. These rods tend to arrange themselves at right angles, producing characteristic V or Y configurations described as "Chinese characters." *C. diphtheriae* produces a toxin that blocks protein synthesis by causing irreversible inactivation of elongation factor 2 (EF-2). This toxin can produce a pseudomembrane covering the larynx, which is difficult to peel away without causing bleeding, and heart damage with fatty change. *L. monocytogenes* is a short, gram-positive, non-spore-forming bacillus that can produce neonatal disease or can result in stillbirth. Characteristics that are unique to *Listeria* include a tumbling motility on hanging drop and an umbrella-shaped motility pattern when a specimen is stabbed into a test tube agar slant.

105. The answer is a. (*Kumar, pp 375–376, 386–388, 379–380. Mandell, pp 2411–2413.*) Anthrax is caused by infection with *Bacillus anthracis*, a spore-forming gram-positive rod-shaped bacillus. Cultures grow colonies of bacteria that grossly are tangled having a "medusae head" appearance; gram stains reveal parallel chains of boxcar-shaped gram-positive organisms. Histology of the infection reveals severe acute necrotizing hemorrhagic inflammation secondary to vasculitis. Infection with anthrax is associated with sheep farmers, veterinarians, and wool workers. Additionally anthrax has been used as a weapon of biological terrorism.

There are three distinct clinical forms of anthrax depending on how it enters the body. Cutaneous anthrax begins with a small bump and within a few days a painless, open sore develops with a tell-tale black center of dead tissue (malignant pustule). This form of anthrax is highly treatable, but about 20% of untreated patients die. Inhalation anthrax initially has symptoms that are similar to the common cold, but it can rapidly progress to severe pneumonia with difficulty breathing and shock. It is fatal if not treated. If treatment begins in the incubation period (1 to 6 days) before symptoms appear then the mortality can decrease to 1%. Inhalation anthrax is not contagious. Gastrointestinal anthrax begins with loss of appetite, nausea, vomiting, and fever. It progresses to vomiting of blood and severe diarrhea and is fatal in 25 to 60% of cases. This type of anthrax is extremely rare in humans.

Leprosy is caused by infection with *Mycobacterium leprae*. There are two clinical forms of leprosy: lepromatous and tuberculoid leprosy. Nerve involvement is more typical of the lepromatous form. Histologic sections reveal acid-fast bacilli within peripheral nerves. Numerous bacilli in packets within histiocytes (lepra cells) are also found in the lesions of lepromatous leprosy. Polyclonal hypergammaglobulinemia often occurs in lepromatous leprosy, in which patients do not have the adequate cellular immune response of the tuberculoid form. Large amounts of antilepra antibody occur in the lepromatous form with frequent formation of antigen-antibody complexes and resultant disorders such as erythema nodosum. A "clear" zone between infiltrate and overlying epidermis is characteristic of lepromatous leprosy, unlike the encroachment on basal epidermis of the tuberculoid infiltrate.

Yersinia (formerly called Pasteurella) is an important genus of gram-negative bacilli that causes a wide variety of human and animal disease, ranging from plague (*Y. pestis*) to acute mesenteric lymphadenitis (*Y. enterocolitica*) in older children and young adults. Finally, scrofula refers to cervical lymphadenitis caused by infection with *Mycobacterium tuberculosis*. Syphilis, which is caused by infection with *Treponema pallidum*, has many different clinical presentations. For example, primary syphilis is characteristically associated with the development of a primary painless lesion, called a chancre, while secondary and tertiary syphilis are associated with more systemic involvement.

106. The answer is b. (*Schneider, pp 289–290. Kumar, pp 377–378, 380–381, 388–391.*) Bacterial vaginosis (*Gardnerella* vaginitis) is the most common cause of a vaginal discharge. Characteristically the discharge is thin and homogenous and may have a "fishy" smell. Bacterial vaginosis is caused by replacement of the normal vaginal flora (lactobacillus sp) by overgrowth of a polymicrobe group that includes *Gardnerella vaginallis*, a pleomorphic gram variable facultative anaerobic coccobacillus. This change in the vaginal flora results in loss of the normal acidic vaginal environment. A gram stain of the vaginal discharge may reveal squamous epithelial cells that are covered by small gram variable rods. Pap smears may show squamous epithelial cells whose borders are obscured by bacteria and appear fuzzy. These cells are called "clue cells."

Granuloma inguinale is a rare, sexually transmitted disease that is caused by *Calymmatobacterium donovani*, a small, encapsulated gram-negative bacillus. Infection results in a chronic disease that is characterized by superficial ulcers of the genital region. Regional lymph node involvement produces large nodular masses that develop extensive scarring. Specialized culture medium is available, but its use is not practical. Serologic tests are also not useful. Instead, histologic examination is used to demonstrate Donovan bodies, which are organisms within the cytoplasm of macrophages. They are seen best with silver stains or Giemsa stain.

Chancroid is an acute venereal disease that is characterized by painful genital ulcers with lymphadenopathy. It is caused by *Haemophilus ducreyi*, a small, gram-negative bacillus. Gram stains of the suppurative lesions or cultures on specialized media may be used to make the diagnosis. Serologic tests are not useful.

Neisseria gonorrheae, a gram-negative diplococcus, causes gonorrhea, an acute suppurative infection of the genital tract. In males it produces a purulent discharge (urethritis) and dysuria. In women, it may be asymptomatic (50%), or it may produce infection of the cervix with accompanying vaginal discharge, dysuria, and abdominal pain. Ascending infections in women can lead to salpingitis, tuboovarian abscess, and pelvic inflammatory disease (PID). Fitz-Hugh-Curtis syndrome refers to perihepatitis infection. In newborns, infection acquired during birth can produce a purulent conjunctivitis (ophthalmia neonatorum). This disease has been prevented due to prophylactic therapy to newborn infants. A Gram stain of the urethral or cervical exudate may reveal the intracytoplasmic gram-negative diplococci, or the exudate can be cultured on special media. Serologic tests are not useful. Characteristically, *N. gonorrheae* produces acid from glucose, but not from maltose or lactose.

The spirochete *T. pallidum*, the causative agent of syphilis, has not been grown on any culture media; therefore, other means are available to aid in the diagnosis of syphilis. Dark-field or immunofluorescence examination may be used to detect organisms in the genital ulcers of primary syphilis. Antibodies to cardiolipin, a substance in beef heart that is similar to a lipoid released by *T. pallidum*, are used to screen for syphilis. This is the basis of both the VDRL and the rapid plasma reagin (RPR) tests; however, these screening tests are not totally specific. *Chlamydia* species are obligate intracellular parasites that form elementary bodies and reticulate bodies. The former are small, extracellular, and infectious, while the latter are intracellular and noninfectious. Three *Chlamydia* species are *C. psittaci*, *C. pneumoniae*, and *C. trachomatis*. The last causes several human diseases including trachoma, inclusion conjunctivitis, nongonococcal urethritis, and lymphogranuloma venereum (LGV). Specialized culture media and direct examination procedures are available to aid in the diagnosis of these diseases. The regional lymph nodes in patients with LGV have a characteristic histologic appearance typified by necrotizing granulomas forming stellate areas of necrosis. Trachoma is the leading cause of blindness in underdeveloped countries. It is a chronic infection of the conjunctiva that eventually scars the conjunctiva and cornea. LGV is a sexually transmitted disease that is characterized by the formation of a genital ulcer with local necrotizing lymphadenitis. The skin test for LGV is the Frei test, which consists of intradermal injection of LGV antigen. *C. psittaci* is the causative agent of psittacosis (parrot fever). It produces a severe pulmonary disease and should be suspected in patients with a history of bird contact, such as pet shop workers or parrot owners.

107. The answer is a. (*Kumar, pp 351, 392–393, 395, 403–404. Mandell, pp 2507–2510.*) *Babesia microti* causes a malaria-like illness, called babesiosis, while *Plasmodia* species cause malaria itself. Both of these disorders are characterized by signs and symptoms resulting from their infection of red blood cells, such as fever, hemolytic anemia, and hemoglobinuria. *Babesia* infects red blood cells and appears similar to the ring forms of *P. falciparum*. The presence of characteristic tetrads forming Maltese cross forms is diagnostic of babesiosis. *B. microti* is transmitted by the same deer ticks that carry Lyme disease and ehrlichiosis. Lyme disease, first described in the mid-1970s in Connecticut, is caused by a spirochete, *Borrelia burgdorferi*, through the bite of a tick belonging to the genus *Ixodes*. The spirochete-infested ticks reside in wooded areas where there are deer and small rodents. The deer act as a wintering reservoir for the ticks. In the spring the tick larval stage emerges and evolves into a nymph, which is infective for humans if they are bitten. Adult ticks are also capable of transmitting the spirochete during questing. The bite is followed by a rash called erythema chronicum migrans, which may resolve spontaneously. However, many patients have a transient phase of spirochetemia, which may allow the spread of the spirochete to the meninges, heart, and synovial tissue. Originally thought to be confined to New England, Lyme disease has now been shown to be present in Europe and Australia as well.

There are three clinical types of leishmaniasis, the vector of which is the sandfly (phlebotomus). Cutaneous leishmaniasis (oriental sore, Baghdad boil) is caused by *L. tropica*. It is characterized by the formation of an itchy papule that develops into an expanding ulcer. Mucocutaneous leishmaniasis is caused by *L. braziliensis*, while deep visceral leishmaniasis (kala-azar, "black sickness", due to pigmentation of the skin) is caused by *L. donovani*. Finally, *Toxoplasma gondii* is the causative agent of toxoplasmosis. It is acquired through contact with oocyst-shedding cats or by eating under-cooked meat. Most immunocompetent individuals infected with *T. gondii* are asymptomatic and the infection is self-limited.

108. The answer is e. (*Kumar, pp 835, 1309. Braunwald, pp 754–755.*) Seronegative spondyloarthropathies are spondyloarthropathies that lack the rheumatoid factor found in rheumatoid arthritis. These disorders include Reiter syndrome, ankylosing spondylitis, psoriatic arthritis, and enteropathic arthritis. All of these are associated with an increased incidence of HLA-B27. Reiter syndrome refers to the triad of arthritis, nongonococcal urethritis, and conjunctivitis. It may be an autoimmune reaction to previous gastrointestinal or genitourinary infections. Causes of these gastrointestinal infections include *Shigella, Salmonella, Yersinia,* and *Campylobacter.* The organism causing the genitourinary infection is *Chlamydia.*

109. The answer is e. (*Kumar, pp 349–350, 395–397. Damjanov, pp 866–878. Mandell, pp 2035–2040.*) Rickettsia are obligate intracellular parasites that infect endothelial cells and produce symptoms as a result of vasculitis and formation of microthrombi. Serologic tests for rickettsia include complement fixation tests and the Weil-Felix agglutination reaction. The basis for the latter test is the fact that the sera of infected patients can agglutinate strains of *Proteus vulgaris.* There are numerous types of rickettsia that produce many different diseases. Examples include Rocky Mountain spotted fever (RMSF, caused by *R. rickettsii*), epidemic typhus (caused by *R. prowazekii* and spread by the human body louse *Pediculus humanus*), endemic typhus (caused by *R. typhi* and spread by lice), scrub typhus (caused by *R. tsutsugamushi* and spread by mites), ehrlichiosis, and Q fever (caused by *C. burnetii* and spread not by vectors but by inhalation of aerosols). RMSF is found not only in the Rocky Mountains, but also the southeastern and south central United States. The vector in the Rocky Mountains is the wood tick (*Dermacentor andersoni*), while in the southeast it is the dog tick (*D. variabilis*) and in the south central United States it is the Lone Star tick. The animal reservoirs for RMSF are wild rodents and dogs. The rash of RMSF characteristically begins peripherally and spreads centrally to the trunk and face. The pathology involves infection of blood vessels producing thrombosis. Intracellular bacilli form parallel rows in an end-to-end arrangement ("flotilla at anchor facing the wind"). Patients also develop muscle pain and high fever.

Bartonella infections are also characterized by proliferations of blood vessels. Examples of Bartonella include *B. quintana, B. henselae,* and *B. bacilliformis,* the causative agent of Oroya fever. *B. quintana* is spread by the human body louse and is the causative agent of trench fever (seen in the trenches of World War I) and bacillary angiomatosis. This latter term refers to a lesion seen in patients with AIDS consisting of a lobular proliferation of capillaries with abundant leukocytoclastic debris. *B. henselae* is the causative agent of cat-scratch fever. Histologically, this disease is characterized by the formation of stellate microabscesses with necrotizing granulomas.

110. The answer is b. (*Kumar, pp 350, 395, 405.*) Ehrlichiosis is a tick-transmitted disease caused by *Rickettsiales*, which infects either neutrophils (*E. ewingii*) or macrophages (*E. chaffeensis*). Cytoplasmic inclusions within leukocytes are "asterisk"-shaped or "mulberry"-shaped. Clinical symptoms include the abrupt onset of fever, headache, and malaise. The disease may progress to respiratory and renal failure with shock. A rash is less often present than is seen with RMSF. Many patients diagnosed with RMSF who do not have a rash probably have ehrlichiosis.

Psittacosis is a respiratory disorder caused by infection with *Chlamydia psittaci*, an obligate intracellular bacteria. It is primarily an occupational disease of zoo and pet employees and poultry farmers. Tularemia is caused by *Francisella tularensis*. Infection is spread to humans from ticks and rabbits. Three clinical forms of tularemia are typhoidal (with systemic symptoms), pneumonic, and ulceroglandular. Some lesions may develop caseating granulomas. Nocardiosis is caused by the filamentous gram-positive, partially acid-fast, bacteria *N. asteroides*. *Nocardia* infection can involve either the lungs (producing progressive pneumonia) or skin (producing mycetoma). Patients who develop nocardiosis are often immunosuppressed. Finally, *Trypanosoma brucei* is the cause of African trypanosomiasis, which is characterized by fever, lymphadenopathy, splenomegaly, and brain dysfunction ("sleeping sickness"). The disease is spread by tsetse flies (genus *Glossina*).

111. The answer is d. (*Kumar, pp 381–388, 748–751.*) Tuberculosis (TB) is caused by infection with *M. tuberculosis*. Mycobacteriaceae are slow-growing aerobic rods with cell walls rich in glycolipids, true waxes, and long-chain fatty acids called mycolic acids. The lipid-rich mycolic acid–containing cell wall is responsible for the unique staining properties of the mycobacteria, namely their impermeability to most basic dyes and their resistance to acid decolorization (acid-fast staining). Infection with *M. tuberculosis* occurs either as a primary infection or a secondary reactivation or reinfection. The initial infection of primary tuberculosis, the Ghon complex, consists of a subpleural lesion near the fissure between the upper and lower lobes and enlarged caseous lymph nodes that drain the pulmonary lesion. The histologic lesions of TB reveal caseating granulomas with Langerhans giant cells. Although primary pulmonary tuberculosis is usually asymptomatic, systemic and localizing symptoms can occur. These symptoms include malaise, anorexia, weight loss, fever, night sweats, cough, and hemoptysis. The pulmonary lesion of secondary tuberculosis is usually located in the apex of one or both lungs. Progressive pulmonary tuberculosis may result in cavitary fibrocaseous tuberculosis, miliary tuberculosis, or tuberculous bronchopneumonia. Miliary tuberculosis consists of multiple small yellow-white lesions scattered throughout the entire lung. These lesions are the result of erosion of a granulomatous lesion into a blood vessel with subsequent lymphohematogenous dissemination. While TB is often asymptomatic, the resultant hypersensitivity reaction is a marker for infection in those individuals without clinically apparent disease. The TB skin test is called the Mantoux test and is performed by intradermally injecting purified protein derivative (PPD). An area of induration ½ cm or more in diameter at 48 h is a positive result. The diagnosis of TB depends upon the clinical picture and chest x-ray. Acid-fast stains of sputum are followed with culture, not only to identify the species of mycobacterium but to determine the pattern of antibiotic sensitivity. Treatment is isoniazid (INH) combined with other antibiotics.

K. pneumoniae is a cause of bacterial pneumonia in debilitated and malnourished individuals, such as chronic alcoholics. Patients develop production of thick, gelatinous sputum. This bacterial infection has a greater mortality than pneumococcal pneumonia. Legionnaires' disease is a form of bronchopneumonia that is caused by the gram-negative bacillus *L. pneumophila*. This organism is almost ubiquitous in water and is spread by inhalation of contaminated airborne droplets. Infection results in a patchy bronchopneumonia, and microscopically the alveolar spaces are filled with an inflammatory exudate of neutrophils and macrophages. There may be multiple small areas of necrosis and abscess. Organisms cannot be visualized by routine stains, so instead a Dieterle silver stain is used.

112. The answer is a. (*Kumar, pp 246, 386. Damjanov, pp 850–854.*) There are several types of mycobacteria that are not *M. tuberculosis*. These organisms are called atypical mycobacteria, or mycobacteria other than tuberculosis (MOTT). They are separated into different classes (Runyon classes) based on several culture characteristics, such as pigment production, colony morphology, and rate of growth. Examples of MOTT include

M. avium, M. intracellulare, M. marinum, and *M. leprae,* which is the causative agent of leprosy. M. avium complex (MAC) consists of two separate species, *M. avium* and *M. intracellulare.* Clinical infections with MAC is rare except that it is an important cause of infection in patients with AIDS. Histologic sections in these immunosuppressed patients do not reveal granulomas because the cellular immune reactions of these patients are defective. Instead numerous organisms can be seen with special stains. Differentiating MAC from infection with *M. tuberculosis* can be difficult, but the presence of a histiocytic proliferation with poorly formed or no granulomas and numerous intracellular bacilli favors the diagnosis of MAC. Definitive mycobacterial cultures usually take 10 to 21 days for growth.

In comparison to MAC, *M. marinum* can cause superficial disease or skin and subcutaneous disease. It inhabits marine organisms, grows in water, and can be obtained from infected aquariums or swimming pools. *M. fortuitum* is a very rare cause of disease, but localized skin or bone lesions can occur after trauma.

113. The answer is c. (*Kumar, pp 754–756. Mandell, pp 2746–2755.*) In the approximate center of the photomicrograph is the classic refractile, double-walled spherule of the deep fungus *Coccidioides immitis,* which is several times the diameter of the largest inflammatory cell nearby. Coccidioidomycosis is endemic in California, Arizona, New Mexico, and parts of Nevada, Utah, and Texas, where it resides in the arid soils and is contracted by direct inhalation of airborne dust. If inhaled, it produces a primary pulmonary infection that is usually benign and self-limiting in immunologically competent persons, often with several days of fever and upper respiratory flulike symptoms. However, certain ethnic groups, such as some African Americans, Asians, and Filipinos, are at risk of developing a potentially lethal disseminated form of the disease that can involve the central nervous system. If the large, double-walled spherule containing numerous endospores can be demonstrated outside the lungs (e.g., in a skin biopsy), this is evidence of dissemination. Antibodies of high titers are detectable by means of complement fixation studies in patients undergoing spontaneous recovery. Amphotericin B is usually reserved for treating high-risk and disseminated infection. The cultured mycelia of the organism on Sabouraud's agar present a hazard for laboratory workers.

114. The answer is b. (*Rubin, pp 336, 434–443. Kumar, pp 754–755.*) The deep fungal infections produce characteristic morphologic features in tissue sections. The two basic morphologic types of fungi are yeasts, which are oval cells that reproduce by budding, and molds, which are filamentous colonies consisting of branched tubules called hyphae. Some yeasts produce buds that do not detach. Instead they form long structures that resemble hyphae and are called pseudohyphae. This is characteristic of *Candida* species. *Blastomyces*, in contrast, is a larger, double-contoured yeast that is characterized by broad-based budding. Aspergillus is characterized by septate hyphae with acute-angle branching of the filamentous colonies and occasional fruiting bodies. Irregular, broad, nonseptate hyphae with wide-angle branching are seen with mucormycosis (zygomycosis). Large spheres with external budding, referred to as a "ship's wheel," are seen with Paracoccidioides, while large spheres with endospores are seen with coccidiomyces infection.

115. The answer is c. (*Kumar, pp 399, 1378. Rubin, pp 436–438.*) Cryptococcosis is caused by Cryptococcus neoformans, an encapsulated yeast (not dimorphic) that infects the central nervous system, primarily in immunocompromised patients. The soil-dwelling yeast is inhaled, but lung involvement tends to be mild in individuals who are not immunodeficient. Diagnosis of cryptococcal meningitis is achieved by finding encapsulated yeasts in CSF preparations. The capsule can be seen with a mucicarmine stain, or it can be negatively stained using India ink. The CSF and serum should also be tested for cryptococcal antigen by the latex cryptococcal agglutination test (LCAT), which is positive in more than 90% of cases. Cryptococcal meningitis varies from a chronic inflammatory and granulomatous infection to a noninflammatory meningitis with numerous yeasts massed, sometimes forming cystic "soap bubble" lesions in the brain. Do not confuse *Cryptococcus* with *Cryptosporidium*. *Cryptosporidium parvum* is a protozoan parasite that may cause a transient diarrhea in immunocompetent individuals or a chronic diarrhea in patients with AIDS (cryptosporidiosis). Histologically, sporozoites may be found attached to the surface of intestinal epithelial cells. They are best seen with an acid-fast stain.

Chromomycosis is a chronic infection of the skin that is produced by an organism that appears as a brown, thick-walled sphere ("copper penny") in tissue sections. Coccidioidomycosis is a mycotic infection caused by inhalation of the arthrospores of the dimorphic fungus *C. immitis*. Within the lung the spores enlarge to form large spherules (sporangia) that become filled with many small endospores. The cyst ruptures, releasing the endospores. Unruptured spherules incite a granulomatous reaction, while the endospores cause a neutrophilic response. Paracoccidioidomycosis (South American blastomycosis) is a chronic granulomatous infection caused by *Paracoccidioides brasiliensis*, a dimorphic fungus seen in tissues as a large central organism having peripheral oval budding. This histologic appearance is described as being similar to a mariner's wheel.

116. The answer is b. (*Kumar, pp 359, 406–407, 839. Rubin, pp 475–476.*) Intestinal tapeworm (cestode) infections result from eating improperly prepared meat. *T. saginata* is acquired from ingesting contaminated beef, *T. solium* is acquired from contaminated pork, and *D. latum* is obtained from contaminated fish. The life cycles of these tapeworms involve larval stages in animals and worm stages in humans. If the contaminated meat contains the larval forms of these organisms, then they may develop into adult worms in the intestines of infected humans. These individuals generally remain asymptomatic, except that *D. latum* may cause a vitamin B_{12} deficiency. A very different disease results from humans eating the eggs of *T. solium*, which may be found in human feces. In this case, the eggs hatch into larva, which then penetrate the gut wall and disseminate via the bloodstream to lodge in different organs. There they encyst and differentiate into cysticerci. Multiple cysticerci in the brain produce a "Swiss cheese" appearance grossly, and microscopically a scolex (the head of the worm) is found with hooklets. This disease is called cysticercosis. Another cestode, *E. granulosa*, is the cause of hydatid disease in humans. Individuals become infected by eating the tapeworm eggs. Patients are usually sheep herders who get the eggs from their dogs. Larvae released from the eggs disseminate most often to the liver (75%), but they may also travel to the lungs or skeletal muscle. They form large, slowly growing, unilocular cysts that contain multiple scolices. *Toxocara* species, such as *T. canis* and *T. cati*, are one cause of visceral larval migrans. This disease is characterized by infection of visceral organs by helminthic larvae. The typical patient is a young child who develops hypereosinophilia and hypergammaglobulinemia. Ocular manifestations of toxocariasis are common, especially the loss of vision in one eye in a child. Note that this disease is different from cutaneous larva migrans, which is caused by the larval forms of the hookworms and *Strongyloides stercoralis*.

117. The answer is d. (*Mandell, pp 2888–2892. Damjanov, pp 987–988.*) *G. lamblia*, a flagellate protozoan, is the most common cause of outbreaks of waterborne diarrheal disease in the United States and is seen frequently in Rocky Mountain areas. Ingestion of cysts from contaminated water results in trophozoites in the duodenum and jejunum. Identification of the trophozoite stage is done by duodenal aspiration or small-bowel biopsy; identification of the cyst stage (intermittent) is done by examination of stool. The trophozoite may appear as a pear-shaped, binucleate organism ("two eyes"). Giardiasis may cause malabsorption but is often asymptomatic. Duodenal aspiration, immunofluorescence, and ELISA testing for *Giardia* antigens are diagnostic and therapy with metronidazole or quinacrine is effective.

118. The answer is c. (*Kumar, p 838. Damjanov, pp 1013–1018. Ravel, pp 438–441.*) Anal pruritus in a child is suggestive of infection with *Enterobius vermicularis* (pinworm). The "Scotch tape" (cellulose-tape) slide test can be used to help identify perianal eggs. Enterobius worms often attach themselves to the fecal mucosa and contiguous regions, and they can even be a cause of acute appendicitis. More commonly, however, they are an incidental finding. In histologic sections of tissue they can be recognized by their distinctive lateral alae.

Cryptosporidiosis is caused by *Cryptosporidium parvum*, a very small protozoa (2–4 μm) that attaches to colonic surface epithelial cells. It typically produces profuse, watery, nonbloody diarrhea in immunosuppressed patients (AIDS). Outbreaks in Wisconsin in rainy years are due to water run-off from dairy farms. The organism is best visualized with an acid-fast stain of a colon biopsy or a stool specimen. Infection with the fish tapeworm *D. latum* can cause a deficiency of vitamin B_{12}. Finally, two tests used in the diagnosis of malabsorption include quantitative fecal fat determination (steatorrhea) and D-xylose absorption. The latter test can help to define the cause of the malabsorption. It is most likely to be abnormal with sprue-type diseases.

119. The answer is d. (*Kumar, pp 359, 401–403. Mandell, pp 2824–2825.*) Malaria results from infection with one of four species of plasmodia, namely *P. falciparum, P. vivax, P. ovale, and P. malariae.* Malarial organisms (sporozoites) are released into the blood after the bite of an affected *Anopheles* mosquito. These sporozoites then enter the hepatocyte via a hepatocyte receptor for the serum proteins thrombospondin and properdin. In the liver, they multiply asexually to form numerous merozoites, which are released when the hepatocyte ruptures. These merozoites then infect erythrocytes and form either gametocytes, which are taken up and fertilized in the mosquito, or trophozoites, which become schizonts that develop into merozoites that infect other red cells. In the blood, *P. falciparum* merozoites bind to gly-cophorin molecules on red blood cells, while *P. vivax* merozoites bind to Duffy antigens on red blood cells. (Note that patients who are Duffy antigen-negative are resistant to *P. vivax* infection.) *P. vivax* infects only young ery-throcytes (reticulocytes), while *P. malariae* infects only old erythrocytes. Within the red cells, merozoites mature to form schizonts, which then secrete proteins that form knobs on the surface of the red cells. Sequestrins form on top of these knobs and then bind to endothelial cells via ICAM-1, the thrombospondin receptor, and CD46, causing thrombosis.

Clinically, patients with malaria develop recurrent bouts of chills and high fever (paroxysms) that result from rupture of infected erythrocytes. These symptoms cycle at different time intervals depending upon the type of malaria. For example, infection with *P. malariae* causes symptoms to cycle every 72 h, and thus it is called quartan or malarial malaria. The remaining plasmodia cause symptoms that cycle every 48 h. The disease produced by *P. falciparum*, however, is much more serious and is called malignant tertian malaria. *P. falciparum* malaria is more serious because it alters RBCs, making them more adherent to endothelial cells. This in turn leads to capillary plug-ging and obstruction. In the brain this is called cerebral malaria, while in the kidney the disease produces acute renal failure (called blackwater fever). In contrast, *P. vivax* malaria is called benign tertian malaria, and the disease caused by *P. ovale* is similar to that caused by *P. vivax*.

Babesiosis is caused by *B. microti*. It is somewhat similar to malaria, except that it is transmitted by the hard-shell tick (ixodid) and it infects individuals living on islands off the New England coast, such as Martha's Vineyard. Patients develop the sudden onset of chills and fever due to destruction of erythrocytes. The disease is usually self-limited, but patients may develop hemoglobinemia, hemoglobinuria, and renal failure.

120. The answer is a. (*Damjanov, pp 714–716. Kumar, pp 447–449.*) Protein-energy malnutrition (PEM) in underdeveloped countries leads to a spectrum of symptoms from kwashiorkor at one end to marasmus at the other. Marasmus, caused by a lack of caloric intake (i.e., starvation), leads to generalized wasting, stunted growth, atrophy of muscles, and loss of subcuta-neous fat. There is no edema or hepatic enlargement. These children are alert, not apathetic, and are ravenous. In contrast, children with kwashiorkor, which is characterized by a lack of protein despite adequate caloric intake, have peripheral edema, a "moon" face, and an enlarged, fatty liver. The peripheral edema is caused by decreased albumin and sodium retention, while the fatty liver is caused by decreased synthesis of the lipoproteins necessary for the normal mobilization of lipids from liver cells. Additionally, these children have "flaky paint" areas of skin and abnormal pigmented streaks in their hair ("flag sign"). In children with marasmus, the skin is inelastic due to loss of subcutaneous fat. In either severe kwashiorkor or marasmus, thymic atrophy may result in the reduction in number and function of circulating T cells. B cell function (i.e., immunoglobulin production) is also depressed, so that these children are highly vulnerable to infections.

121. The answer is c. (*Kumar, pp 450–452. Goldman, pp 1172, 2177.*) The fat-soluble vitamins include vitamin A, D, E, and K, all of which are stored in the body. Therefore, with malabsorption causing a loss of fat in the stool, deficiencies of these vitamins can occur. Deficiencies of vitamin A result in squamous metaplasia of mucus membranes. Squamous metaplasia of the respiratory tract leads to increased numbers of pulmonary infections due to lack of the normal protective mucociliary "elevator." Squamous metaplasia of the urinary tract leads to increased numbers of urinary tract stones, while such metaplasia in sebaceous and sweat glands of dry skin causes follicular hyperkeratosis and predisposes to acne. There are numerous eye changes produced by a vitamin A deficiency. These changes include dry eyes (xerophthalmia), soft cornea (keratomalacia), and elevated white plaques of keratin debris on the conjunctiva (Bitot's spots). Because vitamin A is important in the normal function of rhodopsin, a visual pigment important for vision in dim light, a deficiency of vitamin A is associated with poor vision in dim light. This night blindness is usually the first symptom seen in patients with a vitamin A deficiency.

In contrast, megaloblastic anemia is associated with a deficiency of either vitamin B_{12} or folate, while decreased mineralization of bones (soft bones) can be caused by a deficiency of vitamin D. Perifollicular hemorrhages are seen with a deficiency of vitamin C, while alopecia can be caused by excess storage of vitamin A.

122. The answer is a. (*Kumar, pp 452–455. Wilson, pp 1317–1320.*) A deficiency of vitamin D leads to decreased intestinal absorption of calcium, inadequate serum calcium and phosphorus, and impaired mineralization of the osteoid of bone, which leads to soft, easily deformed bones. Because there is no decreased production of osteoid matrix, a relative excess of woven bone or osteoid with wide osteoid seams results. The causes of vitamin D deficiency are many and include dietary deficiency, decreased synthesis, and malabsorption. Decreased vitamin D synthesis can occur in the northern latitudes or in patients with inherited deficiencies of renal 1-α-hydroxylase, the enzyme that catalyzes the final step in the activation of vitamin D. Individuals with renal disease can also develop deficiencies of the active metabolite of vitamin D.

In contrast, 5-α-reductase converts testosterone into dihydrotestosterone (DHT), while 7-α-hydroxylase is the rate-limiting enzyme of bile acid synthesis. 11-hydroxylase and 21-hydroxylase are both important enzymes involved in the biosynthesis of steroids in the adrenal cortex. Deficiencies of either of these two enzymes can produce congenital adrenal hyperplasia.

123. The answer is c. (*Kumar, pp 456–459. Henry, p 555. Hoffman, pp 437–438.*) Pyridoxine is a cofactor that participates in transamination reactions, decarboxylation reactions, and transsulfuration reactions. It is important in the synthesis of γ-aminobutyric acid (GABA) and delta-aminolevulinic acid (d-ALA). Deficiencies of pyridoxine can lead to decreased synthesis of GABA, which can cause convulsions in infants or a polyneuropathy in adults. Patients also develop cheilosis (inflammation and fissuring of the lips), angular stomatitis (cheilosis occurring at the corners of the mouth), glossitis (atrophy of the mucosa of the tongue), and seborrheic dermatitis. Patients also can develop a sideroblastic anemia. Approximately one-third of the normoblasts in normal bone marrow contain ferritin granules and are called sideroblasts. The iron in these cells is normally located in the cytoplasm away from the nucleus. Sideroblasts that have distinctive rings of Prussian blue–positive granules around their nuclei are abnormal and are called ring sideroblasts. In these cells iron accumulates within mitochondria without any progression into hemoglobin. Ring sideroblasts are seen in sideroblastic anemia, the types of which include hereditary, acquired, and idiopathic forms. The hereditary form of sideroblastic anemia is an X-linked recessive disorder (usually seen in younger males) that is associated with a deficiency of the enzyme 5-aminolevulinic acid synthetase. Acquired sideroblastic anemia may be caused by exposure to toxins or drugs, such as alcohol, lead, or isoniazid (these producing a deficiency of pyridoxine), or it may be caused by a nutritional deficiency, such as a deficiency of folic acid or copper. It can even be caused by excess zinc. The idiopathic form of sideroblastic anemia (usually seen in individuals over the age of 65) is one of the myelodysplastic syndromes. Individuals with sideroblastic anemia should first be treated with a trial therapy of pyridoxine (vitamin B_6) as some of the individuals with the hereditary form or the acquired form of sideroblastic anemia will respond to this therapy.

In contrast to pyridoxine, biotin (vitamin H) is an important cofactor for multisubunit enzymes that catalyze carboxylation reactions, an example of which is the synthesis and oxidation of fatty acids. A deficiency of biotin can lead to multiple symptoms, including depression, hallucinations, muscle pain, and dermatitis. Biotin is present in dietary food and is also produced by intestinal bacteria. Deficiencies of biotin are quite rare, but can occur in people who consume raw eggs. This is because egg white contains a heat-labile protein, avidin, which combines very tightly with biotin and prevents the absorption of biotin. Cyanocobalamin is vitamin B_{12}, a deficiency of which causes megaloblastic anemia. A deficiency of riboflavin (vitamin B_2) is characterized by changes that occur around the mouth, namely cheilosis, angular stomatitis, and glossitis. Additionally, patients may develop seborrheic dermatitis of the face or genitalia, or blindness, which is the result of vascularization of the cornea (interstitial keratitis). Selenium is an antioxidant that is part of glutathione peroxidase, an enzyme that is found in red cells and white cells. As such, it prevents oxidative damage to both red blood cells and white cells. A deficiency of selenium leads to a form of dilated cardiomyopathy in children. This deficiency has been described in China and is called Keshan disease.

124. The answer is b. (*Kumar, pp 456–457. Chandrasoma, pp 160–162. Rubin, pp 348–349.*) A deficiency of vitamin B_1 (thiamine) may produce the central nervous system (CNS) symptoms of Wernicke-Korsakoff syndrome. Wernicke's encephalopathy consists mainly of foci of hemorrhages and necrosis in the mammillary bodies and about the ventricular regions of the thalamus and hypothalamus, about the aqueduct in the midbrain, and in the floor of the fourth ventricle. Symptoms of Wernicke's syndrome include progressive dementia (confusion), ataxia, and paralysis of the extraocular muscles—often with bilateral lateral rectus, or sixth nerve, palsies (ophthalmoplegia). Korsakoff psychosis is a thought disorder that produces retrograde memory failure and confabulation. In contrast, hemorrhage into the CNS in the sites listed as possible answers to this question are not associated with specific etiologies.

125. The answer is c. (*Kumar, pp 453–454, 458–459. Chandrasoma, pp 160–162. Rubin, pp 349–350.*) Deficiencies of niacin (vitamin B₃) produce pellagra, a disease that is characterized by the triad of dementia, dermatitis ("glove" or "necklace" distribution), and diarrhea. Decreased levels of niacin may result from diets that are deficient in niacin, such as diets that depend on maize (corn) as the main staple, because niacin in maize is bound in a form that is not available. Part of the body's need for niacin is supplied by the conversion of the essential amino acid tryptophan to NAD, and therefore a deficiency of tryptophan can also produce symptoms of pellagra. Deficiencies of tryptophan can be seen in individuals with Hartnup disease, which is caused by the abnormal membrane transport of neutral amino acids and tryptophan in the small intestines and kidneys. Deficiencies of tryptophan can also be found in individuals whose diets are high in leucine (an amino acid that inhibits one of the enzymes necessary to convert tryptophan to NAD), in patients with carcinoid tumors (tumors that can convert tryptophan into serotonin), or in patients with tuberculosis who receive isoniazid therapy (because isoniazid is a pyridoxine antagonist and pyridoxine is also necessary for the conversion of tryptophan to NAD).

In contrast to pellagra, beriberi is due to a deficiency of thiamine (vitamin B₁), which has three important functions. It participates in oxidative decarboxylation of α-keto acids, participates as a cofactor for transketolase in the pentose phosphate path, and participates in maintaining neural membranes. Thiamine deficiency mainly affects two organ systems, the heart and the nervous system. If the heart is affected in a patient with beriberi, it may become dilated and flabby. Patients may also develop peripheral vasodilation that leads to a high-output cardiac failure and marked peripheral edema. This combination of vascular abnormalities is called wet beriberi. The peripheral nerves in beriberi may be damaged by focal areas of myelin degeneration, which leads to footdrop, wristdrop, and sensory changes (numbness and tingling) in the feet and lower legs. These symptoms are referred to as dry beriberi. The causes of thiamine deficiency include poor diet, deficient absorption and storage, and accelerated destruction of thiamine diphosphate. This deficiency may be seen in alcoholics and prisoners of war because of poor nutrition, or it may be seen in individuals who eat large amounts of polished rice. (Polishing rice removes the outer, thiamine-containing portion of the grain.) Finally, marasmus is due to a deficiency of calories, rickets is due to a deficiency of vitamin D in children, and scurvy is due to a deficiency of vitamin C.

126. The answer is e. (*Kumar, pp 458–459, 650.*) Vitamin C (ascorbic acid) is a water-soluble vitamin that is important in many body functions, such as the synthesis of collagen, osteoid, certain neurotransmitters, and carnitine. In the synthesis of collagen, vitamin C functions as a cofactor for the hydroxylation of proline and lysine and for the formation of the triple helix of tropocollagen. Patients with decreased vitamin C (scurvy) have abnormal synthesis of connective tissue due to abnormal synthesis of collagen along with abnormal synthesis of osteoid. The former leads to impaired wound healing. In addition, previous wounds may reopen. Because the synthesis of collagen is abnormal, the blood vessels are fragile, leading to bleeding gums, tooth loss, subperiosteal hemorrhage, and petechial perifollicular skin hemorrhages. Abnormal synthesis of osteoid (unmineralized bone) leads to decreased amounts of osteoid in the bone and increased calcification of the cartilage. Vitamin C also functions as an antioxidant and is important in neutrophil function and iron absorption in the gut. These functions are also decreased in patients with scurvy. This syndrome is common in elderly people living on a diet deficient in milk, fruits, and vegetables.

In contrast to scurvy, which is caused by a deficiency of vitamin C, rickets is caused by a deficiency of vitamin D. Rickets is characterized by a lack of calcium. In this abnormality the osteoblasts in bone continue to synthesize osteoid, but this material is not mineralized. This results in increased amounts of osteoid (unmineralized bone) and decreased mineralized bone. In adults this produces osteomalacia and bone pain. Histologically, the bone osteoid seams are markedly increased in thickness. In children this produces rickets, a disease that is characterized by increased osteoid at normal growth centers of bone, which produces wide epiphyses at the wrists and knees and leads to growth retardation. Thiamine deficiency causes beriberi and niacin deficiency causes pellagra.

127. The answer is e. (*Kumar, pp 442–444.*) Wounds can be classified as being either open wounds, in which the skin is torn or cut, or closed wounds, in which the skin remains intact. A laceration is a linear or stellate-shaped open wound that is caused by tearing or ripping forces. Characteristically lacerations have strands of fibrous tissue or blood vessels that can be seen crossing the wound. These strands of tissue are not seen with incisions, which are a type of open wound caused by a sharp-edged object such as a knife or a piece of glass. An abrasion (scrape) is caused by injury to the skin when the superficial layers are rubbed off by friction, such as occurs with sliding on a rough surface. Types of closed wounds include contusions and hematomas. Contusions (bruises) result from blunt trauma to the skin that damages the underlying tissue and causes bleeding within the interstitium, while hematomas result from damage to a blood vessel such that the bleeding into tissue produces a mass of blood. Finally the term avulsion means "tearing away" and refers to removal or amputation of tissue, such as with damage to bone or a nerve.

128. The answer is a. (*Kumar, pp 432–433. Ayala, p 189.*) The major organs affected by lead poisoning are the blood, nervous system, gastrointestinal tract, and kidneys. Many times the early signs and symptoms of lead poisoning are seen only in the blood. These changes include a hypochromic and microcytic anemia with basophilic stippling of the red blood cells. Lead interferes with aminolevulinic acid dehydratase (ALA-D) and ferroketolase (heme synthetase), two enzymes involved in the production of hemoglobin. As a result of decreased activity of both of these enzymes in red cells, iron is displaced from heme, forming increasing blood levels of zinc protoporphyrin and its product, free erythrocyte protoporphyrin (FEP). Also as a result of decreased activity of erythrocyte ALA-D, urinary delta-aminolevulinic acid is increased. Children exposed to lead are vulnerable to CNS damage, which can decrease mental abilities, while adults can develop a peripheral demyelination neuropathy that produces a wrist- and footdrop. GI symptoms include severe, poorly localized abdominal pain, which is called lead colic. In the kidney, damage to the proximal tubular epithelial cells causes Fanconi's syndrome, which consists of the triad of amino aciduria, glycosuria, and hyperphosphaturia. Increased reabsorption of urinary proteins leads to large eosinophilic, acid-fast intranuclear droplets in the tubular epithelial cells. Lead may also be deposited in the gums (forming a blue line along the margins of the gums called Bruton's line) or in the epiphyses of children (which may be seen on x-ray). In contrast, increased urinary levels of hydroxy-indoleacetic acid can be seen with the carcinoid syndrome, while increased urinary levels of N-formiminoglutamate (FIGlu) with folate deficiency, and vanillylmandelic acid with a pheochromocytoma.

129. The answer is e. (*Kumar, pp 424, 432–434, 1400. Braunwald, pp 160, 164–165.*) Many environmental chemicals are potential causes of quite serious human diseases. Methanol, originally called wood alcohol, is metabolized in the body by the enzyme alcohol dehydrogenase to formaldehyde and formic acid. These metabolites cause necrosis of retinal ganglion cells, which leads to a metabolic acidosis and blindness. It is interesting to note that the treatment for acute methanol ingestion is IV ethyl alcohol, because it is also metabolized by alcohol dehydrogenase and therefore ties up this enzyme. Cadmium, which can be found in tobacco smoke, has been implicated in producing not only an acute form of pneumonia, but, with chronic exposure to small concentrations of cadmium vapors, diffuse interstitial pulmonary fibrosis and an increased incidence of emphysema as well.

In contrast, cobalt poisoning can produce a dilated cardiomyopathy, while mercury toxicity damages the kidneys and the brain. The neurologic symptoms include a tremor due to cerebellar abnormalities and mental changes. Historically the use of mercury in the hat-making industry caused these symptoms and resulted in the expression "mad as a hatter." A famous widespread outbreak of mercury poisoning occurred in the Minamata coastal region of Japan (and led to the term Minamata disease).

130. The answer is d. (*Rubin, pp 326–332. Kumar, pp 430, 1400. Braunwald, pp 159, 161–162.*) Cyanide causes cellular damage by binding to cytochrome oxidase and inhibiting cellular respiration. Cyanide is used in industry; an industrial accident in India in 1984 killed more than 2000 people. Cyanide is also a component of amygdalin, which is found in the pits of several fruits, such as apricots and peaches. It is also found in laetrile, a drug that is used outside of the United States. Cyanide poisoning produces a cherry-red color of the skin and also produces the odor of bitter almonds on the breath.

In contrast, acute arsenic toxicity causes central nervous toxicity and renal tubular necrosis. Chronic arsenic exposure causes GI disturbances, peripheral neuropathies, and skin changes (thick areas of skin with increased pigmentation called arsenical keratosis). Arsenic is also associated with cancers of the skin, respiratory tract, and liver (angiosarcomas). Arsenic accumulates in the hair and nails (forming transverse ridges called Mees' lines). Carbon monoxide is a colorless, odorless gas that is produced by natural gas heaters and is found in car exhaust. It replaces oxygen in hemoglobin, causing the formation of carboxyhemoglobin. This results in extreme cyanosis and anoxia. It produces a characteristic cherry-red color of the skin and blood. Finally, carbon tetrachloride can produce liver damage (with steatosis), while ethylene glycol, commonly used as an antifreeze, is toxic to humans (and cats and dogs) because it causes a metabolic acidosis and acute tubular necrosis in the kidney, as ethylene glycol is metabolized to calcium oxalate (polarizable crystals), which are deposited in the renal tubules.

131. The answer is e. (*Warren, pp 1892–1896. Kumar, pp 449, 462–463. Braunwald, pp 236–238.*) Exercise-associated loss of normal cyclic menstrual periods in women may result from excess weight loss and hypothalamic dysfunction producing hypogonadotropic hypogonadism. One hypothesis concerning the pathogenesis of this abnormality is that a decrease in the amount of total body fat will decrease serum levels of leptin, a substance that is thought to normally stimulate gonadotropin release from the pituitary. Therefore, decreased levels of leptin will decrease serum follicle stimulating hormone (FSH) and luteinizing hormone (LH) levels. As a result, serum estrogen levels will also be decreased.

Weight-loss induced amenorrhea is also seen with anorexia nervosa, which refers to self-induced starvation, usually in previously healthy young females. The clinical findings with anorexia nervosa are similar to those in severe protein-energy malnutrition (PEM). Decreased gonadotropin-releasing hormone (GnRH) decreases levels of both LH and FSH, which leads to amenorrhea. Decreased thyroid hormone leads to signs and symptoms of hypothyroidism, which include cold intolerance, bradycardia, constipation, and skin and nail changes. Decreased estrogen can produce osteoporosis, while cardiac arrhythmias may result from hypokalemia and may cause sudden death. Compare anorexia nervosa to bulimia, which refers to binge eating followed by induced vomiting, usually in previously healthy young females. Bulimia is also associated with menstrual irregularities; complications include electrolyte abnormalities (hypokalemia) and aspiration of gastric contents.

132. The answer is b. (*Kumar, pp 475–476, 1276–1277. Sadler, pp 106–107.*) Abnormalities of genes that control normal morphogenesis during embryonic development are associated with the development of congenital malformations. Two important types of genes associated with morphogenesis include homeobox (HOX) genes and paired box (PAX) genes. HOX genes act in temporal or spatial combinations and play an important role in the patterning of limbs, vertebrae, and craniofacial structures. Mutations of HOX genes may cause extra digits (synpolydactyly) or short digits (brachydactyly). It is interesting to note that vitamin A is an upstream regulator of HOX genes, and the use of retinoic acid during pregnancy may produce congenital abnormalities. Mutations of certain PAX genes are associated with malformations. Mutations of PAX-3 are seen in Waardenburg syndrome (congenital pigment abnormalities and deafness), while PAX-6 mutations may be seen with aniridia, and PAX-2 may be involved with Wilms syndrome. In contrast, the Sonic Hedgehog gene participates in the anterior-posterior symmetry of initial limb bud development and also in brain development, while the Cdx-1 gene is a murine gene expressed in cells participating in gastrulation. The receptor for the Sonic Hedgehog gene protein is probably the patched receptor.

133. The answer is e. (*Kumar, pp 389, 391, 477, 480. Rubin, pp 221–223.*) TORCH is an acronym referring to a group of microorganisms that produce similar changes during fetal or neonatal infection. The T stands for toxoplasma, the O for others, the R for rubella, the C for cytomegalovirus, and the H for herpes simplex virus. The "others" include syphilis, tuberculosis, and many other microorganisms. Manifestations of the TORCH complex include brain lesions, such as encephalitis and intracranial calcifications; ocular defects, including chorioretinitis; and cardiac abnormalities. Children born with congenital syphilis, caused by maternal infection with *T. pallidum*, initially show changes typical of the TORCH complex, but later they may develop characteristic lesions including flattening of the nose (saddle nose), notched incisors (Hutchinson's teeth), malformed molars (mulberry molars), outward bowing of the anterior tibias (saber shins), and progressive vascularization of the cornea (interstitial keratitis). The combination of deafness, interstitial keratitis, and notched incisors is referred to as Hutchinson's triad.

134. The answer is e. (*Kumar, pp 485–486.*) Hemolytic disease of the newborn (HDN) is a type of isoimmune hemolytic anemia that is caused by maternal antibodies that react against fetal red blood cells. Once the maternal antibodies cross the placenta, the fetal red cells are destroyed, leading to a hemolytic anemia. The breakdown of hemoglobin leads to hyperbilirubinemia (jaundice), which is due to severe unconjugated hyperbilirubinemia, as the released heme is not easily conjugated by the immature newborn liver, which is deficient in glucuronyl transferase. The unconjugated bilirubin is water-insoluble and has an affinity for lipids. In an infant with a poorly developed blood-brain barrier, the bilirubin may bind to the lipids in the brain and produce kernicterus. The severe anemia may result in congestive heart failure, which, together with hypoproteinemia may lead to generalized edema (anasarca), which in its most severe form is called hydrops fetalis. In the peripheral blood of the newborn, many immature red blood cells may be found (nucleated RBCs or normoblasts). This condition is called erythroblastosis and led to another name for HDN being erythroblastosis fetalis.

In order for the mother to make antibodies that are directed against fetal erythrocyte antigens, she must lack the erythrocyte antigens that the child has, which were inherited from the father. The most important erythrocyte antigens involved in HDN are the Rh and the ABO antigens. The most important Rh antigen is the D antigen. Therefore, for Rh incompatibility, the mother must be Rh negative (d), the child Rh positive (D). For ABO incompatibility, the mother must be type O (lacking the A and B antigens), the child type A or B. ABO incompatibility is the most common cause of hemolytic disease of the newborn. Usually the disease is less severe than HDN due to Rh incompatibility because there is poor expression of blood group antigens A and B on neonatal red cells.

135. The answer is d. (*Behrman, pp 577–578, 1358–1359. Damjanov, pp 1473–1483. Kumar, pp 481–483. Ravel, pp 549–550.*) Hyaline membrane disease (HMD), which accounts for 20% of all deaths in the first 28 days of life, is basically a disease of premature infants; most affected infants weigh 1000 to 1500 g. Contributing factors in the development of HMD include diabetes in the mother (maternal diabetes with increased glucose causes increased fetal secretion of insulin, which inhibits the effects of steroids such as lung maturation and production of surfactant) and cesarean section. Infants who develop HMD appear normal at birth, but within minutes to hours their respirations become labored. Grossly the lungs are a mottled, red-purple color, while microscopically there are hyaline membranes in air spaces, similar to those of acute respiratory distress syndrome (ARDS).

Two defects have been identified in infants with HMD. One is a deficiency of pulmonary surfactant. Surfactant, a lipid consisting of dipalmitoyl phosphatidylcholine, reduces the surface tension in air-fluid interfaces by getting between the molecules in the liquid and reducing their attraction to each other. This reduces the tendency for the alveoli to collapse after birth on expiration. Synthesis of surfactant increases throughout fetal development, but becomes maximal at 34 to 36 weeks. With a deficiency of surfactant, the lungs tend to collapse on expiration (atelectasis) and become stiff. The other defect is increased pulmonary epithelial permeability. This accounts for the protein-rich edema fluid in the alveoli and also for the formation of hyaline membranes. The most reliable test to determine pulmonary maturity is the ratio of lecithin to sphingomyelin (L/S), both of which are phospholipids. The production of lecithin (phosphatidylcholine) begins at 5 months of gestation, but secretion begins at 7 months of gestation, and levels rise sharply at 34 to 36 weeks of gestation. The level of sphingomyelin does not change during this time. An L/S ratio of about 2 indicates fetal maturity, 1.2 indicates a possible risk, and below 1 indicates a definite risk.

Mild cases of HMD can be treated with oxygen, while moderate cases can be treated with continuous positive airway pressure (CPAP). Severe cases may need to be treated with a ventilator with the administration of artificial surfactant.

136. The answer is c. (*Behrman, pp 2113–2114. Kumar, p 482. Rubin, pp 1556–1557.*) Retinopathy of prematurity (ROP), also called retrolental fibroplasia (because of the formation of a fibrovascular mass behind the lens), is a cause of blindness in premature infants that is related to the therapeutic use of high concentrations of oxygen. Immature blood vessels in the retina, particularly in the peripheral portion of the temporal retina, are prone to injury with high-dose oxygen, which inhibits the production of vascular endothelial growth factor (VEGF). This inhibition causes apoptosis of vascular endothelial cells with subsequent constriction and obliteration of the retinal blood vessels. This initial stage of ROP is referred to as the vaso-obliterative phase. Withdrawal of oxygen therapy stimulates VEGF production and results in a marked increase in the proliferation of vascular endothelial cells with new blood formation (neovascularization). This phase of ROP is called the vasoproliferative phase. The incidence of this complication has been markedly reduced due to close clinical monitoring of the concentration of administered oxygen. In contrast, accumulation of abnormal material in the ganglion cells of the retina is seen clinically as a "cherry-red macula," while fibrous obliteration of the canal of Schlemm is a cause of closed-angle glaucoma. Lipid accumulation at the periphery of the cornea produces corneal arcus, a commonly found aging change. Degeneration of the macula occurs most often due to age-related maculopathy, but it can also be caused by inherited disorders or drugs, such as chloroquine.

137. The answer is e. (*Kumar, p 473.*) Various drugs taken during pregnancy can be teratogenic and cause congenital abnormalities (although most congenital abnormalities result from genetic causes). Thalidomide was once used as a tranquilizer but was found to frequently cause limb

defects during pregnancy. These defects, called phocomelia, are characterized by underdeveloped limbs forming short stumps without fingers or
toes ("seal flippers"). 13-cis-retinoic acid is also associated with an
extremely high risk for birth defects, which include central nervous system, cardiac, and craniofacial defects. This drug may interfere with HOX
genes. Diethylstilbestrol (DES) can cause clear cell carcinoma of the vagina
in daughters of women exposed to DES during pregnancy, while tetracy-
clines can cause pigmentation of bone and teeth. ACE inhibitors can cause
renal damage, while iodide use can cause congenital goiter or hypothyroidism. Finally, alcohol may be one of the most common causes of congenital malformations in United States. Alcohol, which may inhibit cell
migration, is associated with prenatal (low birth weight) and postnatal
developmental retardation (mental retardation). Other congenital features
of alcohol use during pregnancy include microcephaly, facial abnormalities
(maxillary hypoplasia and microphthalmos), and short palpebral fissures.
This constellation of features is referred to as the fetal alcohol syndrome.

138. The answer is d. (*Kumar, pp 500–504.*) Neuroblastomas are malignant tumors of the adrenal medulla that occur in very young patients who
present with an abdominal mass. Histologically, these tumors are composed of small cells forming Homer-Wright rosettes, which are groups of
cells arranged in a ring around a central mass of pink neural filaments.
Electron microscopy reveals neurosecretory granules within the cytoplasm
of the tumor cells, while immunohistochemical stains are positive for
neuron-specific enolase (NSE). These highly aggressive tumors are unique
because some spontaneously regress and some dedifferentiate into benign
tumors, such as ganglioneuromas. Three distinct chromosomal abnormalities are associated with neuroblastomas. These abnormalities include near-
terminal deletion of part of the short arm of chromosome 1 (partial
monosomy 1), homogeneously staining regions (HSRs) of chromosome 2,
and multiple double minute chromatin bodies. The latter two are the result
of amplification of the oncogene N-*myc*. The number of N-*myc* copies correlates with the aggressiveness of the tumor. Dedifferentiation of a neuroblastoma into a benign ganglioneuroma is associated with a marked
reduction in this gene amplification. In contrast, deletion of chromosome
11 is associated with nephroblastoma (Wilms' tumor), a malignant tumor
of the kidney found in young patients. This chromosome abnormality is
associated with deletion of WT1, a tumor suppressor gene.

139. The answer is b. (*Henry, pp 259, 409. Kumar, pp 84, 574. Goldman, p 253.*) C-reactive protein (CRP) is an acute phase reactant that is made in the liver and is increased in several disorders. CRP levels can be used to differentiate bacterial infection (elevated CRP) from viral infection (decreased CRP). It can be used to monitor autoimmune disorders and also determine the risk of developing cardiovascular diseases and complications. For example, increased CRP levels are associated with increased risk for stroke or myocardial infarction. Some studies indicate that it may be a marker that is independent of serum lipid levels. Aspirin and statin therapy may also reduce the risk of cardiovascular complications in patients with elevated CRP levels.

140. The answer is b. (*Goldman, pp 294, 298. Henry, pp 295–296, 895, 902–903. Scheider, p 146. Kumar, p 557.*) Some myocytes located within the atrium have specific granules that are the storage sites for atrial natriuretic peptide (ANP). The actions of ANP include natriuresis, diuresis, and vasodilation. ANP is increased in patients with hypertension and congestive heart failure. In the latter it may counteract the effects of the renin-angiotensin-aldosterone (RAA) and sympathetic systems. B-type natriuretic peptid levels are sensitive and specific markers of congestive heart failure and serial measurements may help in the clinical management of congestive heart failure.

Lactate dehydrogenase (LDH) is an enzyme that is found in the heart, skeletal muscle, red blood cells, the lung, and the liver. There are five isoenzymes of LDH. Liver cells contain higher proportions of LDH4 and LDH5 than do myocardium or red blood cells, both of which contain greater relative amounts of LDH1 and LDH2. Increased levels of LDH5 suggest acute hepatocellular damage. Lung tissue is high in LDH3, and brain tissue contains only small amounts of LDH5. During the LDH increase following a myocardial infarction, levels of LDH1 are usually higher than those of LDH2. This pattern is called a "flipped" LDH.

Mannan binding protein (MBP) is part of the mannan-binding lectin (MBL) pathway of complement regulation, while serum amyloid A (SAA) is an acute phase reactant that increases with inflammation and tissue injury. Finally 5'-nucleotidase (5'-NT) can be used to determine the source of an elevated serum alkaline phosphatase. 5'-NT is more commonly elevated with liver and biliary tract disease. It is also increased with ovarian carcinoma and rheumatoid arthritis.

141. The answer is b. (*Henry, pp 138–147.*) Diagnostic specificity is defined as the probability of a negative diagnostic test (true negatives) in the absence of the disease (true negatives and false positives), or simply, it is the ability of a test to correctly identify a person who is free of the specific disease. Specificity can be calculated using the formula true negatives/(true negatives + false positives). Diagnostic sensitivity is defined as the probability of a positive diagnosis (true positives) in patients with the disease the test is designed to detect (true positives and false negatives). Sensitivity can be calculated using the formula true positives/(true positives + false negatives). The results of a laboratory test for a certain disease in a population can be related to the prevalence of that disease in the population being studied to find the positive predictive values and negative predictive values for that laboratory test.

Cardiovascular System

Questions

DIRECTIONS: Each item below contains a question or incomplete statement followed by suggested responses. Select the **one best** response to each question.

142. A 30-year-old man presents because of a swelling involving the posterior distal portion of his right leg. Physical examination finds a single tumor nodule in his right Achilles tendon that is consistent with a xanthoma. Pertinent medical history is that his father died of a myocardial infarct before the age of 40. Laboratory evaluation finds elevated serum cholesterol and normal serum triglycerides. His serum HDL levels are found to be decreased in amount. The signs and symptoms in this individual, who has familial hypercholesterolemia, most likely resulted from an abnormality involving the receptor for which one of the following substances?

a. Apoprotein CI
b. Beta-myosin
c. Chylomicron remnants
d. Lipoprotein lipase
e. Low-density lipoproteins

143. A 37-year-old obese man presents with signs and symptoms of hyperglycemia. After appropriate workup, he is diagnosed as having type II diabetes mellitus, which is due in part to insulin resistance. Laboratory evaluation of his serum also finds hypertriglyceridemia, which is due to his diabetes. The most common type of secondary hyperlipidemia associated with diabetes mellitus is characterized by elevated serum levels of which one of the following substances?

a. Chylomicrons
b. High-density lipoproteins
c. Intermediate-density lipoproteins
d. Low-density lipoproteins
e. Very-low-density lipoproteins

144. The presence of lipoprotein(a) is associated with an increased risk for the development of coronary and cerebral vascular disease. One possible reason for this relates to the fact that lipoprotein(a) has kringle regions, which are regions that have structural homology with which one of the following substances?

a. Cardiolipin, and this homology increases the formation of clots on cardiac valves
b. Fibrinogen, and this homology increases the formation of fibrin thrombi
c. Hepatic lipase, and this homology decreases the formation of low-density lipoproteins
d. Lipoprotein lipase, and this homology decreases the ability to metabolize chylomicrons
e. Plasminogen, and this homology decreases the ability to clear thrombi

145. A 60-year-old man died secondary to coronary artery disease. At the time of autopsy marked atherosclerotic changes were present within his coronary arteries. Sections from these abnormal areas revealed complicated atherosclerotic plaques with calcification and hemorrhage. Within these plaques were cellular zones, composed of smooth-muscle cells and macrophages, and a central core with foam cells and cholesterol clefts. These foam cells are smooth-muscle cells or macrophages that have phagocytized lipid. Which one of the following substances promotes atherosclerosis by stimulating smooth-muscle cells to proliferate, phagocytize lipid, and excrete extracellular matrix material?

a. Alpha-interferon
b. Beta-transforming growth factor
c. Interleukin 1
d. Platelet-derived growth factor
e. Tumor necrosis factor

146. A 51-year-old woman presents with a long history of poorly controlled hypertension, diabetes mellitus, and signs of renal failure. During the workup of her disease, a renal biopsy is performed and reveals the lumens of the small blood vessels to be narrowed by uniform, homogenous, pink deposits within the walls of the vessels. No "onionskinning" or necrosis of blood vessels is seen. What is the best diagnosis?

a. Medial calcific sclerosis
b. Arteriosclerosis obliterans
c. Hyperplastic arteriolosclerosis
d. Hyaline arteriolosclerosis
e. Thromboangiitis obliterans

147. An 82-year-old woman presents with headaches, visual disturbances, muscle pain, and tenderness over her right temporal artery. Describe the microscopic appearance of the temporal artery biopsy shown in the associated photomicrograph.

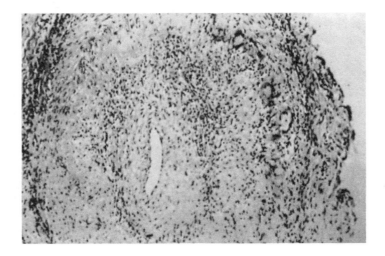

a. Acute inflammation with fragmentation of neutrophils
b. Chronic inflammation with scattered giant cells
c. Luminal thrombosis with microabscesses
d. Subacute inflammation with focal aneurysmal dilation
e. Transmural inflammation with fibrinoid necrosis

148. A 27-year-old man presents with fever, abdominal pain, muscle pain, and multiple tender cutaneous nodules. No pulmonary signs are found. A biopsy from one of the skin lesions is seen in the photomicrograph below. Involvement of small vessels by inflammation is not found. Laboratory tests are negative for P-ANCAs and C-ANCAs. Which of the following is most likely to be present in this patient's serum?

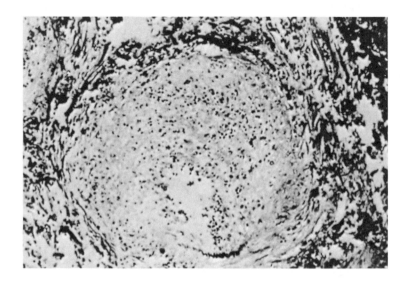

a. CMV antigen
b. *Cryptococcus* antigen
c. Hepatitis B antigen
d. *Histoplasma* antigen
e. *Pneumocystis* antigen

149. In a patient with vasculitis, the finding of serum antineutrophil cytoplasmic autoantibodies (ANCAs) that react by immunofluorescence staining in a perinuclear pattern (P-ANCAs) is most suggestive of which one of the following diseases?

a. Giant cell arteritis
b. Classic polyarteritis nodosa
c. Wegener's granulomatosis
d. Churg-Strauss syndrome
e. Microscopic polyangiitis

150. A 38-year-old woman presents with the new onset of multiple purpuric skin lesions. Two years ago she developed late-onset asthma and mild hypertension. Laboratory examination reveals an increase in the number of eosinophils in the peripheral blood (peripheral eosinophilia), and a biopsy from one of the purpuric skin lesions reveals leukocytoclastic vasculitis. No perivascular IgA deposits are found, and no antineutrophil cytoplasm autoantibodies are present. Which of the following is the most likely diagnosis?

a. Churg-Strauss syndrome
b. Henoch-Schönlein purpura
c. Macroscopic polyarteritis nodosa
d. Microscopic polyangiitis
e. Wegener's granulomatosis

151. A 30-year-old male smoker presents with gangrene of his extremities. Which one of the following histologic findings from a biopsy of the blood vessels supplying this area would be most consistent with a diagnosis of Buerger's disease?

a. Granulomatous inflammation with giant cells
b. Fibrinoid necrosis with overlying thrombosis
c. Focal aneurysmal dilation
d. Fragmentation of neutrophils
e. Thrombosis with microabscesses

152. During a routine physical examination, a 60-year-old man is found to have a 5-cm pulsatile mass in his abdomen. Angiography reveals a marked dilation of his aorta distal to his renal arteries. Which of the following is the most likely cause of this aneurysm?

a. Atherosclerosis
b. A congenital defect
c. Hypertension
d. A previous syphilitic infection
e. Trauma

153. A 56-year-old man presents with the sudden onset of excruciating pain. He describes the pain as beginning in the anterior chest, radiating to the back, and then moving downward into the abdomen. His blood pressure is found to be 160/115. Your differential diagnosis includes myocardial infarction; however, no changes are seen on electrocardiogram (ECG), and you consider this to be less of a possibility. You obtain an x-ray of this patient's abdomen and discover a "double-barrel" aorta. Which of the following is the basic cause of this abnormality?

a. A microbial infection
b. Loss of elastic tissue in the media
c. A congenital defect in the wall of the aorta
d. Atherosclerosis of the abdominal aorta
e. Abnormal collagen synthesis

154. A 2-year-old girl is being evaluated for progressive swelling of her neck. Physical examination finds a nontender, ill-defined, loculated mass in the left side of her neck. During the workup of this patient, a karyotype reveals that she is monosomic for the X chromosome. Which of the following is the cause of the swelling of this patient's neck?

a. Bacillary angiomatosis
b. Cystic hygroma
c. Glomus tumor
d. Nevus flammeus
e. Spider angioma

155. A 6-month-old boy is being evaluated for a lesion on his chin. Physical examination finds a raised, nontender, bright red strawberry-colored vascular lesion measuring approximately 4 mm in greatest dimension. At this time, which of the following is the best therapy for this infant?

a. Leave alone and follow up on a routine basis
b. Photocoagulation with yellow-green laser light
c. Repeated injections with steroids
d. Shave biopsy with frozen section diagnosis
e. Wide local excision with sentinel node sampling

156. A 23-year-old man who is HIV-positive presents with an irregular, slowly enlarging, 1-cm brown lesion located on his left forearm. Physical examination finds several similar lesions on his trunk. Which of the following histologic changes is most likely to be seen in a biopsy specimen taken from one of these skin lesions?

a. Irregular vascular spaces lined by nests of uniform cells
b. Multiple dilated endothelial-lined vessels that lack red blood cells
c. Numerous neutrophils, nuclear dust, and purple granules
d. Proliferating blood vessels, endothelial cells, and fibroblasts
e. Proliferating spindle stromal cells with slit-like spaces and extravasation of erythrocytes

157. A 56-year-old woman dies in a hospital where she is being evaluated for shortness of breath, ankle edema, and mild hepatomegaly. Because of the gross appearance of the liver at necropsy, which is seen in the photograph below, which of the following abnormalities is most likely present?

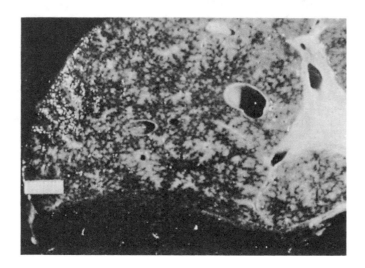

a. A pulmonary saddle embolus
b. Right heart failure
c. Portal vein thrombosis
d. Biliary cirrhosis
e. Splenic amyloidosis

158. A 59-year-old man presents with increasing shortness of breath and problems sleeping. He has a long history of poorly controlled hypertension. Physical examination finds distention of his neck veins, crepitant rales in both lower lungs, and bilateral edema of his feet. A chest x-ray reveals his heart to be dilated and enlarged. Which of the following is the basic defect that caused these clinical signs?

a. Decreased peripheral resistance caused low-output cardiac failure
b. Decreased viscosity of blood caused decreased diastolic filling of his heart
c. Increased afterload caused systolic dysfunction of his heart
d. Increased contractility of cardiac muscle caused high-output cardiac failure
e. Increased preload caused diastolic dysfunction of his heart

159. A 64-year-old man presents with recurrent chest pain that develops whenever he attempts to mow his yard. He relates that the pain goes away after a couple of minutes if he stops and rests. He also states that the pain has not increased in frequency or duration in the last several months. Which of the following is the most likely diagnosis?

a. Stable angina
b. Unstable angina
c. Atypical angina
d. Prinzmetal's angina
e. Myocardial infarction

160. A 50-year-old man presents to the emergency room with severe "crushing" substernal chest pain that began approximately 5 h prior. He states that sometimes the pain extends into his left arm, and during the past hour he has become quite nauseated. Physical examination finds this man to be sweating profusely and in moderate distress. An ECG finds abnormal Q waves in several of the anterior leads. Which of the following substances is most likely to be elevated in this individual?

a. Alkaline phosphatase
b. Aspartate aminotransferase
c. Lactate dehydrogenase
d. Myoglobin
e. Troponin

161. A 59-year-old man develops intense substernal, crushing chest pain that is not relieved by nitroglycerin. He is admitted to the MICU, where ECGs find evidence of myocardial infarction with ST-segment elevation. His condition rapidly worsens as he develops severe heart failure and dies 2 days later. At autopsy a large necrotic area is found that involves the anterior left ventricle. What is the most likely cause of this patient's myocardial infarction?

a. Coronary artery embolism
b. Coronary artery thrombosis
c. Coronary artery vasospasm
d. Coronary amyloid deposition
e. Coronary macroscopic arteritis

162. Arrange the following numbered statements in the correct order of the expected sequence of events that normally occur during healing of a myocardial infarction.

1 = Collagen is deposited, forming a fibrous scar
2 = Flocculent densities form within mitochondria
3 = Granulation tissue begins to form
4 = Macrophages begin to arrive at the area of coagulative necrosis
5 = Neutrophils begin to arrive at the area of coagulative necrosis

a. 2, then 3, then 4, then 5, then 1
b. 2, then 4, then 5, then 3, then 1
c. 2, then 5, then 4, then 3, then 1
d. 4, then 5, then 3, then 2, then 1
e. 5, then 4, then 3, then 2, then 1

163. Several days following a myocardial infarction, a 51-year-old man develops the sudden onset of a new pansystolic murmur along with a diastolic flow murmur. Workup reveals increased left atrial pressure that develops late in systole and extends into diastole. Which of the following is the most likely cause of the abnormalities present in this individual?

a. Aneurysmal dilation of the left ventricle
b. Obstruction of the aortic valve
c. Rupture of the left ventricle wall
d. Rupture of a papillary muscle
e. Thrombosis of the left atrial cavity

164. Three weeks following a myocardial infarction, a 54-year-old man presents with fever, productive cough, and chest pain. The pain is worse with inspiration, better when he is sitting up, and not relieved by nitroglycerin. Physical examination finds a friction rub along with increased jugular venous pressure and pulsus paradoxus (excess blood pressure drop with inspiration). Which of the following is the most likely explanation for these findings?

a. Caplan's syndrome
b. Dressler's syndrome
c. Ruptured papillary muscle
d. Ruptured ventricular wall
e. Ventricular aneurysm

165. A 59-year-old woman presents with increasing shortness of breath. Physical examination reveals signs of left heart failure. She is admitted to the hospital to workup her symptoms, but she dies suddenly. A section from her heart at the time of autopsy reveals marked thickening of the wall of the left ventricle, but the thickness of the right ventricle is within normal limits. Many of the nuclei of the myocytes in the wall of the left ventricle have a "box car" appearance. The endocardium does not appear to be increased in thickness or fibrotic, and the cardiac valves do not appear abnormal. The left ventricular cavity is noted to be decreased in size. What is the most likely cause of this cardiac pathology?

a. Carcinoid heart disease
b. Cor pulmonale
c. Eccentric hypertrophy
d. Systemic hypertensive
e. Volume overload

166. A 71-year-old woman presents with increasing chest pain and occasional syncopal episodes, especially with physical exertion. She has trouble breathing at night and when she lies down. Physical examination reveals a crescendo-decrescendo midsystolic ejection murmur with a paradoxically split second heart sound (S$_2$). Pressure studies reveal that the left ventricular pressure during systole is markedly greater than the aortic pressure. Which of the following is the most likely diagnosis?

a. Aortic regurgitation
b. Aortic stenosis
c. Constrictive pericarditis
d. Mitral regurgitation
e. Mitral stenosis

167. A 63-year-old man presents with signs of congestive heart failure, including shortness of breath, cough, and paroxysmal nocturnal dyspnea. Physical examination reveals a hyperdynamic, bounding, "water-hammer" pulse and a decrescendo diastolic murmur. His hyperdynamic pulse causes "bobbing" of his head. Which of the following is the most frequent cause of the cardiac valvular abnormality present in this individual?

a. Aortic dissection
b. Infective endocarditis
c. Latent syphilis
d. Marfan syndrome
e. Rheumatic fever

168. Physical examination of an asymptomatic 29-year-old woman with a history of rheumatic fever during childhood finds an early diastolic opening snap with a rumbling late diastolic murmur. Which of the following is the most likely diagnosis?

a. Aortic regurgitation
b. Aortic stenosis
c. Mitral regurgitation
d. Mitral stenosis
e. Pulmonic stenosis

169. A 7-year-old boy presents with the acute onset of fever, pain in several joints, and a skin rash. Physical examination finds an enlarged heart, several subcutaneous nodules, and a skin rash on his back with a raised, erythematous margin. Laboratory tests find an elevated erythrocyte sedimentation rate and an elevated antistreptolysin O titers. Within the past month, this boy most likely had which one of the following abnormalities?

a. Anitschkow cells develop in the lungs
b. Aschoff bodies develop in the skin
c. Beta-hemolytic streptococci infection of the pharynx
d. *Pseudomonas aeruginosa* infection of the aorta
e. Stenosis of the mitral valve

170. An autopsy done on a 23-year-old man who died suddenly with no previous medical history reveals the right ventricle to be dilated with near total transmural replacement of the right ventricle (RV) free-wall myocardium by fat and fibrosis. No skin or hair abnormalities are seen. What is the best diagnosis?

a. Arrhythmogenic RV cardiomyopathy
b. Endocardial fibrosis
c. Hyper-serotonin RV syndrome
d. Loeffler endomyocarditis
e. Naxos syndrome

171. A 31-year-old woman presents with fever, intermittent severe pain in the left upper quadrant of her abdomen, and painful lesions involving her fingers and nail beds. History reveals that she had acute rheumatic fever as a child and that when she was around 20 years of age she developed a new cardiac murmur. At the present time one of three blood cultures submitted to the hospital lab grew a specific bacteria. Which of the following is the most likely cause of her disease?

a. *Staphylococcus aureus*
b. α-hemolytic viridans streptococci
c. Candida species
d. Group A streptococci
e. *Pseudomonas* species

172. A 23-year-old woman develops the sudden onset of congestive heart failure. Her condition rapidly deteriorates and she dies in heart failure. At autopsy, patchy interstitial infiltrates composed mainly of lymphocytes are found, some of which surround individual myocytes. Which of the following is the most likely cause of this patient's heart failure?

a. Autoimmune reaction (to group A β-hemolytic streptococci)
b. Bacterial myocarditis (due to *S. aureus* infection)
c. Hypersensitivity myocarditis (due to an allergic reaction)
d. Nutritional deficiency (due to thiamine deficiency)
e. Viral myocarditis (due to coxsackievirus infection)

173. At the time of autopsy of a 39-year-old woman who died of complications of systemic lupus erythematosus, several medium-sized vegetations are found on both sides of the mitral valve and tricuspid valve. Which of the following is the basic abnormality that produced these cardiac vegetations?

a. Turbulent blood flow through an incompetent mitral valve
b. Excess secretion of a vasoactive amine
c. Presence of an anticardiolipin antibody
d. Cachexia produced by a hypercoagulable state
e. Bacterial colonization of an abnormal valve

174. A 37-year-old woman presents with prolonged cramps, nausea, vomiting, diarrhea, and episodic flushing of the skin. Additionally, she develops pearly white, plaque-like deposits on the tricuspid valve leaflets. Which of the following disorders is most likely to be present in this individual?

a. Rheumatic heart disease
b. Amyloidosis
c. Iron overload
d. Hypothyroidism
e. Carcinoid heart disease

175. A 59-year-old patient receiving chemotherapy with the anthracycline Adriamycin develops severe heart failure. Sections from an endocardial biopsy specimen reveal vacuolization of the endoplasmic reticulum of the myocytes. Adriamycin therapy most frequently causes what type of cardiomyopathy?

a. Dilated cardiomyopathy
b. Hyperplastic cardiomyopathy
c. Hypertrophic cardiomyopathy
d. Obliterative cardiomyopathy
e. Restrictive cardiomyopathy

176. A 3-month-old girl is being evaluated for feeding difficulty and failure to thrive. Physical examination finds pallor, peripheral cyanosis, tachypnea, and fine expiratory wheezing. Chest x-ray shows cardiac enlargement. She is admitted to the hospital, quickly develops severe cardiac failure, and dies 3 days after admission. At the time of autopsy the endocardium is found to have a "cream cheese" gross appearance. Histologic sections from this area reveal thickening of the endocardium due to a proliferation of fibrous and elastic tissue. Which of the following is the most likely diagnosis?

a. Dilated cardiomyopathy
b. Hypertrophic cardiomyopathy
c. Infective endocarditis
d. Libman-Sachs endocarditis
e. Restrictive cardiomyopathy

177. A 17-year-old high school student dies suddenly while playing basketball. At autopsy, his heart had abnormal findings similar to those seen in the associated gross picture of the heart. Histologic sections from this area reveal disorganization of the myofibers, which are thicker than normal and have hyperchromatic nuclei. Which of the following statements best describes the familial form of the cardiac disease that caused the death of this individual?

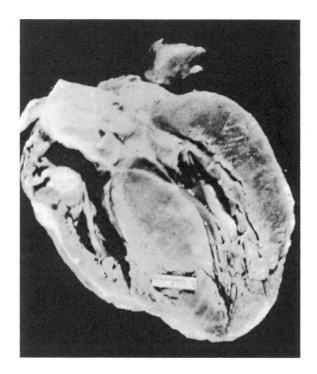

a. An autosomal dominant disorder associated with an abnormal fibrillin gene
b. An autosomal dominant disorder associated with an abnormal β-myosin gene
c. An autosomal recessive disorder associated with decreased acid maltase formation
d. An X-linked recessive disorder associated with an abnormal dystrophin gene
e. An X-linked recessive disorder associated with decreased NADPH oxidase formation

178. A 49-year-old man 7 days after being admitted to the hospital for an inferior wall, transmural myocardial infarction suddenly becomes short of breath. Physical examination reveals hypotension, elevated jugular venous pressure, and muffled heart sounds. His systemic blood pressure drops 13 mmHg with inspiration. Which one of the following pathologic processes produced these clinical findings?

a. Acute inflammation of the pericardium due to an autoimmune reaction
b. Acute mitral regurgitation due to rupture of a papillary muscle
c. Acute suppurative inflammation of the pericardium due to bacterial infection
d. Blood accumulation in the pericardial cavity due to rupture of the ventricular wall
e. Serous fluid accumulation in the pericardial cavity due to congestive heart failure

179. A 35-year-old man presents with weight loss, fever, and fatigue. Physical examination finds signs and symptoms of mitral valve disease. Further workup finds a pedunculated mass in the left atrium. The tumor is resected and histologic sections reveal stellate cells in a loose myxoid background. Which of the following is the most likely diagnosis?

a. Chordoma
b. Fibroelastoma
c. Leiomyoma
d. Myxoma
e. Rhabdomyoma

180. A 2-year-old girl is being evaluated for growth and developmental delay. She has had several past episodes when she would suddenly have trouble breathing, become blue, and then assume a squatting position to catch her breath. Workup finds a defect in the wall of the ventricular septum, increased thickness of the right ventricle, and dextroposition of the aorta. Which of the following cardiovascular abnormalities is most likely to be present in this child?

a. Coarctation of the aorta
b. Incompetence of the mitral valve
c. Patency of the foramen ovale
d. Persistence of the AV canal
e. Stenosis of the pulmonic valve

181. A 2-month-old girl is being examined for a routine checkup. She was born at term, and there were no problems or complications during the pregnancy. The baby appeared normal at birth and has been asymptomatic. Physical examination at this time finds a soft systolic murmur with a systolic thrill. No cyanosis is present, and her peripheral pulses are thought to be within normal limits. An ECG reveals slight left ventricular hypertrophy. Which of the following is the most likely diagnosis?

a. Coarctation of the aorta
b. Patent ductus arteriosus
c. Persistent truncus arteriosus
d. Tetralogy of Fallot
e. Ventricular septal defect

182. Which one of the following statements correctly describes the flow of blood in an individual with an atrial septal defect who develops Eisenmenger's syndrome?

a. Aorta to pulmonary artery to lungs to left atrium to left ventricle to aorta
b. Left atrium to right atrium to right ventricle to lungs to left atrium
c. Left ventricle to right ventricle to lungs to left atrium to right ventricle
d. Right atrium to left atrium to left ventricle to aorta to right atrium
e. Right ventricle to left ventricle to aorta to right atrium to right ventricle

183. Prior to surgery, which of the following is the best medical therapy for a newborn infant with transposition of the pulmonary artery and aorta?

a. Give prostaglandin E_2 to keep the ductus arteriosus open
b. Give prostaglandin F_2 to close the ductus arteriosus
c. Give oxygen to keep the ductus arteriosus open
d. Give indomethacin to keep the ductus arteriosus open
e. Give indomethacin to close the ductus arteriosus

Cardiovascular System

Answers

142. The answer is e. (*Goldman, pp 1093–1095. Kumar, pp 156–158.*) Lipids are transported in the blood complexed to proteins called apo-lipoproteins. Abnormalities of this lipid transport or metabolism result in hyperlipoproteinemias, which are responsible for most syndromes of premature atherosclerosis. The primary hyperlipidemias are divided into five distinct electrophoretic patterns. Type I hyperlipoproteinemia, caused by a mutation in the lipoprotein lipase gene, results in increased chylomicrons and triglycerides. Type II hyperlipoproteinemia, perhaps the most frequent Mendelian disorder, is caused by a mutation in the low-density lipoprotein (LDL) receptor gene. This results in increased LDL and cholesterol. Homozygotes for this gene defect have markedly increased plasma cholesterol levels and develop severe atherosclerosis at an early age. Xanthomas of the Achilles tendon are somewhat specific for this disorder. Mutations in the apolipoprotein E gene result in type III hyperlipoproteinemia, which is characterized by increased intermediate-density lipoproteins (IDLs), triglycerides, and cholesterol. Type IV hyperlipoproteinemia causes increased very-low-density lipoproteins (VLDLs) and triglycerides. The genetic defect causing this abnormality is a mutation in the lipoprotein lipase gene. Type V hyperlipoproteinemia, caused by a mutation in apolipoprotein CII, results in increased VLDLs, chylomicrons, triglycerides, and cholesterol.

143. The answer is e. (*Goldman, pp 1284–1285. Kumar, p 521.*) Increased serum lipids (hyperlipidemia) may be a primary genetic defect or may be secondary to another disorder, such as diabetes mellitus, alcoholism, the nephrotic syndrome, or hypothyroidism. Secondary hypertriglyceridemia in patients with diabetes mellitus usually occurs secondary to increased blood levels of VLDL. The reason for this is that with decreased levels of insulin with diabetes mellitus there is increased mobilization of free fatty acids from adipose tissue (increased lipolysis). This increases delivery of free fatty acids to the liver, which increases production and secretion of VLDL by the liver. This is a type IV hyperlipidemia pattern. Ethanol can also produce a type IV pattern due to increased VLDL. This is because ethanol also increases lipolysis of adipose tissue, which increases delivery of free fatty acids to the liver. Ethanol also increases the esterification of fatty acid to triglycerides in the liver and inhibits the release of lipoproteins from the liver.

144. The answer is e. (*Kumar, pp 521, 523. Damjanov, pp 1405–1406.*) There are various risk factors that predispose individuals to the development of atherosclerosis and ischemic heart disease. These risk factors are either quite significant (major factors) or less significant (minor factors). Major factors include diet and hyperlipidemia (hypercholesterolemia and hypertriglyceridemia), hypertension, cigarette smoking, and diabetes mellitus. Minor risk factors include obesity, lack of physical exercise, male gender, stress, oral contraceptives (birth control pills), and hyperhomocystinemia. Another minor risk factor is the presence in the serum of lipoprotein(a), which is an altered form of LDL, that contains the apoprotein B100 linked to apoprotein(a). This special type of apoprotein has structural homology to plasminogen. These similar areas are called kringles because they resemble a type of Danish pastry. It is thought that, because of the similarity of structure, Lp(a) competes with plasminogen in clots and decreases the ability to form plasmin and clear clots.

145. The answer is d. (*Kumar, p 523–525. Rubin, pp 492–495.*) The pathogenesis of atherosclerosis depends in part on the inflammatory function of macrophages, which involves the release of numerous cytokines. Platelet-derived growth factor (PDGF) is mitogenic and chemotactic for smooth-muscle cells. This may explain the recruitment and proliferation of smooth-muscle cells in atherosclerosis. Other macrophage products participate in the pathophysiology of atherosclerosis by other means. Interleukin 1 (IL-1) and tumor necrosis factor (TNF) transform the normally anticoagulant endothelial surface into a procoagulant surface by stimulating endothelial cells to produce platelet-activating factor (PAF), tissue factor (TF), and plasminogen activator inhibitor (PAI). Interferon alpha and transforming growth factor beta inhibit cell proliferation. This could explain the failure of endothelial cells to repair endothelial defects. These defects could then either provide entry areas for lipoproteins and plasma-derived factors or serve as an area where thrombi are formed.

146. The answer is d. (*Kumar, pp 529–530, 1006–1008.*) Hypertension is associated with two forms of damage to small blood vessels: hyaline arteriolosclerosis and hyperplastic arteriolosclerosis. Hyaline arteriolosclerosis, which is also a vascular complication of patients with diabetes mellitus, is presumably caused by leakage of plasma components across the endothelium. Microscopic examination will reveal the lumens of small arterioles to be narrowed by homogenous pink (hyaline) deposits in the walls. These changes within the kidney are referred to as benign nephrosclerosis, in which the decreased blood supply causes loss of nephrons and a characteristic finely granular appearance to the kidney surface. Hyaline arteriolosclerosis is associated with benign hypertension.

In contrast, hyperplastic arteriolosclerosis is associated with malignant hypertension, which refers to dramatic elevations in systolic and diastolic blood pressure often resulting in early death from cerebral and brainstem hemorrhages. Pathologically, the renal vessels demonstrate a concentric obliteration of arterioles by an increase in smooth-muscle cells and protein deposition in a laminar configuration (onionskining) that includes fibrin material, which leads to total and subtotal occlusion of the vessels. These changes are called hyperplastic arteriolosclerosis.

Medial calcific sclerosis (Mönckeberg's arteriosclerosis) is characterized by dystrophic calcification in the tunica media of muscular arteries. There is no narrowing of the lumen of the affected vessels. Thromboangiitis obliterans (Buerger's disease) is occlusion by a proliferative inflammatory process in arteries of heavy cigarette smokers and is often associated with HLA-A9,B5 genotypes. Finally, the term "ateriosclerosis obliterans" refers to arteriosclerosis of the extremities (peripheral vascular disease).

147. The answer is b. (*Kumar, pp 534–542. Rubin, pp 516–517.*) Giant cell arteritis (temporal arteritis) is an important disease to consider in the differential diagnosis of older individuals who present with a constellation of symptoms that may include migratory muscular and back pains (polymyalgia rheumatica), dizziness, visual disturbances, headaches, weight loss, anorexia, and tenderness over one or both of the temporal arteries. The cause of the arteritis is unknown, but the dramatic response to corticosteroids suggests an immunogenic origin. The disease may involve any artery within the body, but involvement of the ophthalmic artery or arteries may lead to blindness unless steroid therapy is begun. The workup should include evaluation of the erythrocyte sedimentation rate (ESR), which usually is markedly elevated, and a biopsy of the temporal artery, which may show chronic granulomatous inflammation with giant cells or breaks in internal elastic lamina. Many times, however, biopsies do not show inflammatory changes as the temporal artery may be segmentally involved. Therefore, initiation of therapy may have to be based only on clinical suspicion.

The other listed microscopic appearances are suggestive of other disease processes. Transmural inflammation of blood vessels with fibrinoid necrosis and possible overlying thrombosis or focal aneurysmal dilation may be seen with polyarteritis nodosa (PAN). Acute inflammation with fragmentation of neutrophils is characteristic of hypersensitivity angiitis (leukocytoclastic vasculitis), while thrombosis with microabscesses formation is seen with thromboangiitis obliterans (Buerger's disease), a disorder that is linked to cigarette smoking.

148. The answer is c. (*Damjanov, pp 1429–1431. Kumar, p 539.*) Classic PAN is a systemic disease characterized by necrotizing inflammation of small or medium-sized muscular arteries, typically involving the visceral vessels but sparing the small blood vessels of the lungs and kidneys. Histologically, there is intense localized acute inflammation and necrosis of vessel walls with fibrinoid necrosis and often thrombosis of the vessel with ischemic infarcts of the affected organ. Healed lesions display fibrosis in the walls of affected blood vessels with focal aneurysmal dilations. Clinically, PAN is a protracted, recurring disease that affects young adults. It is a multisystem disease affecting many organs of the body, and this makes it difficult to diagnose unless the vasculitis is recognized by biopsy. Symptoms include fever, weight loss, malaise, abdominal pain, headache, and myalgia. Skin involvement results in palpable purpura. The etiology is not known, but 30% of patients with classic PAN have circulating hepatitis B antigen in their serum.

149. The answer is e. (*Kumar, pp 536–541. Rubin, pp 515–516. Damjanov, pp 1429–1431.*) Antineutrophil cytoplasmic antibodies (ANCAs) may be found in patients with certain inflammatory vascular diseases or glomerular diseases, and their presence is of clinical importance for diagnosing these diseases. Immunofluorescence reveals ANCAs to have two different patterns. One is directed toward myeloperoxidase of neutrophils and is found in a perinuclear location (P-ANCAs). This pattern is seen in patients with microscopic PAN or idiopathic crescentic glomerulonephritis without systemic disease. Microscopic PAN commonly involves glomerular and pulmonary capillaries and may produce hematuria, hemoptysis, and renal failure. Histologic sections reveal segmental fibrinoid necrosis. The other

ANCA pattern reveals the antibodies to be directed against neutral leukocyte protease (proteinase 3) and results in a cytoplasmic staining pattern (C-ANCAs). This pattern is seen in patients with Wegener's granulomatosis or Churg-Strauss syndrome.

150. The answer is a. (*Kumar, pp 536–541. Rubin, pp 515–516. Damjanov, pp 1429–1431.*) Leukocytoclastic angiitis refers to the histologic finding of fragmented neutrophils surrounding small blood vessels. The differential diagnosis of leukocytoclastic vasculitis includes microscopic PAN and three other disorders: Henoch-Schönlein purpura, Wegener's granulomatosis, and Churg-Strauss syndrome. Henoch-Schönlein purpura is a disorder of children who present with hemorrhagic urticaria and hematuria following an upper respiratory infection. The pathology of this disease involves the deposition of immunoglobulin A (IgA) immune complexes in small vessels of the skin. Because the antibody is IgA, the alternate complement pathway is activated in these patients. Wegener's granulomatosis (WG) is characterized by acute necrotizing granulomas of the upper and lower respiratory tract, focal necrotizing vasculitis affecting small- to medium-sized vessels, and renal disease. Histologically there is fibrinoid necrosis of small arteries, early infiltration by neutrophils, and granuloma formation with giant cells. The peak incidence is in the fifth decade, and many patients have C-ANCAs. The disease is highly fatal, with death occurring within 1 year, unless recognized and treated with immunosuppressive agents. Churg-Strauss syndrome (allergic vasculitis) is a form of necrotizing vasculitis with granulomas of the respiratory tract and asthma. The disorder is associated with increased serum IgE and peripheral eosinophilia.

151. The answer is e. (*Kumar, pp 542–543. Rubin, pp 519–520.*) Buerger's disease (thromboangiitis obliterans) is characterized by segmental acute and chronic inflammation of intermediate and small arteries. This disorder almost always occurs in cigarette smokers at a young age (usually below 35 years) and is often associated with HLA-A9,B5 genotypes. It used to be found exclusively in men, but recently there has been an increase in the number of reported cases in women. The vessels primarily affected are in the extremities, and this leads to painful ischemia and gangrene of the legs and arms due to thrombosis. Histologic sections reveal an acute inflammatory infiltrate involving the entire wall of the vessel. In contrast to atherosclerosis, small microabscesses may be seen within thrombi. The inflammation leads to intimal proliferation that obliterates the lumen and causes pain. The disease may regress on cessation of smoking. In contrast, granulomatous inflammation with giant cells involving blood vessels can be seen with temporal arteritis or Takayasu's arteritis. Fragmentation of neutrophils surrounding blood vessels is called leukocytoclastic vasculitis, the differential for which includes microscopic PAN, Henoch-Schönlein purpura, Wegener's granulomatosis, and Churg-Strauss syndrome.

152. The answer is a. (*Kumar, pp 530–532. Rubin, pp 520–522.*) An aneurysm is an abnormal dilation of any vessel. The causes of aneurysms are many, but the two most important ones are atherosclerosis and cystic medial necrosis. Atherosclerotic aneurysms, the most common type of aortic aneurysms, usually occur distal to the renal arteries and proximal to the bifurcation of the aorta. Many atherosclerotic aneurysms are asymptomatic, but if they rupture they produce sudden, severe abdominal pain, shock, and a risk of death. Prior to rupture, physical examination reveals a pulsatile mass in the abdomen. Cystic medial necrosis refers to the focal loss of elastic and muscle fibers in the media of vessels and is seen in patients with hypertension, dissecting aneurysms, and Marfan's syndrome. Trauma may also lead to the formation of dissecting aneurysms.

Berry aneurysms, found at the bifurcation of arteries in the circle of Willis, are due to congenital defects in the vascular wall. Syphilitic (luetic) aneurysms are caused by obliterative endarteritis of the vasa vasorum of the aorta. These aneurysms are part of the tertiary manifestation of syphilis and become evident 15 to 20 years after persons have contracted the initial infection with *Treponema pallidum*. Elastic tissue and smooth-muscle cells of the media undergo ischemic destruction as a result of the treponemal infection (obliterative endarteritis). As a consequence of ischemia in the media, musculoelastic support is lost and fibrosis occurs. Grossly, the aorta has a "tree-bark" appearance. Luetic aneurysms almost always occur in the thoracic aorta and may lead to luetic heart disease by producing insufficiency of the aortic valve (aortic regurgitation).

153. The answer is b. (*Kumar, pp 532–534. Rubin, pp 522–524.*) Dissecting aneurysms are usually the result of cystic medial necrosis of the aorta. This abnormality results from loss of elastic tissue in the media and is associated with hypertension and Marfan's syndrome. Most cases of dissecting aneurysms involve a transverse tear in the intima and are located in the ascending aorta, just above the aortic ring. The pain caused by a dissecting aneurysm is similar to the pain caused by a myocardial infarction, but it extends into the abdomen as the dissection progresses. Additionally, the blood pressure is not decreased with a dissecting aneurysm unless the aorta itself has ruptured.

In contrast, berry aneurysms, found at the bifurcation of arteries in the circle of Willis, are due to congenital defects in the vascular wall. Rupture of these aneurysms may produce a fatal subarachnoid hemorrhage. Berry aneurysms have been noted in about one-sixth of patients with adult polycystic renal disease and account for death in about 10% of patients with this type of polycystic renal disease. Syphilitic (luetic) aneurysms occur in the thoracic aorta and may lead to luetic heart disease by producing insufficiency of the aortic valve. Mycotic (infectious) aneurysms result from microbial infection during septicemia, usually secondary to bacterial endocarditis. They are prone to rupture and hemorrhage. The Ehlers-Danlos syndromes (EDSs) are a group of eight syndromes characterized by defects in collagen synthesis. In EDS IV there is deficient synthesis of type III collagen and a tendency to rupture of muscular arteries, including dissecting aneurysms of the aorta.

154. The answer is b. (*Kumar, pp 545–548. Rubin, pp 526–527.*) Benign tumors of vessels may originate from either blood vessels or lymphatics. Lymphangiomas are tumors that are derived from lymphatic vessels. Histologically they reveal dilated vessels lined by endothelial cells, but they lack red blood cells in their lumen. The absence of red blood cells helps to distinguish these lesions from hemangiomas. Cystic hygromas are cystic lymphangiomas that typically occur in the neck or axilla. They may grow to such a large size that the neck is deformed. These lesions may be found in patients with Turner's syndrome, an abnormality that results from complete or partial monosomy for the X chromosome. Swelling of the neck in these individuals occurs because of dilated lymphatic vessels. With time the swelling decreases, but patients may develop bilateral neck webbing and loose skin on the back of the neck.

In contrast, dilated blood vessels (vascular ectasia) may be congenital or acquired. "Birthmarks" may be caused by congenital vascular ectasia (nevus flammeus) or capillary hemangiomas. "Port-wine stains" are similar lesions that may be caused by vascular ectasia or cavernous hemangiomas of the skin. Spider angiomas are acquired vascular ectasias that are the result of increased estrogen levels. They are associated with pregnancy and liver disease. Bacillary angiomatosis is a nonneoplastic proliferation of blood vessels that is found in immunocompromised patients, particularly patients with AIDS. Histologically, there are proliferating capillaries that are lined by protuberant endothelial cells. Additionally, numerous neutrophils are present along with nuclear dust and purple granules. These latter granules are Rickettsia-like bacteria that are the cause of this lesion, which responds to erythromycin.

155. The answer is a. (*Kumar, pp 545–547. Behrman, p 1726.*) Hemangiomas are benign tumors of blood vessels that histologically reveal the presence of red blood cells (erythrocytes) within the lumen of the proliferating vessels. Hemangiomas may be subclassified as capillary or cavernous. The juvenile (strawberry) hemangioma is a fast-growing lesion that appears in the first few months of life, but most completely regresses by the age of 5 years. Unless near the eye, definitive therapy is usually not indicated, as the possible techniques, such as surgery, cryotherapy, laser therapy, and injection of sclerosing drugs, all cause more scarring than is produced by spontaneous resolution.

156. The answer is e. (*Kumar, pp 548–551. Rubin, pp 528–529.*) Kaposi's sarcoma (KS) comprises four distinct forms. The classic, or European, form has been known since 1862. It occurs in older men of Eastern European or Mediterranean origin (predominantly Italian or Jewish) and is characterized by purple maculopapular skin lesions of the lower extremities and visceral involvement in only 10% of cases. The African form occurs in younger people and is more aggressive; it often involves lymph nodes in children. The rare form in immunosuppressed recipients of renal transplants often regresses when immunosuppression stops. In the epidemic form associated with AIDS, skin lesions may occur anywhere and disseminate to the mucous membranes, gastrointestinal (GI) tract, lymph nodes, and viscera. Histologic determination is difficult, but all four clinical types appear similar. In the early stages, irregular, dilated epidermal vascular spaces, extravasated red cells, and hemosiderin are characteristic. This histologic appearance is very similar to that of granulation tissue or stasis dermatitis. Later in the disease process, more characteristic lesions show spindle cells around slit spaces with extravasation of erythrocytes. In contrast, irregular vascular spaces lined by nests of uniform cells describe the histologic appearance of a glomus tumor, while multiple dilated endothelial-lined vessels that lack red blood cells describe the histologic appearance of lymphangiomas. Numerous neutrophils, nuclear dust, and purple granules characterize bacillary angiomatosis, while proliferating blood vessels, endothelial cells, and fibroblasts suggest granulation tissue.

157. The answer is b. (*Kumar, pp 122, 563, 918. Rubin, pp 283–284.*) The photograph shows the classic pattern of hepatic congestion around central veins, which leads to necrosis and degeneration of the hepatocytes surrounded by pale peripheral residual parenchyma. This is the pattern arising in the liver from chronic passive congestion as a result of right heart failure ("nutmeg liver"). Mitral stenosis with consequent pulmonary hypertension leads to right heart failure, as does any cause of pulmonary hypertension, such as emphysema (cor pulmonale). Right heart failure also leads to congestion of the spleen and transudation of fluid into the abdomen (ascites) and lower-extremity soft tissues (pitting ankle edema) as a result of venous congestion. Portal vein thrombosis is most often seen in association with hepatic cirrhosis.

158. The answer is c. (*Kumar, pp 560–563. McPhee, pp 272–279.*) The heart will eventually fail to maintain cardiac output if it is forced to work in an abnormal state for a prolonged period of time. The symptoms produced by congestive heart failure relate to whether the failure involves the left side of the heart or the right side of the heart. Symptoms of acute left ventricular failure include pulmonary edema, pulmonary hemorrhage, and hypoxia, while chronic left ventricular failure will produce dyspnea on exertion, orthopnea (trouble breathing when lying down), paroxysmal nocturnal dyspnea, and eventually right heart failure.

There are many causes of congestive heart failure, but basically they produce either systolic dysfunction or diastolic dysfunction. Systolic dysfunction may result from increased preload, increased afterload, or decreased contractility. Causes of increased preload (volume overload) include regurgitation (mitral and aortic regurgitation), anemia, hyperthyroidism, and beriberi. Note that diseases with increased cardiac output, such as anemia, hyperthyroidism, and beriberi, are classified as high-output failure diseases. In contrast, diseases that decrease cardiac output are called low-output failure diseases. Causes of increased afterload (pressure overload) include hypertension, aortic stenosis, and hypertrophic cardiomyopathy. Decreased contractility can result from myocardial infarction, myocardial ischemia, drugs, and certain infections. Diastolic dysfunction results from decreased filling of the ventricles during diastole. Examples of this include mitral stenosis, infiltrative diseases such as amyloidosis, and constrictive pericardial diseases.

159. The answer is a. (*Kumar, p 575. McPhee, pp 292–294.*) One of the consequences of myocardial ischemia is chest pain, which is called angina. Angina is caused by a mismatch between the myocardial oxygen demand and the myocardial blood flow. There are three main types of angina. Typical angina (stable angina) is the most common type and is characterized by pain that results from exercise, stress, or excitement. The pain is promptly relieved by rest (which decreases oxygen demand) or nitroglycerin. Nitroglycerin is converted to nitric oxide, which is a vasodilator that increases perfusion to the heart. ECG changes in patients with stable angina are nonspecific and include T-wave inversion and ST-segment depression, which occurs secondary to ischemia of the subendocardium of the left ventricle. The second type of angina, Prinzmetal's angina (atypical angina), is caused by coronary artery vasospasm and is characterized by pain occurring at rest. This pain may be relieved by calcium channel blockers or nitroglycerin. ECG in these patients reveals ST-segment elevation, which is the result of transmural ischemia. The third type of angina is unstable angina, which is characterized by increasing frequency of pain, increased duration of pain, or pain that is produced by less physical exertion. This final type of angina indicates that a myocardial infarction (MI) may be near, most likely due to the formation of a thrombus over an area of coronary artery atherosclerosis. In contrast to an MI, with angina there is no actual necrosis (infarction) of myocardial tissue, and therefore there are no increased cardiac enzymes, such as lactate dehydrogenase (LDH) and creatine phosphokinase (CPK), in the serum. Also, the pain of angina is not made worse with deep inspiration, a sign that is suggestive of pleural disease.

160. The answer is e. (*Kumar, pp 583–584. Henry, pp 296–300.*) The clinical diagnosis of MI depends on correlating clinical symptoms, ECG findings, and serum cardiac enzyme changes. The classic description of the pain produced by an MI is crushing, substernal pain that may radiate down the patient's left arm. This pain may be associated with sweating, nausea, and vomiting. ECG findings associated with MI include ST-segment elevation (which may return to normal), inverted T waves, and abnormal Q waves. Serum enzymes that may be elevated after an MI include troponin, CPK, SGOT (AGT), and LDH, which are increased temporally in that order. The troponin complex is made up of three protein subunits: troponin I (Tn-I), troponin T, and troponin C. There are three isoforms of Tn-I: two in skeletal muscle and one in cardiac muscle (cTn-I). cTn-I levels begin to increase 4 to 6 h after the onset of chest pain, reach maximal serum concentration in about 12 to 24 h, and remain elevated for about 3 to 10 days. CPK exists in three isoenzymes, MM, MB, and BB, where M stands for muscle and B stands for brain. Elevation of the CPK MB isoenzyme is seen following an MI. Levels begin to rise at 4 to 8 h, peak at 12 to 24 h, and return to normal in 3 to 4 days. LDH exists in five isoenzyme forms. Normally serum LDH2 is greater than LDH1, but following an MI this ratio is flipped, that is, LDH1 is greater than LDH2. LDH1 levels begin to rise at 10 to 12 h, peak at 2 to 3 days, and return to normal in 7 to 10 days.

Finally note that new cardiac markers use monoclonal antibodies directed against myoglobin, CK-MB mass assay, and cardiac troponin levels. Myoglobin is a small monomer with a rapid rise and fall in serum (narrow window) that may be used to test the effect of "clot-busting" drugs, especially with rapid serial detection.

161. The answer is b. (*Kumar, pp 572–576. Goldman, p 410. Rubin, pp 556–557.*) The term "acute coronary syndrome" encompasses several clinical disorders including unstable angina (UA), subendocardial (nontransmural) myocardial infarction (non-ST-segment elevation myocardial infarction or NSTEMI), and transmural myocardial infarction (ST-segment elevation myocardial infarction or STEMI). Most cases of STEMI are caused by thrombosis of a coronary artery overlying a previously stable atherosclerotic plaque. Atherosclerosis, however, does not affect the coronary arteries equally. Generally atherosclerosis affects the proximal 2 cm of the left anterior descending (LAD) and left circumflex artery, and the proximal and distal one-third of the right coronary artery. Anterior infarcts (such as infarction of the anterior left ventricle) result from occlusion of the LAD, as this artery normally supplies the anterior left ventricle, the apex, and the anterior two-thirds of the interventricular septum.

About 10% of transmural myocardial infarcts (STEMIs) are not caused by thrombosis overlying an atherosclerotic plaque. Less frequent causes of MI in these cases include coronary artery vasospasm (sometimes seen in association with cocaine use), coronary artery embolism (possibly in association with atrial fibrillation), coronary arteritis, or deposition of amyloid in the walls of the coronary arteries.

162. The answer is c. (*Kumar, pp 578–581. Rubin, pp 557–561.*) Areas of myocardial infarction (MI) undergo a series of changes that consists of typical ischemic coagulative necrosis followed by inflammation and repair. MIs less than 6 to 12 h old are not apparent on gross examination. By 12 to 24 h, there is pallor in the area of infarction, which is due to the trapped blood. On days 1 to 3, grossly the infarct develops a hyperemic (red) border and then becomes pale yellow over the next several days (days 4 to 7). By 7 to 14 days, the area of necrosis is surrounded by a hyperemic red-purple border of highly vascularized granulation tissue. Over the next few weeks, the area of necrosis changes to a gray-white fibrotic scar. Electron microscopic (EM) changes in MI can be seen at 20 to 40 min, but routine histologic changes are first seen at 1 to 3 h. These EM findings consist of signs of reversible injury (mitochondrial swelling and distortion of cristae) and signs of irreversible injury (mitochondrial amorphous densities called flocculent densities). The earliest histologic change is the formation of wavy fibers. These wavy fibers result from the pulling of the noncontractile necrotic fibers by adjacent viable fibers. Histologic features of coagulation necrosis are seen at 12 to 24 h. An acute inflammatory response consisting mainly of neutrophils is most pronounced on days 2 to 3, while macrophages predominate during days 4 to 7. The ingrowth of highly vascularized granulation tissue begins around day 7 and is maximal at 2 to 4 weeks. Note that at about days 4 to 10 the infarcted tissue becomes quite soft, and there is a risk of cardiac rupture. These events within the first few weeks are followed by scarring (fibrosis), which is well developed by the sixth week and is irreversible.

163. The answer is d. (*Kumar, pp 578–581. Rubin, pp 557–561.*) Cardiac rupture, whether of free wall, septum, or papillary muscle, occurs in only 1% to 5% of cases following acute MI. It occurs usually within the first week of infarction, when there is maximal necrosis and softening (4 to 5 days) and is very rare after the second week. Rupture of the free wall results in pericardial hemorrhage and cardiac tamponade. Rupture of the interventricular septum causes a left-to-right shunt. Serious mitral valve incompetence results from rupture of anterior or posterior papillary muscles. This valve incompetence can produce signs of mitral regurgitation, including a new pansystolic murmur along with a diastolic flow murmur. Indeed, the onset of a new murmur following a MI should raise the possibility of papillary rupture.

Other common complications of MI include arrhythmias such as heart block, sinus arrhythmias, or ventricular tachycardia or fibrillation. These occur in 90% of complicated cases. Next in importance, but not in frequency (only 10%), is cardiogenic shock from severe left ventricular contractile incompetence. Milder left ventricular failure with lung edema occurs in 60% of these cases, while mural thrombosis with peripheral emboli may occur in up to 40%. Ventricular aneurysm forms a "bulge" of the left ventricular chamber; it consists of scar tissue and does not rupture, but may contain a thrombus. Sudden cardiac death occurs within 2 h in 20% of patients with acute MI.

164. The answer is b. (*Kumar, pp 562–563. Rubin, pp 584–586.*) Cardiac rupture is most frequent at 4 to 7 days post-MI, while fibrinous pericarditis usually develops around day 2 to 3. Pericarditis that develops approximately 1 to 3 weeks following an MI is called Dressler's syndrome. This is an autoimmune disorder. Pericarditis refers to inflammation of the pericardium. Patients develop severe retrosternal chest pain that is typically worse with deep inspiration or coughing. Physical examination reveals the characteristic pericardial friction rub. ECG changes and pulsus paradoxus are also present. Pericarditis developing after a myocardial infarct is usually either serous or serofibrinous. Serous pericarditis contains few inflammatory cells and may also result from uremia or autoimmune diseases such as systemic lupus erythematosus (SLE). Serofibrinous pericarditis has a fibrinous exudate mixed with the serous fluid and may result from uremia or viral infections. Other types of pericarditis include purulent (suppurative) pericarditis with many inflammatory cells (seen with bacterial infections) or hemorrhagic pericarditis (seen with carcinoma or tuberculosis).

165. The answer is d. (*Kumar, pp 560–562, 587–588. Abenhaim, pp 609–616. Connolly, pp 581–588.*) Hypertensive heart disease (HHD) can be divided into systemic HHD and pulmonary HHD. Systemic HHD is the result of systemic hypertension, which causes left ventricular (LV) hypertrophy. There is by definition no other cardiac disease present that could cause LV hypertrophy, such as aortic stenosis. Hypertension is a pressure overload on the heart, and as such it causes concentric LV hypertrophy without dilation. This type of hypertrophy is characterized by a parallel deposition of sarcomeres. Histologic sections may show myocytes with hyperchromatic and rectangular ("box-car") nuclei. In contrast, eccentric hypertrophy is the result of volume overload on the heart. In systemic HHD the LV is stiff, as there is decreased LV compliance.

Pulmonary HHD refers to right ventricular hypertrophy that is the result of pulmonary disease. By definition, this type of heart disease is called cor pulmonale. Pulmonary diseases that can cause cor pulmonale include diseases of the lung parenchyma, such as chronic obstructive pulmonary disease and interstitial fibrosis, and diseases of the pulmonary vessels, such as multiple pulmonary emboli and pulmonary vascular sclerosis. The latter has been associated with the use of the combination of diet drugs fenfluramine and phentermine. (This combination has been referred to as Fen-Phen.)

166. The answer is b. (*Kumar, pp 588–591. McPhee, pp 281–283.*) Aortic stenosis (AS) is usually the result of a bicuspid aortic valve (AV), degenerative calcification of a bicuspid valve, or rheumatic heart disease. Patients with aortic stenosis may present with angina (chest pain), syncopal episodes with exertion, and heart failure. Angina results from the mismatch between increased oxygen demand of the hypertrophied left ventricle (LV) and decreased blood flow, while syncope results from the inability to increase stroke volume as necessary with a stenotic AV. AS is the most common valvular disease that is associated with angina and syncope. The characteristic heart murmur of AS is a crescendo-decrescendo midsystolic ejection murmur that has a paradoxically split S_2. In order to pump the blood into the aorta across a stenotic AV, the pressure in the LV must be much greater than the resultant pressure in the aorta. In order to produce this increased pressure, the LV undergoes concentric hypertrophy, which increases contractility. This concentric hypertrophy also makes the wall of the LV stiffer (decreased compliance). This stiff LV is unable to dilate until the time the LV starts to fail.

167. The answer is e. (*Damjanov, pp 1257–1272. McPhee, pp 283–286.*) Clinical manifestations of aortic regurgitation (AR) include exertional dyspnea, angina, and left ventricular failure. Owing to the rapidly falling arterial pressure during late systole and diastole, there is often wide pulse pressure,

Corrigan's "water-hammer" pulse, capillary pulsations at the nail beds, and a pistol-shot sound over the femoral arteries. A blowing diastolic murmur is heard along the left sternal border. Volume overload of the heart is the basic defect and results in left ventricular dilation and hypertrophy. AR is rheumatic in origin in approximately 70% of cases. Much less frequently it is due to syphilis, ankylosing spondylitis (rarely), infective endocarditis, aortic dissection, or aortic dilation from cystic medial necrosis. Congenital forms of aortic stenosis occur fairly frequently, but AR is rarely congenital in origin.

168. The answer is d. (*Kumar, pp 591–592. McPhee, pp 286–289.*) The normal mitral valve (MV) is a bicuspid valve with the anterior cusp approximately twice the area of the posterior cusp. The MV area is normally 5 to 6 cm². Clinically significant mitral stenosis (MS) usually results when the valve area decreases to less than 1 cm². MS most commonly develops as a consequence of rheumatic heart disease. It may also develop due to congenital abnormalities or calcium deposition. In patients with MS there is decreased flow across the MV due to the stenosis of the valve. In order to move the blood into the left ventricle (LV), the left atrial (LA) pressure during diastole is greater than normal and greater than the LV pressure. Instead of producing changes in the LV, MS causes the left atrium to hypertrophy and dilate. These changes predispose patients with MS to arrhythmias (which are felt as palpitations) and to the development of LA thrombi (which may lead to systemic emboli). The hypertrophied left atrium may also compress the esophagus (resulting in dysphagia, or problems swallowing food) or irritate the recurrent laryngeal nerve (producing hoarseness). The increased LA pressure also causes a mid-diastolic murmur and can be reflected back into the lungs and to the right ventricle. In the lungs this produces venous congestion and hemorrhage, which cause dyspnea, fatigue, and hemoptysis.

169. The answer is c. (*Kumar, pp 592–595. Rubin, pp 566–570.*) Rheumatic fever (RF) is a systemic autoimmune disease that usually develops 10 days to 6 weeks after a pharyngeal infection with group A beta-hemolytic streptococci. This autoimmune disorder results from cross-reactions between cardiac antigens and antibodies evoked by one of the many streptococcal antigens, e.g., streptococcal M protein. Rheumatic fever produces both acute and chronic manifestations. The major findings

[handwritten: characteristic or diagnostic of a specific disease]

of acute RF include migratory polyarthritis of large joints, carditis, erythema marginatum of skin (although skin involvement is not very common), subcutaneous nodules, and Sydenham chorea. The acute cardiac lesions of rheumatic fever (carditis) are characterized by the accumulation of modified tissue monocytes (called Anitschkow myocytes) around areas of fibrinoid necrosis. This entire area is called an Aschoff body. The nuclei of the Anitschkow cells are long, slender, wavy ribbons that resemble a caterpillar (hence the name "caterpillar cells"). Occasional multinucleated giant cells (Aschoff cells) may be seen. The Aschoff body, which is pathognomonic for acute rheumatic fever, may be found in any of the three layers of the heart (pancarditis). In the pericardium, there is a fibrinous pericarditis, which is called a "bread and butter" pericarditis. The endocardial response in acute rheumatic fever is characterized by the formation of small friable vegetations (verrucae) along the lines of closure of the valves.

In contrast, chronic RF mainly produces damage to cardiac valves. The mitral valve is most commonly involved, followed by the aortic valve. The stenotic valve has the appearance of a "fish mouth" or "buttonhole." An additional finding in chronic RF is a rough portion of the endocardium of the left atrium, called a MacCallum's patch.

170. The answer is a. (*Kumar, pp 604, 606–607.*) Arrhythmogenic right ventricular cardiomyopathy or dysplasia (ARVD) is a disorder characterized by an abnormal right ventricle that is dilated and has a thin wall that has been replaced by fat and fibrous tissue. Complications of ARVD include exercise-induced arrhythmias and sudden death. Some cases are related to mutations in the genes coding for either plakoglobin, desmoplakin (DSP), or plakophilin-2 (PKP2). Naxos syndrome (so named because it occurs only on the Greek island Naxos) is a similar disorder that is also associated with abnormalities of the gene coding for plakoglobin (gamma-catenin), an intracellular protein that links adhesion molecules in desmosomes to desmin. The clinical signs of Naxos syndrome are similar to arrhythmogenic RV cardiomyopathy, but hyperkeratoses of the plantar and palmar skin are also present.

Endocardial fibrosis (EF) and Loeffler endomyocarditis (LEM) are two types of restrictive cardiomyopathies that are also associated with fibrosis of the ventricular endocardium. EF is primarily a disease of children and younger adults in tropical areas, while LEM is not restricted to these areas.

[handwritten: site on cell surface used to maintain cohesion w/ an adjacent cell]

In addition, LEM is often associated with an eosinophilic leukemia. It is thought that the release of major basic protein from these neoplastic eosinophils initiates the endocardial damage that leads to fibrosis.

171. The answer is b. (*Kumar, pp 595–598. Chandrasoma, pp 349–353.*) Infective endocarditis is the result of microorganisms growing on any of the heart valves. These organisms may have either high virulence or low virulence. Highly virulent organisms, such as *S. aureus* and group A streptococci, infect previously normal valves and produce severe symptoms within 6 weeks. This abnormality is referred to as acute bacterial endocarditis. In contrast, organisms of low virulence, such as α-hemolytic viridans streptococci and *Staphylococcus epidermidis*, infect previously damaged valves, such as valves damaged by rheumatic fever. These organisms produce symptoms that last longer than 6 weeks. This abnormality is referred to as subacute bacterial endocarditis. Infective endocarditis in IV drug abusers, which normally occurs on the tricuspid valve, is caused by *S. aureus*, group A streptococci, Candida species, and gram-negative bacilli such as *Pseudomonas* species. Symptoms in patients with infective endocarditis are the result of bacteremia, emboli from the vegetations, immune complexes, and valvular disease. Bacteremia produces fever, positive blood cultures (several of which may be needed for confirmation), abscesses, and osteomyelitis. *infection of bone or bone marrow* Embolization of parts of the large, friable vegetations can produce Roth spots in the retina, splinter hemorrhages in nail beds, and infarcts of the brain, heart, and spleen. Splenic infarcts produce left upper quadrant (LUQ) abdominal pain. Immune complexes can deposit in multiple areas of the body and cause glomerulonephritis, vasculitis, tender nodules in the fingers and toes (Osler's nodes), and red papules in the palms and soles (Janeway lesions). Valvular disease can also result in perforation and valvular regurgitation.

172. The answer is e. (*Kumar, pp 603, 607–609. Rubin, pp 575–576.*) Inflammation of the myocardium (myocarditis) has numerous causes, but most of the well-documented cases of myocarditis are of viral origin. The most common viral causes are coxsackieviruses A and B, echovirus, and influenza virus. Patients usually develop symptoms a few weeks after a viral infection. Most patients recover from the acute myocarditis, but a few may die from congestive heart failure or arrhythmias. Sections of the heart show patchy or diffuse interstitial infiltrates composed of T lymphocytes and macrophages. There may be focal or patchy acute myocardial necrosis. Bacterial infections of the myocardium produce multiple foci of inflammation composed mainly of neutrophils. Giant cell myocarditis, which was previously called Fiedler's myocarditis, is characterized by granulomatous inflammation with giant cells and is usually rapidly fatal. In hypersensitivity myocarditis, which is caused by hypersensitivity reactions to several drugs, the inflammatory infiltrate includes many eosinophils, and the infiltrate is both interstitial and perivascular. Beriberi, one of the metabolic diseases of the heart, is a cause of high-output failure and is characterized by decreased peripheral vascular resistance and increased cardiac output. Patients have dilated hearts, but the microscopic changes are nonspecific. Hyperthyroid disease and Paget's disease are other causes of high-output failure.

173. The answer is c. (*Kumar, pp 133, 234, 598–599. Rubin, pp 570–573.*) Plaques or vegetations are found in characteristic locations within the heart in several different disorders. Vegetations can occur in acute rheumatic fever as small masses found in a row along the lines of closure of the valves. In contrast, the vegetations of infective endocarditis are large, irregular masses that extend beyond the valves onto the chordae. Nonbacterial thrombotic (marantic) endocarditis, which is associated with prolonged debilitating diseases and cachexia, may produce one or two small, sterile vegetations at the line of valve closure. In patients with SLE, medium-sized vegetations (Libman-Sacks endocarditis) may occur on either or both sides of the valve leaflets, typically on the mitral valve and the tricuspid valve. The development of Libman-Sacks endocarditis is associated with the presence of the lupus anticoagulant (antiphospholipid syndrome), an antibody that makes platelets "sticky" and increases the chance of thrombosis.

174. The answer is e. (*Kumar, pp 599–600, 866–868.*) White plaques involving the right side of the heart are associated with the carcinoid syndrome. This syndrome is characterized by episodic flushing, diarrhea, bronchospasm, and cyanosis. These symptoms are caused by the release of vasoactive amines, such as serotonin, from carcinoid tumors. These substances are inactivated by enzymes such as monoamine oxidase (MAO) in the liver, lung, and brain. MAO-A degrades norepinephrine and serotonin, while MAO-B degrades dopamine. Cardiac symptoms are found in patients with liver metastases, which bypass the inactivation by the liver itself. The cardiac lesions producing carcinoid heart disease are found on the right side of the heart because these active metabolites are inactivated in the lung. The cardiac lesions consist of fibrous plaques found on the tricuspid and pulmonic valves. Microscopic sections of these plaques reveal smooth-muscle cells and sparse collagen fibers in an acid mucopolysaccharide matrix. Similar lesions can develop with the use of certain diet suppressants or with ergotamine therapy for migraine headaches. Diet suppressants associated with these lesions include dexfenfluramine (Redux) and Fen-Phen (fenfluramine and phentermine). Redux increases serotonin levels by increasing release and decreasing uptake of serotonin in the central nervous system (CNS) (supposedly this increases satiety). Phentermine decreases the appetite center in the brain by increasing norepinephrine levels by increasing the release and decreasing the uptake of norepinephrine.

In contrast to the case with carcinoid heart disease, plaques in the left atrium are seen in chronic rheumatic heart disease and are called MacCallum's patches. Vegetations also occur in rheumatic heart disease; these are small and are found in a row along the lines of closure of the valves. Amyloid deposits may be found in the heart secondary to multiple myeloma or as an isolated event, such as in senile cardiac amyloidosis. Grossly the walls of the heart may be thickened, and there may be multiple small nodules on the left atrial endocardial surface. Iron overload can affect the heart as a result of hereditary hemochromatosis or hemosiderosis. Grossly the heart is a rust-brown color and resembles the heart in idiopathic dilated cardiomyopathy. In hypothyroidism the heart is characteristically flabby, enlarged, and dilated, which results in decreased cardiac output. This reduced circulation results in a characteristic symptom of hypothyroidism, cold sensitivity. Histologically there is an interstitial mucopolysaccharide edema fluid within the heart.

175. The answer is a. (*Kumar, pp 601–604. Rubin, pp 577–579.*) The cardiomyopathies (CMPs) may be classified into primary and secondary forms. The primary forms are mainly idiopathic (unknown cause). Most of the secondary cardiomyopathies result in a dilated cardiomyopathy that is characterized by congestion and four-chamber dilation with hypertrophy. The walls are either of normal thickness or they may be thinner than normal. This results in a flabby, globular, banana-shaped heart that is hypocontracting. The microscopic appearance is not distinctive. The ventricles may contain mural thrombi. The causes of secondary dilated CMP are many and include alcoholism (the most common cause in the United States), metabolic disorders, and toxins. Examples of the latter include cobalt, which has been used in beer as a foam stabilizer; anthracyclines; cocaine; and iron, the deposition of which is seen in patients with hemochromatosis. The anthracycline Adriamycin, which is used in chemotherapy, causes lipid peroxidation of myofiber membranes. One final form of DCM develops in the last trimester of pregnancy or the first 6 months after delivery. About half of these patients recover full cardiac function.

Other forms of cardiomyopathies include a hypertrophic form, a restrictive form, and an obliterative form. In hypertrophic CMP the major gross abnormality is within the interventricular septum, which is usually thicker than the left ventricle. Constrictive (restrictive) CMP is associated with amyloidosis, sarcoidosis, endomyocardial disease, or storage diseases. These abnormalities produce a stiff, hypocontracting heart.

176. The answer is e. (*Kumar, pp 606–607. Rubin, pp 581–583.*) Restrictive (constrictive) cardiomyopathy is associated in the United States with amyloidosis and endocardial fibroelastosis. The latter disorder is so named because of the infiltration and deposition of material in the endomyocardium and the layering of collagen and elastin over the endocardium. This deposition affects the ability of the ventricles to accommodate blood volume during diastole. Grossly this abnormality has a "cream cheese" appearance. Endocardial fibroelastosis occurs mainly in infants during the first 2 years of life; there may be associated aortic coarctation, ventricular septal defects, mitral valve defects, and other abnormalities. In contrast, endomyocardial fibrosis (not fibroelastosis) is a form of restrictive cardiomyopathy that is found mainly in young adults and children in Southeast Asia and Africa. It differs from endocardial fibroelastosis in the United States in that elastic fibers are not present.

177. The answer is b. (*Kumar, pp 604–606. Rubin, pp 579–581.*) The cardiomyopathy shown in the photograph is designated hypertrophic cardiomyopathy with the synonyms of idiopathic hypertrophic subaortic stenosis (IHSS), hypertrophic obstructive cardiomyopathy, and asymmetric septal hypertrophy (ASH). It is characterized by a prominent and hypertrophic interventricular septum that is out of proportion to the thickness of the left ventricle. Histologically the myocardial fibers exhibit disarray, caused by wide fibers with unusual orientation, and prominent hyperchromatic nuclei. There is an increased incidence of hypertrophic cardiomyopathy within families, and there is evidence that it may be an autosomal dominant disorder. The disease is thought to result from a mutation in the cardiac β-myosin heavy-chain gene. (In contrast, an abnormal fibrillin gene is associated with Marfan's syndrome, decreased acid maltase is associated with Pompe's disease, an abnormal dystrophin gene is associated with Duchenne muscular dystrophy, and decreased NADPH oxidase is associated with chronic granulomatous disease.)

Patients with hypertrophic cardiomyopathy may experience dyspnea, light-headedness, and chest pain, especially upon physical exertion; however, many patients appear to be asymptomatic, although sudden, unexpected death occurs not infrequently, especially following or during physical exertion. This risk is increased with factors that either increase the contractility of the heart or decrease the volume of the left ventricle (both of which increase the left ventricular outflow obstruction). Treatment for patients with hypertrophic cardiomyopathy, therefore, is with drugs that decrease contractility. Examples of these types of drugs include beta-adrenergic blockers and calcium channel blockers. In individuals with hypertrophic cardiomyopathy, agents that increase contractility are contraindicated. Examples of these types of drugs include glycosides, such as digitalis. Epinephrine and beta-adrenergic agonists, which increase cardiac output by increasing stroke volume and heart rate, would also be contraindicated. Diuretics would also be dangerous, as they would decrease intravascular volume, and this would accentuate the bad effects of the septal hypertrophy because of the decreased left ventricular volume.

178. The answer is d. (*Kumar, pp 610–613. Rubin, pp 584–585.*) There are several types of pericardial effusions, which refers to the accumulation of excess fluid within the pericardial cavity. Hemopericardium (blood in the pericardial cavity) is most commonly caused by the rupture of a MI. Serous pericardial effusions are caused most often by congestive heart failure, but they can also be caused by renal disease that produces uremia. Serosanguinous effusions are caused by trauma and cardiopulmonary resuscitation (CPR). Chylous effusions are caused by lymphatic obstruction, while cholesterol effusions are seen in patients with myxedema, which is caused by hypothyroidism. Sudden filling of the pericardial space with fluid is called pericardial tamponade. The three classic signs of pericardial tamponade, called Beck's triad, include hypotension, elevated jugular pressure, and muffled heart sounds. The latter is due to the damping effect of the pericardial fluid on the heart sounds. Some patients may also demonstrate a decrease in systemic pressure with inspiration, which is called paradoxic pulse. The decrease in cardiac output produces dyspnea (shortness of breath) and hypotension. Decreased atrial filling results in elevated jugular venous pressure.

179. The answer is d. (*Kumar, pp 613–614. Rubin, pp 583–584.*) Most tumors involving the heart are secondary to metastases, most commonly from bronchogenic carcinoma or breast carcinoma, and they usually involve the pericardium. Primary tumors of the heart are quite rare; the most common in the adult is the myxoma. These tumors occur most often in the left atrium, and if pedunculated they may interfere with the mitral valve by a "ball valve" effect. Histologically they are composed of stellate cells in a loose myxoid background. In contrast, rhabdomyomas are the most common primary cardiac tumors in infants and children and often occur in association with tuberous sclerosis. Histologically, so-called spider cells may be seen. Papillary fibroelastomas usually are incidental lesions found at the time of autopsy and are probably hamartomas rather than true neoplasms.

180. The answer is e. (*Kumar, pp 568–569. Rubin, pp 548–549.*) The tetralogy of Fallot consists of subaortic ventricular septal defect, obstruction to right ventricular outflow, aortic overriding of the ventricular septal defect (aortic dextroposition), and moderate right ventricular hypertrophy. The obstruction to right ventricular outflow may be caused by infundibular stenosis of the right ventricle or stenosis of the pulmonic valve. A right-sided aorta occurs in about 25% of cases with this tetralogy. Most patients are cyanotic from birth or develop cyanosis by the end of the first year of life, since even mild obstruction of right ventricular outflow is progressive. The tetralogy of Fallot is the most common cause of cyanosis after 1 year of age and causes 10% of all forms of congenital heart disease. Hypoxic attacks and syncope are serious complications, forming the most common mode of death from this disease during infancy and childhood. Other complications include infectious endocarditis, paradoxical embolism, polycythemia, and cerebral infarction or abscess.

181. The answer is e. (*Kumar, pp 566–568. Rubin, pp 543–544.*) Ventricular septal defects (VSDs) are the most common congenital cardiac anomaly and can occur anywhere in the intraventricular septum. They are classified according to their location (membranous, infundibular, muscular) or to their size (large, medium, small). Small VSDs (<0.5 cm in diameter) are common and are usually located in the muscular septum. This type of defect, which is called Roger's disease, produces a loud pansystolic murmer but causes little functional disturbances. These defects tend to close as the heart enlarges or the muscle hypertrophies. The clinical effects produced by VSDs range in severity according to the volume of blood that crosses the shunt. Patients with severe cases die secondary to left-sided congestive failure, while smaller shunts increase the risk for endocarditis. Otherwise, the classic signs of a VSD include dyspnea, poor growth (no cyanosis), and pansystolic murmur over left lower sternal border with biventricular hypertrophy.

Note that some congenital heart defects involve shunting of blood between the systemic and pulmonary circulations. These shunts may shunt blood from the left side to the right side, or they shunt the blood from the right side to the left side. VSDs initially involve a left-to-right shunt, from the higher-pressure left side to the lower-pressure right side. This type of shunt, also seen with atrial septal defects, patent ductus arteriosus, and persistent truncus arteriosus, is initially acyanotic. This is in contrast to right-to-left shunts, such as the tetralogy of Fallot, which is initially cyanotic.

182. The answer is d. (*Kumar, pp 564–568. Rubin, pp 544–546.*) Left-to-right congenital shunts are not initially cyanotic, but cyanosis may develop later (tardive cyanosis) if the shunt shifts to a right-to-left shunt due to increased pulmonary vascular resistance (Eisenmenger's complex). Atrial septal defects (ASDs) illustrate this pathophysiologic effect well. The shunt with an ASD is initially left-to-right: left atrium to right atrium to right ventricle to lungs to left atrium. Cyanosis does not occur until later, when the shunt reverses, becoming right-to-left. This occurs because with time the pulmonary vessels become hyperplastic and irreversible pulmonary hypertension develops because of the volume overload to the lungs. The blood flow with an ASD that has reversed due to Eisenmenger's complex is right atrium to left atrium (e.g., right-to-left) to left ventricle to aorta and then back to right atrium. An ASD with elevated pulmonary pressures allows emboli to enter the systemic circulation directly (paradoxical embolus). Note that ASDs are the most common type of congenital heart disease that presents in adults; these individuals develop palpitations, exertional dyspnea, systolic flow murmurs, widely split fixed S_2, and right axis deviation.

183. The answer is a. (*Kumar, pp 569–570. Rubin, p 549.*) As the endocardial cushions join to divide the ventricles, the streams of blood from the right and left ventricles are divided as they flow out of the truncus. A spiral septum develops to physically separate the two streams of blood. The fusion of the spiral ridges results in division of the truncus into the pulmonary and aortic arteries. Occasionally the spiral is reversed, resulting in the aorta arising from the right ventricle and the pulmonary artery from the left. This is a complete transposition of the great vessels and produces two completely separate blood systems. This situation obviously is incompatible with life unless some type of mixing of blood can occur between these separate systems. In utero, mixing of blood occurs across the atrial septum and in connections with the placental circulation. Cases that survive to corrective surgery must have a persistent atrial septal defect or patent ductus arteriosus to allow mixing of blood. Therefore, clinical consideration should be to keep the ductus arteriosus open. Usually, at birth, breathing decreases pulmonary resistance and this then reverses flow through the ductus arteriosus. This oxygenated blood (flowing from the aorta into the ductus) inhibits prostaglandin production, which in turn closes the ductus arteriosus. To keep the ductus arteriosus open, prostaglandin E_2 should be given.

Hematology

Questions

DIRECTIONS: Each item below contains a question or incomplete statement followed by suggested responses. Select the **one best** response to each question.

184. A 59-year-old man with a history of coronary artery disease and severe mitral regurgitation has surgery to replace his mitral valve. Postoperatively there were no complications until 6 months after the surgery when he presented with increasing fatigue. Workup finds a normocytic normochromic anemia that is due to fragmentation of red blood cells by his artificial heart valve. Which of the following red cell abnormalities is most indicative of intravascular hemolysis and is most likely to be seen when examining a peripheral blood smear from this patient?

a. Drepanocytes
b. Heinz bodies
c. Pappenheimer bodies
d. Schistocytes
e. Target cells

185. A 51-year-old woman living on Martha's Vineyard off the coast of New England presents with fever and chills, fatigue, malaise, and dark, tea-colored urine. She had a splenectomy when she was 23 years of age due to a motor vehicle accident. Examination of a peripheral blood smear finds intracellular ring forms in erythrocytes. Urinalysis documents the presence of hemoglobinuria, most likely the result of intravascular hemolysis. Markedly decreased blood levels of which of the following substances is the best indicator of free hemoglobin being released into her serum?

a. Alkaline phosphatase
b. Direct bilirubin
c. Haptoglobin
d. Lactate dehydrogenase
e. Myoglobin

186. A 24-year-old man presents with signs and symptoms of mild anemia. Physical examination finds a mildly enlarged spleen. Laboratory examination reveals normal liver serum enzyme levels and a negative direct antiglobulin test. His red blood cells, however, have an abnormal osmotic fragility test, as seen in the associated picture. The shaded area depicts the results of normal red blood cells, while the dashed curve is the result obtained from this man's red blood cells. These results are most commonly caused by an abnormality involving which one of the following substances?

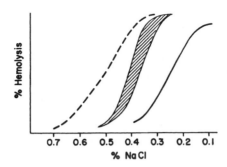

a. Ankyrin
b. Dystrophin
c. Fibrillin
d. Frataxin
e. Merlin

187. Two days after receiving the antimalarial drug primaquine, a 27-year-old African American man develops sudden intravascular hemolysis resulting in a decreased hematocrit, hemoglobinemia, and hemoglobinuria. Examination of the peripheral blood reveals erythrocytes with a membrane defect forming "bite" cells; when crystal violet stain is applied, many Heinz bodies are seen. Which of the following is the most likely diagnosis?

a. Hereditary spherocytosis
b. Glucose-6-phosphate dehydrogenase deficiency
c. Paroxysmal nocturnal hemoglobinuria
d. Autoimmune hemolytic anemia
e. Microangiopathic hemolytic anemia

188. A 7-year-old African American boy presents with a nonhealing ulcer of his left foot. He has a medical history of recurrent infections, several episodes of severe abdominal pain, and a chronic hemolytic anemia. Examination of his peripheral blood reveals abnormal-shaped erythrocytes along with target cells and an occasional Howell-Jolly body. Laboratory examination finds increased amounts of an abnormal hemoglobin in his peripheral blood. Which of the following is the basic defect causing this disorder?

a. A single nucleotide change in a codon
b. A trisomy involving an autosomal chromosome
c. Autoantibodies to red blood cell membrane antigens
d. Expansion of a trinucleotide repeat
e. Genetic imprinting of an autosomal chromosome

189. A 65-year-old woman presents with increasing fatigue and shortness of breath. Physical examination finds decreased vibratory sensation in her lower extremities. Laboratory examination finds pancytopenia while hypersegmented neutrophils and oval macrocytes are seen in her peripheral smear. A gastric biopsy reveals atrophy of the gastric epithelium with numerous chronic inflammatory cells. Neutrophils are not present. Which one of the listed laboratory tests would best help to identify the etiology of her peripheral blood abnormalities?

a. Coombs' test
b. Metabisulfite test
c. Osmotic fragility test
d. Schilling test
e. Sucrose hemolysis test

190. A couple is being evaluated for possible hematologic problems after the mother delivered a stillborn infant at 25 weeks of gestation. A Coombs' test was also performed on cord blood and the mother's blood and was negative on both specimens. The parents, both of whom are Vietnamese and 21 years of age, are found to have mild microcytic anemias with normal serum iron levels. Further workup finds that each parent has α–thalassemia trait, due to the deletion of two α-globin genes on one chromosome 16 (the other chromosome 16 being normal with two α-globin genes). Inheritance of the abnormal chromosome 16 from each parent in a subsequent pregnancy would most likely produce which one of the following disorders?

a. Cooley's anemia
b. Fanconi anemia
c. Hemoglobin H disease
d. Hemolytic disease of the newborn
e. Hydrops fetalis

191. Hemoglobin electrophoresis of the blood from an individual with Cooley's anemia (β–thalassemia major) would most likely show which one of the following combinations of findings?

	Hemoglobin A	Hemoglobin A2	Hemoglobin F
a.	Increased	Increased	Increased
b.	Increased	Increased	Decreased
c.	Increased	Decreased	Increased
d.	Decreased	Increased	Increased
e.	Decreased	Decreased	Decreased

192. A 49-year-old woman presents with signs of anemia and states that every morning her urine is dark. Laboratory studies find anemia, leukopenia, and thrombocytopenia. A bone marrow biopsy is unremarkable, and no morphologic abnormalities of blood cells are seen on the peripheral smear. A Coombs' test is negative, but a Ham's test and sucrose lysis test on erythrocytes is positive. What is the basic abnormality that caused this woman's disease?

a. Deficiency of CD22
b. Mutations involving AIRE-1
c. Mutations involving phosphatidyl glycan A
d. Presence of anti-P antibodies
e. Presence of autoantibodies against red blood cells

193. A 32-year-old woman who has recently started taking α-methyldopa develops dark, tea-colored urine. Physical examination reveals mild scleral icterus, a low-grade fever, and mild hepatosplenomegaly. Examination of her peripheral blood reveals many microspherocytes, while laboratory examination finds a positive Coombs' test. Which of the following is the basic pathomechanism that caused this individual's signs and symptoms?

a. Autoimmune destruction of red blood cells in the spleen
b. Drug-induced destruction of red blood cell precursors in the bone marrow
c. Hyperimmune destruction of neutrophils in the liver
d. Immune complex deposition in the capillaries of the kidneys
e. Isoimmune destruction of red blood cells in the peripheral blood

194. A 25-year-old woman presents with the new onset of severe intermittent pain in her fingers that developed shortly after she recovered from mycoplasma pneumonia. She states the pain occurs when she goes outside in the cold, at which time her fingers turn white and then become numb. Laboratory evaluation finds the presence of an IgM autoantibody that is directed against the I-antigen found on the surface of her red blood cells. Based on these clinical findings, the diagnosis of Raynaud's phenomenon is made. Which of the following disorders is most likely present in this individual?

a. Cold autoimmune hemolytic anemia
b. Isoimmune hemolytic anemia
c. Paroxysmal cold hemoglobinuria
d. Paroxysmal nocturnal hemoglobinuria
e. Warm autoimmune hemolytic anemia

195. A 67-year-old man presents with increasing fatigue and is found to be anemic. Physical examination reveals a hard 1-cm nodule in the left lobe of the prostate. The prostatic-specific antigen (PSA) level is found to be elevated. Examination of the peripheral blood reveals an occasional myelocyte. The erythrocytes are mainly normochromic and normocytic, and teardrop RBCs are not found. There are, however, about two nucleated red blood cells per 100 white cells. Which of the following is the most likely diagnosis?

a. Fanconi anemia
b. Microangiopathic hemolytic anemia
c. Myelophthisic anemia
d. Autoimmune hemolytic anemia
e. Aplastic anemia

196. A 41-year-old woman presents with increasing fatigue, lethargy, and muscle weakness. Her CBC reveals decreased numbers of erythrocytes, leukocytes, and platelets along with an increase in the MCV of the erythrocytes. The associated picture is from a smear of her peripheral blood. Which of the following substances is most likely to be deficient in this individual?

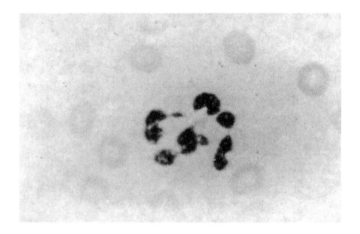

a. Aminolevulinic acid
b. Ascorbic acid
c. Folic acid
d. Retinoic acid
e. Vanillylmandelic acid

197. A 45-year-old woman presents with increasing fatigue, weakness, and tingling of her arms and legs. Physical examination finds numbness and loss of balance, position, and vibratory sense in both of her lower extremities. Histologic examination of a smear made from a bone marrow aspiration reveals asynchrony in red blood cell precursors between the maturation of their nuclei and their cytoplasm. Additional workup discovers achlorhydria, and a biopsy of the antrum of her stomach reveals chronic atrophic gastritis. Which of the following is the most likely diagnosis?

a. Fanconi anemia
b. Leukoerythroblastic anemia
c. Megaloblastic anemia
d. Myelophthisic anemia
e. Sideroblastic anemia

198. A 61-year-old woman presents with increasing fatigue and is found to have hypochromic microcytic red cells in her peripheral smear. Physical examination finds her heart rate and respiratory rate to both be increased in frequency. A bone marrow biopsy stained with a Prussian blue stain reveals absent stainable iron. Which one of the listed sets of laboratory values is most likely to be found in this individual?

	Serum ferritin	Serum iron-binding capacity	Free erythrocyte porphyrin
a.	increased	increased	increased
b.	decreased	increased	increased
c.	decreased	decreased	increased
d.	decreased	decreased	decreased
e.	increased	decreased	decreased

199. An anemic patient has the following red cell indexes: mean corpuscular volume, 70 mm³; mean corpuscular hemoglobin, 22 pg; and mean corpuscular hemoglobin concentration, 34%. Based on these laboratory findings, which of the following is the most likely diagnosis?

a. Folic acid deficiency anemia
b. Iron-deficiency anemia
c. Pernicious anemia
d. Sideroblastic anemia
e. Thalassemia minor

200. An anemic patient is found to have hypochromic, microcytic red cells. Additional tests reveal the serum iron levels, the total iron-binding capacity, and the transferrin saturation to be reduced. A bone marrow biopsy reveals the iron to be present mainly within macrophages. Which of the following is the most likely diagnosis?

a. Iron deficiency
b. Thalassemia trait
c. Anemia of chronic disease
d. Sideroblastic anemia
e. Pernicious anemia

201. A 25-year-old man presents because of a recurrent rash on the sun-exposed areas of his face and arms. He has recently moved to the United States from South Africa, where he has lived all of his life. He states that he has always been sensitive to the light and he says that his face will break out in a rash if he stays in the sun too long. He notes that sometimes alcohol ingestion will make these episodes worse. Pertinent medical history includes episodes of neuropsychiatric changes, including hallucinations and manic-depressive episodes. Physical examination reveals multiple fluid-filled vesicles and bullae on his face and forearms. Laboratory examination reveals elevated levels of delta-aminolevulinic acid and porphobilinogen in the urine. This individual's disorder results from the abnormal synthesis of which one of the following substances?

a. Globin
b. Heme
c. Immunoglobulin
d. Spectrin
e. Transferrin

202. Medical evaluation of a 55-year-old man finds the following laboratory data: increased hematocrit, increased RBC count, and increased serum erythropoietin. Which of the following abnormalities is most likely to be present in this individual?

a. Acute gastroenteritis
b. Pancreatic adenocarcinoma
c. Polycythemia rubra vera
d. Porphyria cutanea tarda
e. Renal cell carcinoma

203. An 8-year-old girl presents with fever and a rash on her legs that developed approximately 2 weeks after she recovered from a sore throat. During this time she also had intermittent pain in her abdomen and her knees and ankles. Physical examination finds multiple palpable hemorrhagic lesions on her legs each measuring about 5 mm in diameter. These lesions do not blanch when pressure is applied. Laboratory examination finds an elevated erythrocyte sedimentation rate. Which one of the following statements best describes the skin lesions in this girl?

a. Bleeding secondary to nutritional deficiency
b. Erythema secondary to active hyperemia
c. Hemorrhage secondary to hypersensitivity vasculitis
d. Telangiectasis secondary to a drug reaction
e. Thrombosis secondary to viral infection

204. A 24-year-old woman presents with multiple pinpoint bleeding spots on both of her legs. She is not currently taking any medications. Physical examination reveals multiple, nonpalpable petechiae on her legs. No enlarged lymph nodes are found, and neither her liver nor the spleen is enlarged. A bone marrow biopsy reveals a normocellular marrow with increased numbers of megakaryocytes, some of which are slightly immature in appearance. What is the correct diagnosis?

a. Disseminated intravascular coagulopathy
b. Immune thrombocytopenic purpura
c. Thrombocytopenia with absent radii
d. Thrombotic thrombocytopenic purpura
e. Waterhouse-Friderichsen syndrome

205. A 37-year-old woman who has a clinical picture of fever, splenomegaly, varying neurologic manifestations, and petechial hemorrhages of her skin is found to have a hemoglobin level of 10.0 g/dL, a mean cell hemoglobin concentration (MCHC) of 48, peripheral blood polychromasia with stippled macrocytes, and schistocytes, with a blood urea nitrogen level of 68 mg/dL. The findings of coagulation studies and the patient's fibrin-degradation products are within normal limits. What is the most likely etiology of this woman's disease?

a. Antibodies to GpIIb/IIIa
b. Antibodies to platelet factor 4
c. Deficiency of ADAMTS 13
d. Infection with *E. coli* strain 0157:H7
e. Mutations in the Tyrp1 gene

206. A 5-year-old child develops the sudden onset of bloody diarrhea, vomiting of blood, hematuria, and renal failure following a flulike gastrointestinal illness. The blood urea nitrogen (BUN) level is markedly increased, but fibrin degradation products and blood clotting times are within normal limits. A peripheral blood smear reveals poikilocytes, schistocytes, and a decrease in the number of platelets. No fever or neurologic symptoms are present. Which of the following is the most likely diagnosis?

a. Autoimmune thrombocytopenic purpura (autoimmune ITP)
b. Disseminated intravascular coagulopathy (DIC)
c. Hemolytic-uremic syndrome (HUS)
d. Isoimmune thrombocytopenic purpura (isoimmune ITP)
e. Thrombotic thrombocytopenic purpura (TTP)

207. A 20-year-old woman presents with excess menstrual bleeding. She has a history of easy bruising and recurrent nosebleeds. Physical examination is essentially unremarkable. No abnormalities involving her joints are found. Laboratory examination reveals a prolonged bleeding time and a slightly prolonged partial thromboplastin time. Quantitative levels of factor VIII and von Willebrand's factor are both decreased. Her platelet count is normal and her platelets are normal in appearance. Which of the following laboratory findings is most likely to be present in this individual?

a. Decreased platelet response to ristocetin
b. Decreased fibrin precipitation with protamine sulfate
c. Increased D-dimer amounts in the serum
d. Increased fibrin incorporation into ethanol gelatin
e. Increased platelet aggregation with collagen

208. A 4-year-old boy is being evaluated for recurrent epistaxis and other abnormal bleeding episodes, including excessive bleeding from the umbilical cord at birth. Laboratory studies reveal the following: decreased hemoglobin (with microcytic hypochromic red cell indices), normal platelet count, normal prothrombin time (PT), and normal partial thromboplastin time (PTT). Platelet aggregation studies reveal a normal platelet response to ristocetin, but with other substances (including collagen, ADP, and epinephrine), this patient's platelets exhibit a primary wave defect. Based on these findings, which of the following is the most likely diagnosis?

a. Afibrinogenemia
b. Bernard-Soulier syndrome
c. Glanzmann's thrombasthenia
d. Gray platelet syndrome
e. Wiskott-Aldrich syndrome

209. A 31-year-old woman presents with the acute onset of pain and swelling in the lower portion of her left leg. An ultrasound of this area finds venous thrombosis, and further laboratory evaluation discovers the presence of the Leiden mutation. This abnormality involves which one of the listed substances?

a. Factor V
b. Factor X
c. Fibrinogen
d. Plasmin
e. Prothrombin

210. A 6-year-old boy whose factor VIII activity is less than 10% of normal is most at risk for developing which one of the following clinical signs?

a. Diffuse petechiae
b. Hemorrhagic urticaria
c. Intramuscular hematomas
d. Perifollicular hemorrhages
e. Small ecchymoses

211. A 27-year-old woman in the last trimester of her first pregnancy presents with the sudden onset of multiple skin hemorrhages. She states that for the past several days she has not felt the baby move. Workup reveals an increase in PT and PTT, while fibrin degradation products (FDPs) are increased in the patient's blood. Her platelet count is found to be 43,000/μL. Which of the following is the most likely diagnosis?

a. Autoimmune thrombocytopenic purpura (autoimmune ITP)
b. Isoimmune thrombocytopenic purpura (isoimmune ITP)
c. Thrombotic thrombocytopenic purpura (TTP)
d. Hemolytic-uremic syndrome (HUS)
e. Disseminated intravascular coagulopathy (DIC)

212. A 45-year-old man with an artificial heart valve is given oral Coumadin (warfarin) to prevent the formation of thrombi on his artificial valve. Which combination of laboratory results is most likely to be associated with this individual?

	Tourniquet Test	Bleeding Time	Platelet Count	PTT	PT
a.	Positive	Prolonged	Normal	Normal	Normal
b.	Normal	Normal	Normal	Prolonged	Normal
c.	Positive	Prolonged	Decreased	Normal	Normal
d.	Normal	Normal	Normal	Normal	Prolonged
e.	Normal	Prolonged	Normal	Prolonged	Normal

213. A person taking an oral sulfonamide is found to have a markedly decreased peripheral blood neutrophil count, but the numbers of platelets and erythrocytes are normal. Further workup finds this peripheral neutropenia to result from the presence of antineutrophil antibodies. Which of the following clinical findings is most likely to be present in this person?

a. An atrophic spleen
b. Decreased vitamin B_{12} levels
c. Hypoplasia of the bone marrow myeloid series
d. Hyperplasia of the bone marrow myeloid series
e. A monoclonal large granular lymphocyte proliferation in the peripheral blood

214. A 28-year-old man presents with vague muscle pain involving his right arm that developed several weeks after eating undercooked pork. Laboratory examination reveals increased serum activity of CPK. A biopsy from the affected muscle reveals rare encysted forms of *Trichinella spiralis*. What type of white blood cell is most likely to be increased in numbers in the peripheral blood of this individual?

a. Basophil
b. Eosinophil
c. Macrophage
d. Neutrophil
e. Lymphocyte

215. A 5-year-old girl presents with a several day history of localized swelling in the right side of her neck. There is no recent history of sore throat. Physical examination finds a low-grade fever, and one very tender, firm, slightly enlarged lymph node is palpated in the right cervical region. A CBC reveals a mild leukocytosis. A fine needle aspiration of the lymph node reveals scattered neutrophils. Which of the following is the most likely diagnosis?

a. Bacterial lymphadenitis
b. Granulomatous lymphadenitis
c. Necrotizing lymphadenitis
d. Toxoplasmic lymphadenitis
e. Tuberculous lymphadenitis

216. A 21-year-old man presents with a 5-day history of malaise, sore throat, and fever. Physical examination finds bilateral cervical lymphadenopathy. Examination of the peripheral blood reveals the presence of atypical lymphocytes with abundant cytoplasm. A monospot test is positive. What histologic change would most likely be seen in a biopsy taken from one of his enlarged lymph nodes?

a. Follicular hyperplasia due to a reactive proliferation of B lymphocytes
b. Interfollicular hyperplasia due to a reactive proliferation of T immunoblasts
c. Nodular hyperplasia due to a neoplastic proliferation of monocytoid B cells
d. Paracortical hyperplasia due to a neoplastic proliferation of T immunoblasts
e. Paracortical hyperplasia due to a reactive proliferation of T lymphocytes

217. A 65-year-old man presents with several enlarged lymph nodes in his left supraclavicular region. Physical examination reveals painless lymphadenopathy in this region. No other abnormalities are found. A biopsy from one of these enlarged lymph nodes, which is shown in the associated picture, reveals effacement of the normal lymph node architecture by numerous nodules of uniform size that are found crowded within the cortex and medulla of the lymph node. Tingible-body macrophages are not seen in these nodules. Which one of the listed chromosomal translocations is most closely associated with this type of lymphoma?

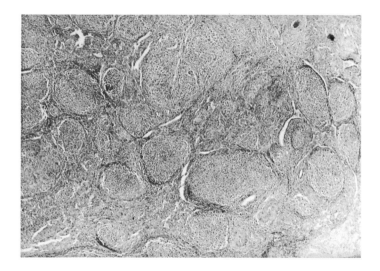

a. t(2;8)
b. t(8;22)
c. t(9;14)
d. t(11;14)
e. t(14;18)

218. A 60-year-old man presents with several enlarged lymph nodes involving his right axilla. A biopsy from one of these enlarged lymph nodes reveals effacement of the normal lymph node architecture by a diffuse proliferation of small, normal-appearing lymphocytes. These same cells are present in the peripheral blood, enough to cause a peripheral lymphocytosis. A bone marrow biopsy reveals a diffuse proliferation of these small lymphocytes. Special stains reveal these cells to be positive for CD5 and CD23. Which of the following is the best classification for this type of lymphoma?

a. A high grade non-Hodgkin's lymphoma (using the Working Formulation)
b. A low grade non-Hodgkin's lymphoma (using the Working Formulation)
c. A precursor B-cell neoplasm (using the REAL classification)
d. A peripheral T-cell neoplasm (using the REAL classification)
e. A poorly differentiated lymphoma (using the Working Formulation)

219. A 66-year-old man presents for his annual physical examination. He is asymptomatic and physical examination is unremarkable. Examination of his peripheral smear, however, reveals the presence of small mononuclear cells with little cytoplasm and a mature nucleus with a prominent nuclear cleft. No "smudge cells" are seen. The presence of these "buttock cells" in the peripheral blood warrants further clinical workup to search for which one of the following malignancies?

a. Chronic lymphocytic leukemia
b. Follicular non-Hodgkin's lymphoma
c. Multiple myeloma
d. Nodular sclerosis Hodgkin's disease
e. Small-cell carcinoma of the lung

220. An 8-year-old African girl develops a rapidly enlarging mass that involves a large portion of the right side of her maxilla. A smear made from an incisional biopsy of this mass reveals malignant cells with cytoplasmic vacuoles that stain positively with oil red O. Histologic sections from this biopsy reveal a diffuse, monotonous proliferation of small, noncleaved lymphocytes. In the background are numerous tingible-body macrophages that impart a "starry-sky" appearance to the slide. Which of the following viruses is most closely associated with this malignancy?

a. Cytomegalovirus (CMV)
b. Epstein-Barr virus (EBV)
c. Herpes simplex virus (HSV)
d. Human immunodeficiency virus (HIV)
e. Human papillomavirus (HPV)

221. A 20-year-old man presents in the emergency room with respiratory distress resulting from a lymphoma involving his mediastinum. These malignant lymphocytes most likely have cell surface markers characteristic of what type of cell?

a. B lymphocytes
b. T lymphocytes
c. Macrophages
d. Dendritic reticulum cells
e. Langerhans cells

222. A 22-year-old woman presents with fever, weight loss, night sweats, and painless enlargement of several supraclavicular lymph nodes. A biopsy from one of the enlarged lymph nodes is shown in the photomicrograph below. The binucleate giant cell with prominent acidophilic "owl-eye" nucleoli shown stains positively with both CD15 and CD30 immunoperoxidase stains. Also present are atypical mononuclear cells that are surrounded by clear spaces (lacunar cells). Which of the following is the most likely diagnosis?

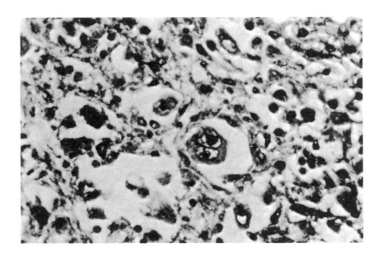

   a. Anaplastic large cell lymphoma
   b. Diffuse non-Hodgkin's lymphoma
   c. Lymphocyte predominate Hodgkin's disease
   d. Nodular sclerosis Hodgkin's disease
   e. Reactive lymph node hyperplasia

223. A 28-year-old man presents with widespread ecchymoses and bleeding gums. Physical examination reveals enlargement of his spleen and liver. Laboratory examination of his peripheral blood reveals a normochromic, normocytic anemia, along with a decreased number of platelets and an increased number of white blood cells. Coagulation studies reveal prolonged prothrombin and partial thromboplastin times and increased fibrinogen degradation products. Examination of the patient's bone marrow reveals the presence of numerous granular-appearing blast cells with numerous Auer rods. These immature cells make up about 38% of the nucleated cells in the marrow. Which of the following is the most likely diagnosis?

a. Acute erythroid leukemia
b. Acute lymphoblastic leukemia
c. Acute monocytic leukemia
d. Acute myelomonocytic leukemia
e. Acute promyelocytic leukemia

224. A 4-year-old girl is being evaluated for the sudden onset of multiple petechiae and bruises. She is found to have a peripheral leukocyte count of 55,000, 86% of which are small, homogeneous cells that have nuclei with immature chromatin. Indistinct nucleoli are also present. Initial tests on these immature cells are as follows: TdT, positive; PAS, positive; acid phosphatase, positive; and myeloperoxidase, negative. Based on these findings, which of the following is the cell of origin of these immature cells?

a. Myeloblasts
b. Monoblasts
c. Megakaryoblasts
d. Lymphoblasts
e. Erythroblasts

225. A 38-year-old man presents with increasing weakness and is found to have a markedly elevated peripheral leukocyte count. Laboratory testing on peripheral blood finds a decreased leukocyte alkaline phosphatase (LAP) score, while chromosomal studies on a bone marrow aspirate find the presence of a Philadelphia chromosome. This abnormality refers to a characteristic chromosomal translocation that involves which oncogene?

a. *bcl-2*
b. *c-abl*
c. *c-myc*
d. *erb*-B
e. N-*myc*

226. A 64-year-old man is being evaluated for pancytopenia. Clinical examination reveals a marked increase in the size of his spleen. A bone marrow biopsy histologically reveals replacement of the normal marrow cells by a diffuse proliferation of small mononuclear cells. There is a clear space around each of these abnormal cells ("fried egg" appearance). These cells stained positively for cytoplasmic acid phosphatase and this staining was not inhibited by treatment with tartrate. A bone marrow aspiration did not reveal any marrow particles. Although his peripheral leukocyte count was decreased, the majority of the cells were lymphocytes. Which of the following is the expected histologic appearance of these lymphocytes?

a. "Cerebriform" lymphocytes
b. "Chicken-footprint" lymphocytes
c. "Cloverleaf" lymphocytes
d. "Hairy" lymphocytes
e. "Smudge" lymphocytes

227. A 72-year-old man presents with increasing fatigue. Physical examination reveals an elderly man in no apparent distress (NAD). He is found to have multiple enlarged, nontender lymph nodes along with an enlarged liver and spleen. Laboratory examination of his peripheral blood reveals a normocytic normochromic anemia, a slightly decreased platelet count, and a leukocyte count of 72,000 cells/μL. An example of his peripheral blood is seen in the picture below. Which of the following is the most likely diagnosis?

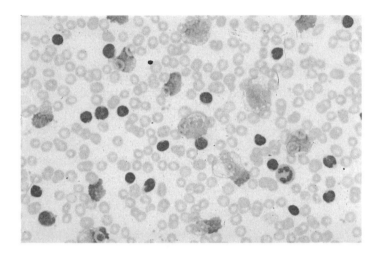

a. Acute lymphoblastic leukemia
b. Atypical lymphocytosis
c. Chronic lymphocytic leukemia
d. Immunoblastic lymphoma
e. Prolymphocytic leukemia

228. A 65-year-old man presents with increasing fatigue and shortness of breath. Examination of his peripheral blood finds pancytopenia, and a few (less than 5%) immature cells are present. Some of the neutrophils are bilobed (Pelger-Huët change) and a dimorphic red blood cell population is seen. A bone marrow biopsy reveals a hypercellular marrow with about 15% of the cells being immature cells. Approximately 20% of the red cell precursors have iron deposits that encircled the nucleus. Which of the following is the most likely cause of these clinical findings?

a. Chronic blood loss
b. Iron deficiency
c. Lead poisoning
d. Myelodysplasia
e. Vitamin B$_{12}$ deficiency

229. Which one of the labeled boxes in the diagram below is most consistent with the expected findings for an individual with polycythemia rubra vera?

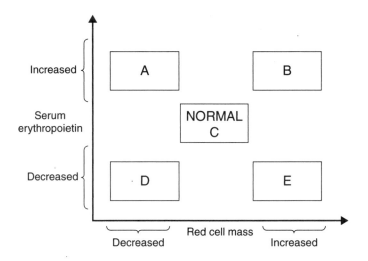

a. Box A
b. Box B
c. Box C
d. Box D
e. Box E

230. A 59-year-old woman presents with increasing fatigue and left-side upper abdominal pain. Physical examination reveals a markedly enlarged spleen. No enlarged lymph nodes are found. A CBC reveals a normocytic normochromic anemia. Myelocytes, nucleated red blood cells, and teardrop-shaped red blood cells are seen in the peripheral smear. A bone marrow aspiration could not be performed due to a "dry tap." The bone marrow biopsy specimen revealed a hypocellular marrow as shown in the picture below. Marrow reticulin was markedly increased in amount. The peripheral leukocyte alkaline phosphatase score was within normal limits. Which of the following clinical findings is most likely to be present in this individual?

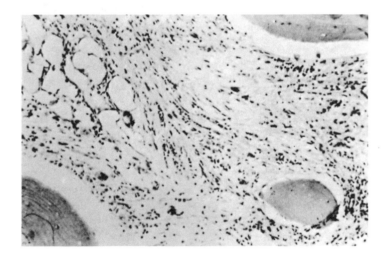

a. Extramedullary hematopoiesis in the spleen
b. Increased total protein in the serum
c. Multiple black stones in the gallbladder ·
d. Multiple lytic lesions in the skull
e. Sequestration of neutrophils in the liver

231. A 70-year-old man presents with increasing weakness and weight loss. Laboratory findings include anemia, hypercalcemia, and increased serum protein. A photomicrograph of the bone marrow aspirate is shown below. Which of the following histologic findings is present in this photomicrograph?

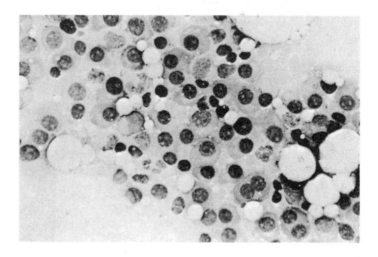

a. Accumulation of glycogen in histiocytes, as seen with Gaucher disease
b. Decreased numbers of myeloid precursors, as seen with aplastic anemia
c. Increased numbers of myeloblasts, as seen in acute myelocytic leukemia
d. Increased numbers of plasma cells, as seen in multiple myeloma
e. Numerous inclusions in erythroid precursors, as seen with parvovirus infection

232. A 54-year-old woman presents with headaches, visual abnormalities, bleeding, and Raynaud's phenomenon. Workup reveals a normal serum calcium, and no lytic lesions are found within the skeleton by x-ray. Serum electrophoresis reveals a single large M spike in the peripheral blood due to a monoclonal proliferation of IgM. Sections from the patient's bone marrow reveal numerous plasma cells, lymphocytes, and plasmacytoid lymphocytes. Which of the following is the most likely diagnosis?

a. IgM multiple myeloma
b. Monoclonal gammopathy of undetermined significance
c. mu heavy-chain disease
d. Plasmacytoid small-cell lymphoma
e. Waldenström's macroglobulinemia

233. A 5-year-old girl is brought to your office by her mother, who states that the girl has been drinking a lot of water lately. Physical examination reveals a young girl whose eyes protrude slightly. Further workup reveals the presence of multiple lytic bone lesions involving her calvarium and the base of her skull. Which of the following is the most likely diagnosis?

a. Letterer-Siwe disease
b. Hand-Schüller-Christian disease
c. Dermatopathic lymphadenopathy
d. Unifocal Langerhans cell histiocytosis
e. Sarcoidosis

234. A 20-year-old woman presents with a 5-day history of fatigue, low-grade fever, and sore throat. Physical examination reveals bilateral enlarged, tender cervical lymph nodes, an exudative tonsillitis, and an enlarged spleen. A complete blood cell count reveals the hemoglobin and platelet counts to be within normal limits. The total white blood cell count is increased to 9200 cells/μL. Examination of the peripheral blood reveals the presence of atypical mononuclear cells with abundant cytoplasm. These cells have peripheral condensation of the cytoplasm, which gives them a "ballerina skirt" appearance. Which of the following laboratory findings is most likely to be present in this individual?

a. Aggregates of mononuclear cells with cytoplasmic Birbeck granules in the liver
b. Elevated levels of delta-ALA in the urine
c. Group A streptococcus in cultures from the tonsillar exudate
d. Heterophil antibodies in the serum
e. M spike in the gamma region of a serum protein electrophoresis

Hematology

Answers

184. The answer is d. (*Henry, pp 505–508.*) Abnormalities of red cells can help to identify the disease process that is present. Schistocytes, which are red cell fragments, indicate the presence of hemolysis, and they can be seen with hemolytic anemia, megaloblastic anemia, or severe burns. Other red cell shapes characteristic of hemolysis include triangular cells and helmet cells. Acanthocytes and echinocytes are considered by some to be fragmented red blood cells. Acanthocytes are irregularly spiculated red cells found in patients with abetalipoproteinemia or liver disease. Echinocytes, in contrast, have regular spicules (undulations) and may either be artifacts (crenated cells) or be found in hyperosmolar diseases such as uremia.

In contrast, drepanocytes are sickle cells, while target cells (red cells with a central dark area) are called dacrocytes. These cells are the result of excess cytoplasmic membrane material and are found in patients with liver disease, such as obstructive jaundice, or in any of the hypochromic anemias. Pappenheimer bodies are red cell inclusions composed of iron, while Heinz bodies are formed by denatured hemoglobin. The latter, which are not seen with routine stains, are found in patients with glucose-6-phosphatase dehydrogenase deficiency and the unstable hemoglobinopathies.

185. The answer is c. (*Kumar, pp 624–625. Hoffman, p 408. Mandell, pp 2899–2902.*) Babesiosis, which is caused by *B. microti*, infects individuals living on islands off the New England coast, such as Martha's Vineyard. Patients develop the sudden onset of chills and fever due to destruction of erythrocytes. The disease is usually self-limited, but patients may develop hemoglobinemia, hemoglobinuria, and renal failure from the destruction of red cells (hemolysis). Recall that hemolysis may occur within the vascular compartment (intravascular hemolysis) or within the mononuclear-phagocyte system (extravascular hemolysis). In both cases, the hemolysis leads to anemia, and the breakdown of hemoglobin leads to jaundice due to increased indirect bilirubin. Intravascular hemolysis releases hemoglobin into the blood (hemoglobinemia); this hemoglobin then binds to haptoglobin. When haptoglobin levels are depleted, free hemoglobin is oxidized to methemoglobin, and then both hemoglobin and methemoglobin are secreted into the urine (hemoglobinuria and methemoglobinuria). Within the renal tubular epithelial cells, hemoglobin is reabsorbed and hemosiderin is formed; when these cells are shed into the urine, hemosiderinuria results. Since extravascular hemolysis does not occur within the vascular compartment, hemoglobinemia, hemoglobinuria, methemoglobinuria, and hemosiderinuria do not occur. The breakdown of the red cells within the phagocytic cells causes anemia and jaundice, just as with intravascular hemolysis, and, since hemoglobin escapes into the blood from the phagocytic cells, plasma haptoglobin levels are also reduced. Unlike the case with intravascular hemolysis, the erythrophagocytosis causes hypertrophy and hyperplasia of the mononuclear phagocytic system, which in turn may lead to splenomegaly.

186. The answer is a. (*Henry, pp 557–559. Kumar, pp 625–627, 1395.*) Hereditary spherocytosis (HS), an autosomal dominant disorder, is characterized by an abnormality of the skeleton of the red cell membrane that makes the erythrocyte spherical, less deformable, and vulnerable to splenic sequestration and destruction (extravascular hemolysis). This mild to moderate hemolytic anemia can lead to splenomegaly, jaundice, and pigmented gallstones. In HS, the most common defect involves mutations in the gene that codes for ankyrin. Less commonly mutations involve either band 3, spectrin, or band 4.2. These mutations decrease the amount of red blood cell membrane and cause the formation of spherocytes (because of the low surface-to-volume ratio). Spherocytes in a peripheral blood smear show a smaller diameter than normal and an apparent increase in hemoglobin concentration because of a decrease in cell surface, with consequent deeper staining for hemoglobin. The increase in hemoglobin concentration within the red cells can be seen clinically as an increase in the mean cell hemoglobin concentration (MCHC). The osmotic fragility test (the shaded area in the graph reflects a normal response to a hypotonic solution) can be used to document the presence of spherocytes in the peripheral blood. Spherocytes lyse at a higher concentration of sodium chloride than do normal red cells. In contrast, flat hypochromic cells, such as those in thalassemia, have a greater capacity to expand in dilute salt solution and thus lyse at a lower concentration (which is seen in the unbroken curve to the far right). The longer the incubation of the red cells in these salt concentrations, the greater the response to osmotic change. The differential diagnosis of spherocytosis in the peripheral blood includes hereditary spherocytosis and autoimmune hemolytic anemia.

In contrast, abnormalities of dystrophin are seen with Duchenne's muscular dystrophy, while abnormalities of fibrillin are seen with Marfan's syndrome. A trinucleotide expansion involving the frataxin gene is seen in individuals with Friedreich's ataxia, while abnormalities of the NF-2 gene, which encodes for a protein called merlin, are associated with neurofibromatosis type 2. Merlin has homology with protein 4.1 of the red cell membrane.

187. The answer is b. (*Kumar, pp 627–628.*) Glucose-6-phosphate dehydrogenase (G6PD) is an enzyme of the hexose monophosphate shunt pathway that maintains glutathione in a reduced (active) form. Glutathione normally protects hemoglobin from oxidative injury. If the erythrocytes are deficient in G6PD, as occurs in G6PD deficiency, exposure to oxidant drugs, such as the antimalarial drug primaquine, denatures hemoglobin, which then precipitates with erythrocytes as Heinz bodies. Macrophages within the spleen remove these bodies, producing characteristic "bite" cells. These red cells then become less deformable and are trapped and destroyed within the spleen (extravascular hemolysis). The gene for G6PD is located on the X chromosome and has considerable pleomorphism at this site. Two variants are the A type, which is found in 10% of African Americans and is characterized by milder hemolysis of younger red cells, and the Mediterranean type, which is characterized by a more severe hemolysis of red cells of all ages.

In contrast, hereditary spherocytosis (HS), an autosomal dominant disorder, is characterized by an abnormality of the skeleton of the red cell membrane that makes the erythrocyte spherical, less deformable, and vulnerable to splenic sequestration and destruction (extravascular hemolysis). In HS, there is a defect in the spectrin molecule, which then is less binding to protein 4.1. This disorder can be diagnosed in the laboratory by the osmotic fragility test. Paroxysmal nocturnal hemoglobinuria (PNH), an acquired clonal stem cell disorder, is characterized by abnormal red cells, granulocytes, and platelets. The red cells are abnormally sensitive to the lytic activity of complement due to a deficiency of glycosyl phosphatidyl inositol (GPI)-linked proteins, namely, decay-accelerating factor (DAF, or CD55), membrane inhibitor of reactive lysis CD59, and a C8 binding protein. Complement is activated by acidosis, such as with exercise or sleep, which can produce red morning urine. Complications of PNH include the development of frequent thromboses and possibly acute leukemia. Autoimmune hemolytic anemia is caused by anti–red cell antibodies and is diagnosed using the Coombs' antiglobulin test. Microangiopathic hemolytic anemia refers to hemolysis of red cells caused by narrowing within the microvasculature and is seen in patients with prosthetic heart valves or those with disseminated intravascular coagulopathy, thrombotic thrombocytopenic purpura, or hemolytic-uremic syndrome.

188. The answer is a. (*Kumar, pp 628–630. Rubin, pp 1079–1082.*) Hemoglobin S (Hb S) is an abnormal form of hemoglobin that is found in individuals with sickle cell disease and sickle cell trait. Hb S is formed by a single nucleotide change in a codon, namely, glutamic acid is replaced by valine in the sixth position in the β chain of hemoglobin. On deoxygenation, this abnormal hemoglobin polymerizes, the red cells sickle, and symptoms result. Because of the content of Hb A, however, these symptoms are much milder in sickle cell trait than in sickle cell disease. The latter is characterized clinically by the triad of chronic hemolytic anemia, vascular occlusion, and vulnerability to infection. The severe chronic hemolytic anemia leads to chronic hyperbilirubinemia (jaundice), which leads to pigmented gallstones. Vascular occlusion results in leg ulcers, renal papillary necrosis, and multiple infarcts, which may cause severe bone pain. Repeated splenic infarcts cause progressive fibrosis and splenic atrophy (autoinfarction). The lack of splenic function along with defects in the alternate complement pathway predispose to infections such as *Salmonella* osteomyelitis and pneumococcal infections. The vaso-occlusive disease also leads to painful crises, hand-foot syndrome in children (consisting of the typical triad of fever, pallor, and symmetric swelling of hands and feet), and infarctive crises. In patients not having yet undergone splenic autoinfarction (usually children), massive splenic sequestration (sequestration crisis) may lead to rapid splenic enlargement, hypovolemia, and shock. Hydroxyurea has recently been approved for the treatment of sickle cell disease because it increases the synthesis of hemoglobin F, thus reducing the severity of the disease.

189. The answer is d. (*Hoffman, pp 536–537. Henry, pp 548, 557–559, 564–566, 581.*) The presence of hypersegmented neutrophils and oval macrocytes in a peripheral smear are consistent with a diagnosis of megaloblastic anemia. The additional finding of neurologic abnormalities (decreased vibratory sensation of the lower extremities) suggests the etiology being a deficiency of vitamin B_{12}, while finding gastric atrophy further suggests the diagnosis of pernicious anemia, which is an autoimmune disorder characterized by a lack of intrinsic factor. The Schilling test, which measures intestinal absorption of vitamin B_{12} with and without intrinsic factor, is used to diagnose pernicious anemia. To perform this test, the patient is first given an intramuscular shot of vitamin B_{12} (to treat the deficiency). Next the patient is given oral radioactive vitamin B_{12} and a 24-hour urine specimen is examined for radioactive vitamin B_{12}. In a patient with pernicious anemia who lacks intrinsic factor, the oral radioactive B_{12} will not be absorbed and will not appear in the urine. To confirm the diagnosis of pernicious anemia, the patient is next given oral intrinsic factor along with radioactive B_{12}. The addition of intrinsic factor will allow for the absorption of the radioactive B_{12}, which will then appear in the urine.

The direct antiglobulin test (DAT), or Coombs' test, is used to differentiate autoimmune hemolytic anemia (AIHA) due to the presence of anti–red cell antibodies from other forms of hemolytic anemia. In this test, antibodies to human immunoglobulin cause the agglutination (clotting) of red cells if these anti–red cell antibodies are present on the surface of the red cells. The metabisulfite test is used to detect the presence of hemoglobin S, but it does not differentiate the heterozygous sickle cell trait from the homozygous sickle cell disease. The test is based on the fact that erythrocytes with a large proportion of hemoglobin S sickle in solutions of low oxygen content. Metabisulfite is a reducing substance that enhances the process of deoxygenation. The osmotic fragility test is a diagnostic test for hereditary spherocytosis. Spherocytes lyse at a higher concentration of salt than do normal cells, thus causing an increased osmotic fragility. Finally, in patients with paroxysmal nocturnal hemoglobinuria, the erythrocytes are excessively sensitive to complement-mediated lysis in low-ionic environments (the basis for the sucrose hemolysis test) or in acidotic conditions, such as sleep, exercise, or the Ham's acid hemolysis test.

190. The answer is e. (*Kumar, pp 635–636. Hoffman, pp 491–495.*) The thalassemia syndromes are characterized by a decreased or absent synthesis of either the α- or the α-globin chain of hemoglobin A (alpha2-beta2). α thalassemias result from reduced synthesis of α-globin chains, while β thalassemias result from reduced production of β-globin chains. The α thalassemias result from deletions of one or more of the total of four α-globin genes, while β thalassemias result from point mutations involving the β-globin gene. There are two α-globin genes on each chromosome 16, and the normal genotype is α,α/. On each chromosome either or both of the α genes can be deleted. Deletion of both genes (— —/) is called alpha thal 1. This genotype is found in individuals in Southeast Asia and the Mediterranean. In contrast, deletion of only one α gene on a chromosome (— α/) is called alpha thal 2 and is found in Africans. The severity of α thalassemia depends on the number of α genes deleted. Deletions of only one gene (— α/α,α) results in a silent carrier. These patients are completely asymptomatic and all laboratory tests are normal. This clinical state can only be inferred from examination of a pedigree. Deletion of two α genes results in alpha thal trait. There are two possibilities for deletion of two α genes: the deletions may be on the same chromosome (— —/α,α, which is called the *cis* type) or the deletions may be on different chromosomes (— α/—α, which is called the *trans* type). The former, which is also called heterozygous alpha thal 1, is more common in Asians, while the latter, which is also called alpha thal 2, is more common in Africans. Clinically this is quite important because the offspring of parents with the *trans* deletions cannot develop H disease or hydrops. Deletion of three α genes (— —/—α) is called hemoglobin H disease. This name results from the fact that excess β chains postnatally form aggregates of β tetramers, which are called hemoglobin H. These aggregates form Heinz bodies, which can be seen with crystal blue stain. The most severe form of α thalassemia, hydrops fetalis, results from deletion of all four α *genes* (— —/— —) (Note that Cooley's anemia is the most severe form of β thalassemia). In hydrops fetalis, which is lethal in utero, no α chains are produced. Staining of the erythrocytes with a supravital stain demonstrates numerous intracytoplasmic inclusions within the red cells, which are aggregates of hemoglobin Bart's (gamma4).

191. The answer is d. (*Kumar, pp 632–635. Rubin, pp 1078–1079.*) β thalassemias result from reduced production of β-globin chains, which results in a relative excess production of α-globin chains. Most of the β thalassemias result from point mutations involving the β-globin gene. The amount of β-globin produced depends upon the location of the point mutation. Promoter region mutations result in decreased production of β-globin. This is called β+ thalassemia. Chain terminator mutations generally produce no functional β-globin. This is called β0 thalassemia. Splicing mutations may result in either β0 *or* β+ thalassemia. In patients with β thalassemia, a deficiency of β-globins causes a deficiency of hemoglobins that have β-globin chains, and at the same time there is an increase in hemoglobins that do not have β-globin chains (due to the excess α chains present). These hemoglobins include hemoglobin A_2 (α2-δ2) and hemoglobin F (α2-δ2). The most severe clinical form of β thalassemia is Cooley's anemia (β thal major), which is characterized by severe, transfusion-dependent anemia. Because of the need for repeated transfusions, over time these patients develop iron accumulation that leads to the formation of hemochromatosis. Indeed, congestive heart failure due to iron deposition within the heart is the major cause of death. Individuals with β thal major have increased reticulocytes, increased hemoglobin A_2, and markedly increased hemoglobin F (90%). In these patients, increased α chains produce intramedullary destruction ("ineffective erythropoiesis"). The resultant increased red marrow produces a "crew-cut" x-ray appearance of the skull and enlarges the maxilla.

192. The answer is c. (*Kumar, pp 636–638. Hoffman, pp 334–336.*) Paroxysmal nocturnal hemoglobinuria (PNH) is an acquired clonal stem cell disorder that is characterized by abnormal red cells, granulocytes, and platelets. The red blood cells (RBCs) are abnormally sensitive to the lytic activity of complement due to a deficiency of glycosyl phosphatidyl inositol (GPI)-linked proteins, which are an important part of the cell membrane of erythrocytes. Proteins are anchored into the lipid bilayer of cell membranes in one of two basic ways. Most have a hydrophobic sequence that spans the cell membrane; these being called transmembrane proteins. The rest are attached to the cell membrane by covalent linkage to a specialized phospholipid called glycosylphosphatidylinositol (GPI). Phosphatidylinositol glycan A (PIGA) is needed for the synthesis of the GPI anchor. Mutations in PIGA result in decreased GPI-linked proteins such as CD55 (decay-accelerating factor), CD59 (membrane inhibitor of reactive lysis), and a C8 binding protein. All of these proteins regulate complement activation and can be abnormal with PNH, but of these three proteins, CD59 is the most important. It is a potent inhibitor of C3 convertase. In contrast, CD22 is an antigen found on the surface of mature B lymphocytes.

Complement is normally activated by acidotic states, such as occur with exercise or sleep. In patients with PNH, the acidotic condition that develops during sleep (which is usually at night) causes hemolysis of red blood cells and results in red urine in the morning. The erythrocytes of these patients lyse in vitro with acid (Ham's test) or sucrose (sucrose lysis test). Complications of PNH include the development of frequent thromboses, particularly of the hepatic, portal, or cerebral veins. Since PNH is a clonal stem cell disorder, patients are at an increased risk of developing aplastic anemia or acute leukemia.

The autoimmune hemolytic anemias are characterized by the presence of autoantibodies against red blood cells. They are important causes of acute anemia in a wide variety of clinical states and can be separated into two main types: those secondary to "warm" antibodies and those reactive at cold temperatures. Warm-antibody autoimmune hemolytic anemias have antibodies that react at 37°C in vitro, are composed of IgG, and do not fix complement. They are found in patients with malignant tumors, especially leukemia-lymphoma; with use of such drugs as α-methyldopa; and in the autoimmune diseases, especially lupus erythematosus. The antibodies found with cold-antibody autoimmune hemolytic anemia reacts at 4 to 6°C, fixes complement, is of the IgM type, and is classically associated with *Mycoplasma* pneumonitis (pleuropneumonia-like organisms). These antibodies are termed cold agglutinins and may reach extremely high titers and cause intravascular red cell agglutination. Cold hemolysins, autoantibodies that hemolyze red blood cells, are found with paroxysmal cold hemoglobinuria (PCH). These autoantibodies are usually directed against the P antigen of red blood cells. Finally, autoimmune polyendocrinopathy syndrome type 1 (APS1) is associated with an abnormal AIRE-1 (autoimmune regulator) gene, which codes for a transcription factor expressed in the thymus, pancreas, and adrenal cortex.

193. The answer is a. (*Kumar, pp 636–638. Rubin, pp 1084–1085.*) The presence of microspherocytes in an individual with a positive Coombs' test is diagnostic for autoimmune hemolytic anemia (AIHA). This type of hemolytic anemia is characterized by the presence of antibodies that destroy red cells. The AIHAs are divided into two main types: those secondary to "warm" antibodies and those secondary to "cold" antibodies. The antibodies seen in warm-antibody autoimmune hemolytic anemias react at 37°C in vitro, are composed of IgG, and do not fix complement. Instead, immunoglobulin-coated red blood cells are removed by splenic macrophages that recognize the Fc portion of the immunoglobulin. These warm IgG antibodies are found in patients with malignant tumors, especially leukemia-lymphoma; they are associated with the use of such drugs as α-methyldopa; and they are also found in the autoimmune diseases, especially lupus erythematosus.

194. The answer is a. (*Kumar, pp 542–543, 636–638. Rubin, pp 1085–1086.*) Cold-antibody autoimmune hemolytic anemia (cold AIHA) is subdivided into two clinical categories based on the type of antibodies involved. These two types of cold antibodies are cold agglutinins and cold hemolysins. Cold agglutinins are monoclonal IgM antibodies that react at 4 to 6°C. They are called agglutinins because the IgM can agglutinate red cells due to its large size (pentamer). Additionally, IgM can activate complement, which may result in IV hemolysis. *Mycoplasma* pneumonitis and infectious mononucleosis are classically associated with cold-agglutinin formation. Vascular obstruction by the red cell agglutination can produce Raynaud's phenomenon, which is characterized by ischemia in the fingers when exposed to the cold.

In contrast to cold agglutinins, cold hemolysins are seen in patients with paroxysmal cold hemoglobinuria (PCH). These cold hemolysins are unique because they are biphasic antierythrocyte autoantibodies. These antibodies are IgG that is directed against the P blood group antigen. They are called biphasic because they attach to red cells and bind complement at low temperatures, but the activation of complement does not occur until the temperature is increased. This antibody, called the Donath-Landsteiner antibody, was previously associated with syphilis, but may follow various infections, such as mycoplasmal pneumonia.

195. The answer is c. (*Kumar, pp 648–649. Hoffman, p 370.*) Myelophthisic anemia results from space-occupying lesions of the bone marrow, such as granulomas or metastatic carcinomas. It is characterized by the presence of leukoerythroblastosis in the peripheral blood. This term refers to finding in the peripheral blood immature white cells, such as myelocytes and metamyelocytes, and immature red blood cells, such as nucleated red blood cells. Metastatic disease in the bone can produce localized bone pain and elevation of alkaline phosphatase that is associated with a normal γ-glutamyl-transferase (GGT) level.

In contrast, microangiopathic hemolytic anemia refers to mechanical destruction (hemolysis) of red cells caused by narrowing within the microvasculature and is seen in patients with prosthetic heart valves or severe calcific aortic stenosis, or in patients having disseminated intravascular coagulopathy, thrombotic thrombocytopenic purpura, or hemolytic-uremic syndrome. In addition to microangiopathic HA, other causes of IV mechanical destruction of red cells include march hemoglobinuria and certain types of infections, such as bartonellosis and malaria. Aplastic anemia is a stem cell disorder of the bone marrow that causes a marked decrease in the production of marrow cells, which results in extreme marrow hypoplasia. Patients present with symptoms related to pancytopenia (anemia, agranulocytosis, and thrombocytopenia). Because their bone marrow cannot respond normally, patients with aplastic anemia have no increased reticulocytes in the peripheral blood (no polychromasia). Aplastic anemia may be inherited (Fanconi anemia) or acquired. The most common cause of aplastic anemia is drugs. Other causes include chemicals (benzene and glue sniffing), radiation, and certain types of infections, such as hepatitis C. There are certain predisposing conditions, such as PNH, that are associated with an increased risk of developing aplastic anemia.

196. The answer is c. (*Kumar, pp 638–639, 642–643. Rubin, pp 1073–1076.*) In contrast to a normal, mature neutrophil, which has from two to five nuclear lobes, the neutrophil shown has at least six lobes and is an illustration of neutrophilic hypersegmentation. Granulocytic hypersegmentation is significant and among the first hematologic findings in the peripheral blood of patients who have megaloblastic anemia in its developmental stages. Neutrophilic hypersegmentation is generally considered a sensitive indicator of megaloblastic anemia, which can be caused by a deficiency in vitamin B_{12}, in folate, or in both. This deficiency impairs DNA synthesis and delays mitotic division, which in turn causes the nuclei to be enlarged. The synthesis of RNA and cytoplasmic elements is not affected, however, so there is nuclear-cytoplasmic asynchrony. These cellular changes affect all rapidly proliferating cells in the body, but in the bone marrow they result in enlarged erythroid precursors, which are referred to as megaloblasts. These abnormal cells produce abnormally enlarged red cells, which are called macroovalocytes. These megaloblasts also undergo autohemolysis within the bone marrow, resulting in ineffective erythropoiesis. Granulocyte precursors are also enlarged and are called giant metamyelocytes. These abnormal cells produce enlarged hypersegmented neutrophils. The megakaryocytes are large and have nuclear abnormalities, but, although the platelet count is decreased, the platelets are not enlarged.

Tetrahydrofolate (FH4) acts as an intermediate in the transfer of one-carbon units from compounds such as formiminoglutamic acid (FIGlu), a breakdown product of histidine. Excess urinary levels of FIGlu are a useful clinical indicator of a folate deficiency. Folate deficiency may result from dietary deficiency, impaired absorption, or impaired utilization. Dietary deficiency most often occurs in chronic alcoholics or the elderly. Impaired absorption occurs in malabsorptive states, while impaired utilization can occur with folate antagonists, an example being methotrexate. Increased requirements for B_{12} and folate may be seen in pregnancy, cancer, and chronic hemolytic anemia; if these needs are not met, deficiency states can result. Note that folate deficiency during pregnancy has been associated with the development of open neural tube defects in the fetus. Folate supplements are recommended for all women prior to and after conception.

197. The answer is c. (*Kumar, pp 212, 638–642. Rubin, pp 1073–1076.*) The combination of clinical signs suggesting damage to both the posterior spinal cord (such as loss of vibratory and position sense) and the lateral spinal cord (such as arm and leg dystaxia and spastic paralysis) are suggestive of subacute degeneration of the spinal cord, a disorder that results from a deficiency of vitamin B_{12}. Loss of vibratory sensation in the lower extremities is the first neurologic manifestation of this disease. These neurologic abnormalities of B_{12} deficiency do not occur with folate deficiency. They are thought to be the result of abnormal myelin production due to either excess methionine or abnormal fatty acid production (fatty acids with an odd number of carbons), such as propionate.

There are many different causes of vitamin B_{12} deficiency, which also results in a megaloblastic anemia. Examples include inadequate diet, impaired absorption, bacterial overgrowth, or competitive parasitic infections. Dietary deficiencies will take years to produce deficiency states since liver stores are so great (recall that vitamin B_{12} is the only water soluble vitamin that is stored in the body). Dietary deficiency is seen only in strict vegetarians (diet with no animal proteins, milk, or eggs). Normally dietary B_{12} binds to salivary R-binders, forming a B_{12}-R complex that is broken down by pancreatic proteases. Free B_{12} then binds to intrinsic factor (IF is secreted by gastric parietal cells) and the B_{12}-IF complex is absorbed by ileal mucosal epithelial cells. B_{12} is then transported in blood bound to transcobalamin II. Impaired absorption occurs with deficiency of intrinsic factor (patients with pernicious anemia or gastrectomy) or malabsorptive states that involve the ileum (such as celiac disease, Crohn's disease, or chronic pancreatitis). Pernicious anemia, an autoimmune disease, is the most common cause of vitamin B_{12} deficiency. Chronic pancreatitis is associated with B_{12} deficiency because pancreatic enzymes are necessary to enzymatically cleave the R factor from B_{12} in the duodenum before IF can attach to B_{12}. Bacterial overgrowth occurs in the blind-loop syndrome or with broad-spectrum antibiotic therapy, while a competitive parasitic infection is the giant fish tapeworm, *Diphyllobothrium latum*.

In contrast, Fanconi anemia is an autosomal recessive disorder characterized by bone marrow failure combined with certain birth defects, such as abnormalities of the radius. Leukoerythroblastic anemia refers to any space occupying lesion of the bone marrow (myelophthisic anemia) that causes immature red blood cells and immature white blood cells to appear in the peripheral blood. Finally sideroblastic anemia is characterized by the presence of numerous sideroblasts in the bone marrow and may be caused by a deficiency of pyridoxine or it may be a form of myelodysplasia.

198. The answer is b. (*Henry, pp 93–94, 544–545. Kumar, pp 643–646.*) Absent iron stores in the bone marrow, demonstrated by the absence of Prussian blue staining, in a patient with a microcytic hypochromic anemia is consistent with the diagnosis of iron deficiency anemia. The normal serum level of iron is about 100 µg/dL. Iron is transported in the plasma bound to transferrin, which is normally about 33% saturated with iron. Therefore, the total iron-binding capacity (TIBC) is normally about 300 µg/dL. The TIBC indicates the blood transferrin levels and is inversely proportional to the total body stores of iron. That is, iron deficiency is associated with increased TIBC (or serum iron-binding capacity), while iron excess is associated with decreased TIBC.

All storage iron is in the form of ferritin or hemosiderin. In the liver, ferritin is found within parenchymal cells, while in the spleen and bone marrow, ferritin is found within macrophages. Very small amounts of ferritin circulate in the plasma, but since it is derived from the storage pool, serum ferritin levels are a good indicator of total body stores. That is, with iron deficiency serum ferritin levels are decreased. Finally, note that in the normal synthesis of heme, iron is inserted into protoporphyrin IX. A deficiency of iron will result in an increase in free erythrocyte porphyrin (FEP). This laboratory test is also increased in lead poisoning and sometimes in sideroblastic anemia. It is not increased with thalassemia.

199. The answer is e. (*Henry, pp 93–94, 542–545, 580. Hoffmann, pp 372–373.*) The differential diagnosis of microcytosis includes β thalassemia (due to a defect in globin chain synthesis) and iron-deficiency anemia. It is important to distinguish between these two disorders because therapy with iron benefits patients with iron-deficiency anemia, but harms patients with thalassemia because these patients are at risk for iron overload. Both thalassemia minor and iron-deficiency anemia are microcytic disorders in which the mean corpuscular hemoglobin is usually found to be reduced. Red blood cell indexes may be useful in differentiating the two disorders because, while the mean corpuscular hemoglobin concentration (MCHC) is often normal or only slightly reduced in association with thalassemia minor, the MCHC is often definitely reduced in association with iron-deficiency anemia. (Both pernicious and folate-deficiency anemias lead to megaloblastic changes in erythrocytes.) The red cell distribution width (RDW) is a measure of variation in the size of the red cells (anisocytosis). The RDW is increased in patients with iron-deficiency anemia, but is normal in patients with β thalassemia. Also unique to the microcytic anemias is the fact that patients with β thalassemia have increased red blood cell counts, while patients with all of the other microcytic anemias have decreased red blood cell counts. This increased red cell count in β thalassemia may be due to the increased hemoglobin F, which shifts the oxygen dissociation curve to the left. This in turn causes an increased release of erythropoietin. Unlike iron-deficiency anemia, β thalassemia begins as a microcytic anemia. In contrast, iron-deficiency anemia progresses through several stages. First, there is decreased storage iron, which is followed by decreased circulating iron. At this time patients are still not clinically anemic. Next, patients develop a normocytic normochromic anemia that transforms into a microcytic normochromic anemia and finally a microcytic hypochromic anemia.

200. The answer is c. (*Henry, pp 542–545, 550–551. Hoffman, pp 415–416.*) The four main causes of microcytic/hypochromic anemias are iron deficiency, anemia of chronic disease (AOCD), thalassemia, and sideroblastic anemia. Additional laboratory tests can differentiate between these four diseases. The serum iron and percentage of saturation are decreased in both iron-deficiency anemia and AOCD, are increased in sideroblastic anemia, and may be normal or increased in thalassemia. The total iron-binding capacity (TIBC) is increased only in iron-deficiency anemia; it is normal or decreased in the other diseases. An additional differentiating test for these four diagnoses is evaluation of the bone marrow iron stores. In iron deficiency, iron stores are decreased or absent. In AOCD, iron is present, but is restricted to and increased within macrophages. It is decreased in amount within marrow erythroid precursors. Marrow iron is increased in patients with sideroblastic anemia. Iron levels in patients with thalassemia trait are generally within normal limits. Approximately one-third of the normoblasts in the normal bone marrow contain ferritin granules and are called sideroblasts. In sideroblastic anemia, because of the deficiency of pyridoxine and ferritin, the production of globin or heme is markedly reduced, and ferritin granules accumulate within the mitochondria that rim the nucleus. This produces the characteristic ring sideroblast.

201. The answer is b. (*Hoffman, pp 431–437. Kumar, pp 1263–1264.*) The porphyrias are inherited or acquired disorders of heme biosynthesis with varied patterns of overproduction, accumulation, and excretion of heme synthesis intermediates. Major characteristics of the porphyrias include intermittent neurologic dysfunction and skin sensitivity to sunlight, but these changes do not occur in all of the different types of porphyria. Neurologic changes, such as hallucinations and manic-depressive episodes, can be seen with acute intermittent porphyria (AIP), hereditary coproporphyria (HCP), and variegate porphyria (VP), while skin changes, such as a bullous photosensitivity, can be seen with porphyria cutanea tarda (PCT), which is the most common type of porphyria, congenital erythropoietic porphyria (CEP), HCP, and VP. That is, AIP produces no skin photosensitivity. Abdominal pain (colic) can be seen with AIP, HCP, and VP. Therefore, the combination of neurologic changes with skin changes and abdominal pain is suggestive of either HCP or VP. These two disorders are clinically similar with increased urinary delta-aminolevulinic acid (ALA) and porphobilinogen (PBG), but VP is quite prevalent in South Africa.

202. The answer is e. (*Kumar, pp 649, 699–700. Ravel, pp 76–77.*) Polycythemia refers to an increased concentration of red blood cells (RBCs) in the peripheral blood. This is manifested by an increase in the red blood cell count, hemoglobin concentration, or hematocrit. The differential diagnosis of polycythemia includes primary polycythemia, which is due to a defect in myeloid stem cells (polycythemia rubra vera), and secondary polycythemia, which is caused by an increase in the production of erythropoietin (EPO). In patients with primary polycythemia, a myeloproliferative disorder, the red cell mass is increased but the levels of EPO are normal or decreased. That is, the abnormality is a primary defect in the red blood cells themselves. In contrast, with secondary polycythemia, the polycythemia is secondary to the increased EPO. This secondary increase in the EPO may be appropriate or inappropriate. Appropriate causes of increased EPO, in which the oxygen saturation of hemoglobin will be abnormal, include lung disease, cyanotic heart disease, living at high altitudes, or abnormal hemoglobins with increased oxygen affinity. Inappropriate causes of increased EPO include EPO-secreting tumors, such as renal cell carcinomas, hepatomas, or cerebellar hemangioblastomas. In contrast, pancreatic adenocarcinoma may be associated with migratory thrombophlebitis (Trousseau's sign).

It is important to understand that an increase in red blood cell count, reported clinically as number of cells per microliter, is not the same thing as the RBC mass, which is a radioactive test that is reported in mL/kg. The RBC count and the RBC mass do not necessarily parallel each other. For example, a decreased plasma volume increases the RBC count but does not affect the RBC mass. An increased red blood cell concentration may be a relative polycythemia or an absolute polycythemia. A relative polycythemia is due to a decrease in the plasma volume (hemoconcentration), causes of which include prolonged vomiting or diarrhea (as seen with acute gastroenteritis), or the excessive use of diuretics.

To summarize these clinical findings, an increased total red cell mass indicates an absolute polycythemia, increased serum EPO indicates a secondary polycythemia, and a normal oxygen saturation of hemoglobin suggests an inappropriate secretion of EPO, such as seen with renal cell carcinoma.

203. The answer is c. (*Kumar, pp 539–541, 650. Goldman, pp 1004, 1526.*) Hemorrhages into the skin may produce lesions of varying sizes. Petechiae measure less than 2 mm in size, purpuric lesions measure 2 mm to 1 cm, and ecchymoses are larger than 1 cm. (Note that erythema and telangiectasis do not involve hemorrhage outside of blood vessels. They can be differentiated from true hemorrhages into the skin by the fact that they blanch if direct pressure is applied to them.) True purpura may be caused by hemostatic or nonhemostatic defects. Hemostatic defects are caused by platelet or coagulation abnormalities, while nonhemostatic defects generally involve the blood vessels. These vascular abnormalities can be separated into palpable and nonpalpable purpura. The latter may be caused by excess corticosteroids (Cushing's syndrome), vitamin C deficiency (scurvy), infectious agents, or abnormal connective tissue diseases (Ehlers-Danlos syndrome). Causes of palpable purpura include diseases that cause cutaneous vasculitis, such as collagen vascular diseases and Henoch-Schönlein purpura. The latter, also known as anaphylactoid purpura, is a type of hypersensitivity vasculitis found in children. It usually develops 1 to 3 weeks following a streptococcal infection, but it may also occur in relation to allergic food reactions.

Cross-reacting IgA or immune complexes are deposited on the endothelium of blood vessels. Patients may develop fever, purpura, abdominal pain, arthralgia, arthritis, and glomerulonephritis.

204. The answer is b. (*Kumar, pp 651–652. Hoffman, pp 2270–2272.*) Petechial hemorrhages result from abnormalities of platelets or blood vessels. A bone marrow biopsy specimen that reveals an increase in the number of megakaryocytes is consistent with increased peripheral destruction of platelets, a major cause of which is immune thrombocytopenic purpura (ITP). Clinically, ITP may be divided into an acute form and a chronic form. The acute form is more commonly seen in children following a viral infection, while the chronic form is more often seen in adult women of childbearing years. Most individuals with ITP are asymptomatic, but if the platelet count drops low enough, they may develop petechial hemorrhages or epistaxis, usually after an upper respiratory infection. Both clinical types of ITP are associated with the development of antiplatelet antibodies, mainly against the platelet antigens GpIIb/IIIa and GpIb/IX. Therefore, ITP is a form of autoimmune destruction of platelets.

There are several therapies for patients with symptomatic ITP. The initial therapy is with corticosteroids, which decrease antibody formation and also inhibit reticuloendothelial function, and high-dose immunoglobulin therapy, which floods the Fc receptors of the splenic macrophages with Ig, making them less likely to bind to antibody-coated platelets. Splenectomy may be beneficial in symptomatic patients with ITP who do not respond to either of these therapies. The rationale for splenectomy is that the spleen is the major site for the production of the autoimmune antiplatelet antibodies in patients with ITP and because the spleen is the site for the removal of the platelets (antibody-coated platelets bind to the Fc receptors of macrophages within the spleen).

In contrast to ITP, disseminated intravascular coagulation (DIC) is characterized by widespread bleeding and thrombosis, while thrombotic thrombocytopenic purpura (TTP) is characterized by thrombocytopenia and a microangiopathic hemolytic anemia, along with other systemic signs. Finally, Waterhouse-Friderichsen syndrome refers to bilateral hemorrhagic necrosis of the adrenal glands associated with infection by *Neisseria meningitidis.*

205. The answer is c. (*Kumar, pp 652–653, 656–658. Rubin, pp 1104–1105.*) The differential diagnosis of a patient with schistocytes in the peripheral blood and petechial hemorrhages includes the thrombotic microangiopathies, a group of disorders characterized by arteriole and capillary occlusions by fibrin and platelet microthrombi. These microangiopathic hemolytic anemias include thrombotic thrombocytopenic purpura (TTP), hemolytic-uremic syndrome (HUS), and disseminated intravascular coagulation (DIC). Additionally, finding abnormal coagulation studies with increased fibrin degradation products favors the diagnosis of DIC, which is associated with several predisposing conditions including malignancy, infection, retained fetus, and amniotic fluid embolism.

In contrast, the presence of deteriorating mental status and renal failure suggests the diagnosis of TTP, a disorder that is associated with a characteristic pentad of clinical signs: fever, microangiopathic hemolytic anemia, thrombocytopenia, renal dysfunction, neurologic abnormalities. TTP is often associated with a deficiency of ADAMTS 13, a metalloprotease that normally processes large von Willebrand's factor (vWF) multimers into small multimers. With TTP there are too many large multimers, which in turn activate platelets and leads to the production of systemic fibrin microthrombi. In contrast, antibodies to GpIIb/IIIa are seen in patients with immune thrombocytopenia purpura (ITP), while mutations in the Tyrp1 (tyrosinase-related protein-1) gene are the cause of some forms of oculocutaneous albinism (OCA) and infection with E. coli strain O157:H7 is seen with HUS. Finally the treatment for TTP may involve the use of plasma exchange, large-volume plasmapheresis, or steroids. Platelets should not be given as this makes the signs and symptoms worse.

206. The answer is c. (*Damjanov, pp 1089, 1716, 1751, 1823. Kumar, pp 652–653, 1009–1011.*) Hemolytic-uremic syndrome (HUS) is similar to thrombotic thrombocytopenic purpura (TTP) in that it produces a microangiopathic hemolytic anemia, but it is distinguished from TTP by the lack of neurologic symptoms and by the severe acute renal failure, which is manifested clinically by a markedly increased serum BUN. Classic HUS is seen in children and is related to infection, usually acquired from contaminated ground meat, by verocytotoxin-producing *Escherichia coli*. This toxin is similar to *Shigella* toxins, which, together with *E. coli* and viruses, are causes of the adult form of HUS. Multiple microthrombi in glomerular capillaries result in renal failure, while systemically the micro-thrombi cause microangiopathic hemolytic anemia. Subsequently thrombocytopenia develops and leads to a bleeding diathesis, seen as vomiting of blood and hematuria. Disseminated intravascular coagulopathy (DIC) is separated from these two thrombotic microangiopathic syndromes by its excessive activation of the clotting system, which results in increased fibrin degradation products (FDP or FSP) and prolonged clotting times (PT and PTT) due to depletion of coagulation factors.

207. The answer is a. (*Kumar, pp 654–655. Henry, pp 624–629, 646–649.*) Platelet aggregation studies are used to evaluate qualitative disorders of platelets. These tests measure the response of platelets to various aggregating agents, such as ADP, epinephrine, collagen, and ristocetin. ADP causes the initial aggregation of platelets (phase I). This is followed by activation of the platelets, which then release their own ADP, which further aggregates the platelets (phase II). Platelet aggregation may be caused by collagen, ADP, or ristocetin. In von Willebrand's disease (vWD), aggregation induced by collagen and ADP is normal, but ristocetin is decreased. vWD is considered to be adhesion defects of platelets. Platelet adhesion refers to attachment of platelets to sites of endothelial cell injury where collagen is exposed. von Willebrand factor (vWF) is a molecular bridge between the subendothelial collagen and platelets through the platelet receptor GpIb. A deficiency of either vWF (vWD) or GpIb (Bernard-Soulier syndrome) results in defective platelet adhesion to collagen (adhesion defects). Cryoprecipitate, which contains vWF, corrects this defect in patients with vWD, but not in patients with Bernard-Soulier syndrome (since the defect involves the receptor for vWF). Clinically, vWD is characterized by mucocutaneous bleeding, menorrhagia, and epistaxis. Milder forms of the disease may not be diagnosed until the patient is older. Factor VIII is a complex of several components that can be discerned electrophoretically. Of all the factor VIII components, factor VIII:R, or ristocetin cofactor, is most apt to be abnormal in vWD. In contrast, increased D-dimers (fibrin split products) can be elevated in the serum with disseminated intravascular coagulation and pulmonary emboli.

208. The answer is c. (*Kumar, pp 649–650, 653. Henry, pp 628–636, 650–651.*) Congenital abnormalities of platelet function are classified into three categories: (1) defective platelet adhesion, (2) defective platelet aggregation, and (3) defective platelet secretion. Platelet aggregation refers to platelets binding to other platelets. One mechanism for this involves fibrinogen, which can act as a molecular bridge between adjacent platelets by binding to GpIIb and GpIIIa receptors on the surface of platelets. Abnormalities of platelet aggregation (aggregation defects or primary wave defects) include Glanzmann thrombasthenia (GT) and abnormalities of fibrinogen. Patients with GT have a deficiency of GpIIb-IIIa and defective platelet aggregation. These patients have a normal prothrombin time (PT) and normal partial thromboplastin time (PTT). In contrast, patients with no fibrinogen (afibrinogenemia) or dysfunctioning fibrinogen (dysfibrinogenemia) characteristically have prolonged PT, PTT, and thrombin time (TT) values: in fact, they are so prolonged they are unmeasurable.

In contrast to platelet aggregation, platelet adhesion refers to platelets binding to subendothelial collagen via von Willebrand's factor (vWF) serving as a molecular bridge between the receptor Gp Ib/IX on platelets to collagen. A deficiency of Gp Ib/IX is seen in Bernard-Soulier syndrome, which has clinical signs similar to von Willebrand's disease. Finally, platelet secretion refers to the secretion of the contents of two types of granules within the platelet cytoplasm. α granules contain fibrinogen, fibronectin, and platelet-derived growth factor, while dense bodies contain ADP, ionized calcium, histamine, epinephrine, and serotonin. Decreased platelet secretion (activation defects) is seen with deficiencies of these granules; these diseases are called storage pool defects. They can involve either α granules (gray platelet syndrome) or dense bodies (Chédiak-Higashi syndrome, Wiskott-Aldrich syndrome, or TAR). Wiskott-Aldrich syndrome is an X-linked disorder that is characterized by eczema, thrombocytopenia (small platelets), and immunodeficiency consisting of decreased levels of IgM and progressive loss of T-cell function. These patients have recurrent infections with bacteria, viruses, and fungi. TAR refers to the combination of thrombocytopenia and absent radii.

209. The answer is a. (*Kumar, p 131. Henry, pp 642–643, 650, 1379–1380. Hoffman, pp 2086–2088, 2206–2208.*) The Leiden mutation of coagulation factor V is the most common inherited predisposition to thrombosis (approximately 2 to 15% of Caucasians have this type of factor V mutation). Normally protein C functions as a potent anticoagulant by inhibiting activated coagulation factors V and VIII. Factor V Leiden mutation results in an abnormal form of factor V that when activated (Va) is resistant to protein C (this abnormality is also referred to as activated protein C resistance). Clinically factor V Leiden mutation is associated with an increased risk for recurrent thromboembolism. Patients usually present because of thrombosis of one leg (often the left leg), but can develop recurrent pulmonary emboli or spontaneous abortions.

In contrast, congenital deficiencies of factor V are quite rare, but mutations in the prothrombin gene are fairly common. Laboratory findings with a deficiency of factor V include a prolonged PTT and PT with a normal TT. Patients with this abnormality have an increased risk of venous thrombosis. A severe deficiency of factor X can lead to hemarthroses, soft tissue hemorrhages, and menorrhagia. Like a deficiency of factor V, the laboratory findings with a deficiency of factor X include a prolonged PTT and PT with a normal TT.

210. The answer is c. (*Kumar, pp 655–656. Henry, pp 649–650, 993–997.*) An X-linked recessive disorder that results from a deficiency of coagulation factor VIII is hemophilia A. Clinically, patients with hemophilia exhibit a wide range of severity of symptoms that depends upon the degree to which factor VII activity is decreased. Petechiae and small ecchymoses are characteristically absent, but large ecchymoses and subcutaneous and intramuscular hematomas are common. Other types of bleeding that are characteristic include massive hemorrhage following trauma or surgery and "spontaneous" hemorrhages in parts of the body that are normally subject to trauma, such as the joints (hemarthroses). Intra-abdominal hemorrhage and intracranial hemorrhage also occur. The latter is a major cause of death for these individuals. Because of the decreased factor VIII activity, patients with hemophilia A have a prolonged PTT, which measures the intrinsic coagulation cascade. Other clinical tests, including bleeding time, tourniquet test, platelet count, and PT, are normal. Treatment is with factor VIII concentrates, but this carries a risk for the transmission of viral hepatitis and AIDS.

In contrast, hemorrhagic urticaria is seen with Henoch-Schönlein purpura, a disorder of children characterized by the deposition of IgA immune complexes in the small vessels of the skin. Perifollicular hemorrhages are seen with scurvy, which is caused by a deficiency of vitamin C. In this disorder the defective synthesis of collagen will increase the fragility of the basement membrane of capillaries causing periosteal and perifollicular hemorrhages.

211. The answer is e. (*Kumar, pp 656–658. Rubin, pp 1107–1109.*) Disseminated intravascular coagulopathy (DIC) is a severe thrombohemorrhagic disorder that results from extensive activation of the coagulation sequence. With DIC there are widespread fibrin deposits in the microcirculation, which leads to hemolysis of the red cells (microangiopathic hemolytic anemia), ischemia, and infarcts in multiple organs. Continued thrombosis leads to consumption of platelets and the coagulation factors, which subsequently leads to a bleeding disorder. The excessive clotting also activates plasminogen and increases plasmin levels, which cleaves fibrin and increases serum levels of fibrin split products. DIC is never a primary disorder, but instead is always secondary to other diseases that activate either the intrinsic or the extrinsic coagulation system. Activation of the intrinsic pathway results from the release of tissue factor into circulation. Examples include obstetric complications (due to release of placental tissue factor) and cancers (due to release of the cytoplasmic granules of the leukemic cells of acute promyelocytic leukemia or to release of mucin from adenocarcinomas). Coagulation may also result from the activation of the extrinsic pathway by widespread injury to endothelial cells, such as with the deposition of antigen-antibody complexes (vasculitis) or endotoxic damage by microorganisms.

212. The answer is d. (*Kumar, pp 450, 456. Henry, pp 642–655.*) Abnormalities of blood vessels (capillary fragility) or platelets can be detected by either the tourniquet test or the bleeding time. These tests do not test the coagulation cascade. In contrast, the platelet count and platelet morphology are both useful in evaluating platelet abnormalities, while the prothrombin time (PT) and the partial thromboplastin time (PTT) measure the coagulation cascade. The PT measures the extrinsic pathway, while the PTT measures the intrinsic coagulation pathway.

An abnormal tourniquet test and bleeding time with a normal PTT and PT may be caused by either blood vessel abnormalities or platelet abnormalities. Blood vessel abnormalities and abnormal platelet function are accompanied by normal platelet counts (choice a in the table). Causes of blood vessel abnormalities include decreased vitamin C (scurvy) and vasculitis, while causes of platelet dysfunction include Bernard-Soulier syndrome and Glanzmann thrombasthenia. A decrease in the platelet count (choice c in the table) indicates thrombocytopenia and can be seen in patients with ITP. Normal platelet counts with normal bleeding times are suggestive of abnormalities of the coagulation cascade. A prolonged PTT only (choice b in the table) is seen with abnormalities of the intrinsic pathway, such as hemophilia A or B. A prolonged PT only (choice d in the table) is seen with abnormalities of the extrinsic pathway, such as a deficiency of factor VII. A prolongation of both PTT and PT is seen with liver disease, vitamin K deficiency, and DIC. Deficiencies of the vitamin K–dependent factors, such as induced with Coumadin therapy or broad-spectrum antibiotic therapy, are associated with a normal tourniquet test, bleeding time, and platelet count, but there is also a markedly increased PT, and the PTT may be increased or normal (also choice d in the table). Therefore, the PT is used as a screening test to monitor patients taking oral Coumadin. A prolonged bleeding time with a normal platelet count, but a prolonged PTT (choice e in the table), is highly suggestive of von Willebrand's disease.

213. The answer is d. (*Kumar, pp 662–663. Rubin, pp 1087–1088.*) Decreased numbers of neutrophils in the peripheral blood (neutropenia) may be due to decreased production of neutrophils in the bone marrow or to increased peripheral destruction of neutrophils. Decreased production may be caused by megaloblastic anemia, certain drugs, or stem cell defects such as aplastic anemia, leukemias, or lymphomas. Drug-induced destruction of neutrophil precursors is the most common cause of peripheral neutropenia. With all of these different causes of decreased neutrophil production, the bone marrow is hypoplastic and there is a decrease in the number of granulocytic precursors. Some causes of neutropenia also cause a decrease in the numbers of platelets and erythrocytes (pancytopenia).

In contrast to decreased production, neutropenia secondary to peripheral destruction causes a hyperplasia of the bone marrow, with an increase in the number of granulocytic precursors. Causes of increased destruction of neutrophils include sequestration in the spleen due to hypersplenism (not splenic atrophy), increased utilization, such as with overwhelming infections, and immunologically mediated destruction (immune destruction). Causes of immune destruction include Felty's syndrome and certain drug reactions, such as to aminopyrine and some sulfonamides. Drugs may cause decreased production or increased destruction of neutrophils. In the latter, antibodies are formed against neutrophils, and then these cells are destroyed peripherally. Felty's syndrome refers to the combination of rheumatoid arthritis, splenomegaly, and neutropenia. A significant number of patients with Felty's syndrome have a monoclonal proliferation of CD8 large granular lymphocytes, unrelated to drug use.

214. The answer is b. (*Kumar, pp 82, 84, 663–665. Rubin, pp 74–75, 1089–1090.*) Leukocytosis (increased numbers of leukocytes in the peripheral blood) is a reaction seen in many different disease states. The type of leukocyte that is mainly increased may be an indicator of the type of disease process present. Eosinophilia can be associated with cutaneous allergic reactions; allergic disorders, such as bronchial asthma or hay fever; Hodgkin's disease; some skin diseases, such as pemphigus, eczema, and dermatitis herpetiformis;

and parasitic infections, such as trichinosis (caused by infection with *Trichinella spiralis*), schistosomiasis, and strongyloidiasis. The most common cause of eosinophilia is probably allergy to drugs such as iodides, aspirin, or sulfonamides, but eosinophilia is also seen in collagen vascular diseases. Marked eosinophilia occurs in hypereosinophilic syndromes (Löffler's syndrome and idiopathic hypereosinophilic syndrome), which may be treated with corticosteroids.

In contrast, neutrophilic leukocytosis (neutrophilia) may be the result of acute bacterial infections or tissue necrosis, such as is present with myocardial infarction, trauma, or burns. Basophilia is most commonly seen in immediate type (type I) hypersensitivity reactions. Both eosinophils and basophils may be increased in patients with any of the chronic myeloproliferative syndromes. Monocytosis is seen in chronic infections, such as tuberculosis, some collagen vascular diseases, neutropenic states, and some types of lymphomas. Lymphocytosis (especially with increased numbers of T lymphocytes) may be seen along with monocytosis in chronic inflammatory states or in acute viral infections, such as viral hepatitis or infectious mononucleosis.

215. The answer is a. (*Kumar, pp 665–666. Chandrasoma, pp 433–443.*) Lymph nodes may be enlarged (lymphadenopathy) secondary to reactive processes, which can be either acute or chronic. Acute reaction (acute nonspecific lymphadenitis) can result in focal or generalized lymphadenopathy. Focal lymph node enlargement is usually the result of bacterial infection (bacterial lymphadenitis). Sections from involved lymph nodes reveal infiltration by neutrophils. In contrast, generalized acute lymphadenopathy is usually the result of viral infections and usually produces a proliferation of reactive T lymphocytes called T immunoblasts. These reactive T cells tend to have prominent nucleoli and can be easily mistaken for malignant lymphocytes or malignant Hodgkin cells.

216. The answer is b. (*Kumar, pp 369–371, 665–666. Rubin, pp 1095–1099. Chandrasoma, pp 433–443.*) Reactive processes involving lymph nodes typically involve different and specific portions of the lymph nodes depending upon the type of cell that is reacting. For example, reactive T lymphocytes typically result in hyperplasia involving the T-cell areas of the lymph node, namely, the interfollicular regions and the paracortex. Examples of clinical situations associated with a T lymphocyte response include viral infections, vaccinations, use of some drugs (particularly

Dilantin), and systemic lupus erythematosus. An example of such a viral infection is infectious mononucleosis, a disorder usually caused by infection with the Epstein-Barr virus (EBV) in young adults. Classic clinical symptoms include fever, cervical lymphadenopathy, and pharyngitis. Atypical lymphocytes are usually found in the peripheral blood, and these same cells, which are reactive T immunoblasts cause enlargement of the cervical lymph nodes.

In contrast to reactive T-cell processes, reactive B lymphocytes typically result in hyperplasia of the lymphoid follicles and germinal centers (follicular hyperplasia). Examples of diseases that are associated with follicular hyperplasia include chronic inflammation caused by organisms, rheumatoid arthritis, and AIDS. Lymph nodes from patients with AIDS undergo characteristic changes that begin with follicular hyperplasia with loss of mantle zones, intrafollicular hemorrhage ("follicle lysis"), and monocytoid B-cell proliferation. Subsequently there is depletion of lymphocytes (CD4 lymphocytes) in both the follicles and the interfollicular areas.

217. The answer is e. (*Kumar, pp 28–30, 670–678, 659–661. Rubin, pp 1131–1132. Hoffman, pp 1313–1314.*) In general, the non-Hodgkin's lymphomas (NHLs) can be divided histologically into nodular forms and diffuse forms. All nodular NHLs, one of which is seen in the picture associated with this question, are the result of neoplastic proliferations of B lymphocytes. Histologically these nodules somewhat resemble the germinal centers of lymphoid follicles, but instead they are characterized by increased numbers (crowding) of nodules, their location in both the cortex and the medulla, their uniform size, and their composition (a monotonous proliferation of cells). These neoplastic B cells express CD19, CD20, CD10 (CALLA), and surface immunoglobulin. In addition, these cells express BCL6, the gene for which is located on chromosome 18. Indeed, the hallmark of follicular non-Hodgkin's lymphoma is a (14;18) translocation, which results in the overproduction of the BCL2 protein, which normally inhibits apoptosis. This product is located on the outer mitochondrial membrane, endoplasmic reticulum, and nuclear envelope. It inhibits apoptosis by blocking bax channels and by binding to and sequestering apoptosis activating factor 1 (Apaf-1). This interferes with one mechanism of apoptosis that involves cytochrome c being released into the cytoplasm from mitochondria via bax channels, these channels being upregulated by p53. Cytochrome c then binds to and activates Apaf-1, which then stimulates a caspase cascade. The end result is that by inhibiting apoptosis, overexpression of BCL2 promotes the survival of the follicular lymphoma cells.

The t(14;18) is also found in a minority of cases of diffuse large B-cell lymphoma (DLBCL). These cases are thought to have arisen from prior follicular lymphomas that became diffuse in appearance. More frequently these DLBCLs are associated with dysregulation of BCL6. In contrast, Burkitt's lymphoma is associated with abnormal expression of the MYC gene, which is located on chromosome 8. Translocations associated with Burkitt's lymphoma involve this gene and include t(2;8), t(8;14), and t(8;22). Finally, t(9;14) is characteristic of lymphoplasmacytic lymphoma and involves the PAX-5 gene on chromosome 9, while t(11;14) is characteristic of mantle cell lymphoma and involves BCL1 (cyclin D1).

218. The answer is b. (*Kumar, pp 667–669, 673–674. Rubin, pp 1133–1136. Hoffman, pp 1268–1270, 1293–1294.*) The Working Formulation divides the non-Hodgkin's lymphomas (NHLs) into low grade, intermediate grade, and high grade based on prognostic criteria. The low-grade NHLs include small-lymphocytic NHL (well-differentiated lymphocytic NHL), follicular small-cleaved NHL, and follicular mixed small-cleaved and large-cell NHL. Small-lymphocytic NHL (SLL), which has only a diffuse pattern, is characterized by a proliferation of small B lymphocytes, which have B-cell markers (such as CD23) and one T-cell marker (CD5). SLL frequently has a leukemic phase and has a propensity for metastasis to the bone marrow and is similar to B-cell chronic lymphocytic leukemia. The intermediate-grade NHLs include follicular large-cell NHL, diffuse small-cleaved NHL, diffuse mixed small-cleaved and large-cell NHL, and diffuse large-cell NHL. The high-grade NHLs include immunoblastic lymphoma, lymphoblastic lymphoma, and small noncleaved NHL (Burkitt's lymphoma).

Compare Working Formulation classification to the newer REAL (revised European-American classification of lymphomas), which was developed to include some recently described lymphomas that did not fit into the Working Formulation. The REAL classification includes precursor B-cell neoplasms (immature B cells), peripheral B-cell neoplasms (mature B cells), precursor T-cell neoplasms (immature T cells), and peripheral T-cell neoplasms (mature T cells). Finally, the Rappaport classification is an old classification (developed in 1966) that was based on the microscopic appearance of tumor cells. That is, the size of the malignant cells was classified as being either lymphocytic or histiocytic, while the tumor growth pattern was nodular or diffuse. Also this classification is called well-differentiated cells being similar to lymphocytes and poorly differentiated cells being angulated (cleaved) or having nucleoli.

219. The answer is b. (*Kumar, pp 674–676. Rubin, pp 1135–1137.*) Some of the non-Hodgkin's lymphomas are associated with involvement of the peripheral blood (leukemic phase). More than half of the patients with small lymphocytic lymphoma (SLL) have involvement of the bone marrow with spillage of neoplastic cells into the peripheral blood, where they appear as mature lymphocytes, many of which are smudged. The clinical picture is then similar to that of chronic lymphocytic leukemia (CLL). Follicular NHLs also commonly involve the bone marrow, but spillage into the peripheral blood is much less common than in SLL. Still, when the malignant small cleaved lymphocytes, which are also called centrocytes, are found within the peripheral blood, they have a characteristic cleaved appearance that is described as "buttock cells." Lymphoblastic lymphoma is another type of lymphoma that frequently involves the bone marrow and peripheral blood. The clinical picture then is similar to that of T-cell acute lymphoblastic leukemia (ALL). In contrast, multiple myeloma and Hodgkin's disease do not have malignant cells in the peripheral blood.

220. The answer is b. (*Henry, pp 612–613. Kumar, pp 677–678.*) Burkitt's lymphoma (small noncleaved non-Hodgkin's lymphoma) is characterized by a rapid proliferation of primitive lymphoid cells with thick nuclear membranes, multiple nucleoli, and intensely basophilic cytoplasm when stained with Wright's stain. The cells are often mixed with macrophages in biopsy, giving a starry sky appearance. The cytoplasmic vacuoles of the lymphoma cells contain lipid, and this would be reflected by a positive oil red O reaction. The African type of Burkitt's lymphoma is the endemic form and typically involves the maxilla or mandible, while the American type of small noncleaved NHL is nonendemic and commonly involves the abdomen, such as bowel, ovaries, or retroperitoneum. The African type is associated with Epstein-Barr virus (EBV) and a characteristic t(8;14) translocation.

221. The answer is b. (*Kumar, pp 670–673. Rubin, pp 1137–1138.*) T-cell lymphomas occurring in the thoracic cavity in young patients usually arise in the mediastinum and have a particularly aggressive clinical course with rapid growth in the mediastinum impinging on the trachea or mainstem bronchi and leading to marked respiratory deficiency, which can in turn lead to death in a relatively short period of time if not treated. These unique lymphomas are characterized by rapid cell growth and spread into the circulation, where they produce elevated total white counts reflected by circulating lymphoma cells. As T cells they have characteristics of rosette formation with sheep blood cells. T cells also have subtypes and subsets, which can be delineated by monoclonal antibodies as CD4 helper and CD8 suppressor (cellular differentiation) T-cell surface antigens. The tumor cells also express IL-2 receptor. Fc receptors occur on B cells and macrophages. Class II HLA antigens can be found on macrophages, Langerhans cells, and dendritic reticulum cells.

222. The answer is d. (*Kumar, pp 686–690. Rubin, pp 1140–1147.*) The diagnosis of Hodgkin's disease (HD) depends on the clinical findings added to the total histologic picture, which includes the presence of binucleated giant cells with prominent acidophilic "owl-eye" nucleoli known as Reed-Sternberg (RS) cells. These malignant cells characteristically stain with both the CD15 and CD30 immunoperoxidase stains. Note that cells similar in appearance to RS cells may also be seen in infectious mononucleosis, mycosis fungoides, and other conditions. Thus, while RS cells are necessary for histologic confirmation of the diagnosis of Hodgkin's disease, they must be present in the appropriate histologic setting of the different types of HD, which includes lymphocyte predominance, nodular sclerosis, mixed cellularity, and lymphocyte depletion. The most common type of HD is the nodular sclerosis variant. This type is characterized morphologically by the presence of the lacunar variant of RS cells and by bands of fibrous tissue that divide the lymph node into nodules. Unlike the other subtypes of Hodgkin's disease, it is more common in females. Young adults are classically affected and the disease typically involves the cervical, supraclavicular, or mediastinal lymph nodes. Involvement of extranodal lymphoid tissue is unusual. Variant RS cells with a multilobed, puffy nucleus ("popcorn" cells) are seen in the lymphocyte-predominant subtype.

223. The answer is e. (*Kumar, pp 692–695. Rubin, pp 1117–1122.*) The leukemias are malignant neoplasms of the hematopoietic stem cells that are characterized by diffuse replacement of the bone marrow by neoplastic cells. These malignant cells frequently spill into the peripheral blood. The leukemias are divided into acute and chronic forms, and then further subdivided based on lymphocytic or myelocytic (myelogenous) forms. Thus, the four basic patterns of acute leukemia are acute lymphocytic leukemia (ALL), chronic lymphocytic leukemia (CLL), acute myelocytic leukemia (AML), and chronic myelocytic leukemia (CML).

Acute leukemias are characterized by a decrease in the mature forms of cells and an increase in the immature forms (leukemic blasts). Acute leukemias (both ALL and AML) have an abrupt clinical onset and present with symptoms due to failure of normal marrow function. Symptoms include fever (secondary to infection), easy fatigability (due to anemia), and bleeding (due to thrombocytopenia). The peripheral smear in patients with acute leukemia usually reveals the white cell count to be increased. The peripheral smear also reveals signs of anemia and thrombocytopenia. More importantly, however, there are blasts in the peripheral smear. The diagnosis of acute leukemia is made by finding more than 30% blasts in the bone marrow.

AML primarily affects adults between the ages of 15 and 39 and is characterized by the neoplastic proliferation of myeloblasts. Myeloblasts, characterized by their delicate nuclear chromatin, may contain three to five nucleoli. Myeloblasts in some cases of AML contain distinct intracytoplasmic rodlike structures that stain red and are called Auer rods. These are abnormal lysosomal structures (primary granules) that are considered pathognomonic of myeloblasts. AML is divided into seven types by the French-American-British (FAB) classification:

M1—myeloblastic leukemia without maturation (cells are mainly blasts)

M2—myeloblastic leukemia with maturation (some promyelocytes are present)

M3—hypergranular promyelocytic leukemia (numerous granules and many Auer rods)

M4—myelomonocytic leukemia (both myeloblasts and monoblasts)

M5—monocytic leukemia (infiltrates in the gingiva are characteristic)

M6—erythroleukemia (Di Guglielmo's disease)

M7—acute megakaryocytic leukemia (associated with myelofibrosis)

Acute promyelocytic leukemia (M3 AML) is characterized by several specific features that are found in no other types of acute leukemia. There are numerous abnormal promyelocytes present that contain numerous cytoplasmic granules and numerous Auer rods. If these numerous granules are released from dying cells, which may occur with treatment, they may activate extensive, uncontrolled intravascular coagulation and cause the development of disseminated intravascular coagulopathy (DIC). This abnormality is characterized by increased fibrin degradation products in the blood. M3 AML is also characterized by the translocation t(15;17), which results in the fusion of the retinoic acid receptor α gene on chromosome 17 to the PML unit on chromosome 15. This produces an abnormal retinoic acid receptor and provides the basis for treatment of these patients with all-*trans*-retinoic acid.

224. The answer is d. (*Kumar, pp 670–673. Rubin, pp 1128–1130.*) Acute lymphoblastic leukemia (ALL) is primarily a disease of children and young adults that is characterized by the presence of numerous lymphoblasts within the bone marrow. These malignant cells may spill over into the blood and other organs. In contrast to myeloblasts, lymphoblasts do not contain myeloperoxidase, but they do stain positively with the PAS stain or acid phosphatase stain and for the enzyme TdT. The FAB classification of ALL divides ALL into three types based on the morphology of the proliferating lymphoblasts. L1-ALL, seen in about 85% of the cases of ALL, consists of small homogeneous blasts. L2-ALL, seen in only 15% of cases of ALL, but more common in adults, consists of lymphoblasts that are larger and more heterogeneous (pleomorphic) than L1 blasts. These cells may also contain nuclear clefts. The final type of FAB ALL is the L3 type, which is seen in less than 1% of the cases of ALL. This form is essentially the leukemic form of Burkitt's lymphoma. Like the malignant cells of Burkitt's lymphoma, these L3-ALL cells are large blasts with cytoplasmic vacuoles that stain positively with the oil red O lipid stain.

In contrast to the FAB classification of ALL, the immunologic classification of ALL is based on the developmental sequence of maturation of B and T lymphocytes. First, it is necessary to determine whether the blasts have B- or T-cell markers. Most cases of ALL are of B-cell origin; that is, the lymphoblasts express both CD19 and DR. A few cases of ALL are of T-cell origin; the lymphoblasts lack CD19 and DR and instead express T-cell antigens CD2, 5, and 7. Many cases of T-ALL involve a mediastinal mass and are clinically similar to cases of lymphoblastic lymphoma. To subclassify B-ALL, first determine if surface immunoglobulin (sIg) is present. Mature B-ALL cells (L3-ALL or Burkitt's lymphoma) have surface immunoglobulin, which is not found in the other types of B-ALL. These mature cells typically lack TdT, which is a marker for more immature cells. Next, determine if there is cytoplasmic μ present. Cytoplasmic μ chains are specific for pre-B-ALL cells, which have a characteristic translocation t(1;19). The B cell ALL cells that lack both surface Ig and cytoplasmic μ are called early pre-B-ALL and are separated into the CALLA (CD10)-positive and CALLA-negative types.

225. The answer is b. (*Kumar, pp 295, 297, 697–698. Rubin, pp 1110–1114.*) Chronic myeloid leukemia (CML) is one of the four chronic myeloproliferative disorders, but, unlike myeloid metaplasia or polycythemia vera, CML is associated with the Philadelphia chromosome translocation t(9;22) in over 90% of cases. This characteristic translocation, which involves the oncogene c-*abl* on chromosome 9 and the breakpoint cluster region on chromosome 22, results in the formation of a new fusion protein (P210) that is a nonreceptor tyrosine kinase. (In contrast, the translocation t(8;14) and the c-*myc* oncogene are associated with Burkitt's lymphoma.) In differentiating CML from a leukemoid reaction, several other features are important in addition to the presence of the Philadelphia chromosome: lack of alkaline phosphatase in granulocytes, increased basophils and eosinophils in the peripheral blood, and, often, increased platelets in early stages followed by thrombocytopenia in late or blast stages. Other well-known features of CML include marked splenomegaly, leukocyte counts greater than 50,000/μL, and mild anemia.

226. The answer is d. (*Kumar, pp 683–686. Rubin, pp 1126–1128.*) Hairy cell leukemia, a type of chronic B-cell leukemia, should be suspected in patients with splenomegaly; pancytopenia, including thrombocytopenia; bleeding; and fatigue. These leukemic lymphocyte-like cells in the peripheral blood demonstrate cytoplasmic projections at the cell periphery ("hairy" cells). These cells stain for acid phosphatase, and the reaction is refractory to treatment with tartaric acid (tartrate-resistant acid phosphatase [TRAP]). These hairy cells also express pan–B-cell markers (CD19 and CD20), the monocyte marker CD11c, and the plasma cell marker PCA-1. The most common sign in these patients is splenomegaly, which is due to leukemic cells infiltrating the red pulp, which is unusual considering that most leukemias preferentially infiltrate the white pulp. Because these neoplastic cells proliferate in the spleen, splenectomy may be a treatment choice. Another treatment option is interferon-alpha and pentostatin; the latter blocks adenine deaminase. The histologic appearance of the bone marrow is that of "fried eggs," but aspiration of the marrow typically produces a dry tap.

227. The answer is c. (*Kumar, pp 673–674. Rubin, pp 1122–1126.*) Chronic lymphocytic leukemia (CLL) is the most common leukemia and is similar in many aspects to small lymphocytic lymphoma (SLL). It is typically found in patients older than 60 years of age. Histological examination of the peripheral smear reveals a marked increase in the number of mature-appearing lymphocytes. These neoplastic lymphocytes are fragile and easily damaged. This fragility produces the characteristic finding of numerous smudge cells in the peripheral smears of patients with CLL. About 95% of the cases of CLL are of B-cell origin (B-CLL) and are characterized by having pan–B-cell markers, such as CD19. These malignant cells characteristically also have the T-cell marker CD5. The remaining 5% of cases of CLL are mainly of T-cell origin. Patients with CLL tend to have an indolent course and the disease is associated with long survival in many cases. The few symptoms that may develop are related to anemia and the absolute lymphocytosis of small, mature cells. Splenomegaly may be noted. In a minority of patients, however, the disease may transform into prolymphocytic leukemia or a large cell immunoblastic lymphoma (Richter's syndrome). Prolymphocytic leukemia is characterized by massive splenomegaly and a markedly increased leukocyte count consisting of enlarged lymphocytes having nuclei with mature chromatin and nucleoli.

228. The answer is d. (*Kumar, pp 695–696. Henry, pp 605–606.*) The myelodysplastic syndromes (MDS) are a group of disorders characterized by defective hematopoietic maturation and an increased risk of developing acute leukemia. These disorders characteristically have hypercellular bone marrows but pancytopenia in the peripheral blood. The two basic types of MDS are an idiopathic (primary) form and a therapy-related (secondary) form. Both have numerous dysplastic features affecting all blood cell lines. Red cell dysplastic features include the presence of ringed sideroblasts, megaloblastoid erythroid precursors, and misshapen erythroid precursors. A dimorphic population of red cells may be seen in the peripheral blood of some patients with some types of MDS. White cell dysplastic features include hypogranular cells or Pelger-Huët white blood cells, which are abnormal appearing neutrophils having only two nuclear lobes. Megakaryocytes may be abnormal and have only a single nuclear lobe or multiple separate nuclei, so-called "pawn ball" megakaryocytes. Chromosomal abnormalities are commonly associated with the MDSs, especially 5q_ and trisomy 8.

Except for chronic myelomonocytic leukemia (CMML), which is characterized by a marked increase in the number of monocytes, the MDSs are subclassified by the number of blasts present within the bone marrow. The

FAB classification of MDS is as follows: if there are less than 5% blasts present, the MDS is either refractory anemia (RA) or RA with ring sideroblasts (RARS). RA with excess blasts (RAEB, pronounced "rab") has between 5 and 20% blasts, while refractory anemia with excess blasts in transformation (RAEBIT, pronounced "rabbit") has between 20 and 30% blasts in the marrow. Acute leukemia is defined as the presence of more than 30% blasts in the marrow. The WHO (World Health Organization) has a similar classification of the MDS except that in their classification the number of blasts in the bone marrow needed for the diagnosis of acute leukemia is only 20%.

229. The answer is e. (*Kumar, pp 699–700. Rubin, 1110–1112.*) Polycythemia rubra vera (PRV) is a myeloproliferative disorder that is characterized by excessive proliferation of erythroid, granulocytic, and megakaryocytic precursors derived from a single stem cell. In PRV, the erythroid series dominates, but there is hyperplasia of all elements. There is plethoric congestion of all organs. The liver and spleen are typically moderately enlarged and may show extramedullary hematopoiesis. Thrombotic complications are an important cause of morbidity and mortality, and major and minor hemorrhagic complications are also frequent. The red cell count is elevated with hematocrit >60% (despite the fact that serum erythropoietin levels are decreased). The white cell count and platelet count are also elevated. Leukocyte alkaline phosphatase (LAP) activity is elevated, in contrast to the case with chronic myeloid leukemia, where it is reduced. Pruritus and peptic ulceration are common, possibly in relation to increased histamine release from basophils.

230. The answer is a. (*Kumar, pp 700–701. Rubin, pp 1114–1116.*) Myeloid metaplasia with myelofibrosis is a myeloproliferative disorder in which the bone marrow is hypocellular and fibrotic and extramedullary hematopoiesis occurs, mainly in the spleen (myeloid metaplasia). Marked splenomegaly with trilineage proliferation of normoblasts, immature myeloid cells, and large megakaryocytes occur. Giant platelets and poikilocytic (teardrop) red cells are seen in the peripheral smear along with immature white blood cells (e.g., myelocytes) and immature red blood cells (e.g., nucleated red blood cells). The bone marrow is fibrotic with increased reticulin and an aspiration of the marrow is usually unsuccessful and results in a "dry tap." Clinically, myeloid metaplasia may be preceded by polycythemia vera or chronic myeloid leukemia. Biopsy of the marrow is essential for diagnosis. In contradistinction to chronic myeloid leukemia, levels of leukocyte alkaline phosphatase are elevated or normal in myeloid metaplasia; in CML, levels are low or absent. In 5 to 10% of cases of myeloid metaplasia, acute leukemia occurs.

In contrast, increased total protein in the serum (with a normal serum albumin and hypercalcemia) is diagnostic of multiple myeloma. Patients also develop multiple lytic bone lesions and their marrow will have increased numbers of plasma cells, some of which may be atypical in appearance. Finally, multiple black gallstones (bilirubin stones) can be seen with any chronic hemolytic anemia.

231. The answer is d. (*Kumar, pp 678–681. Rubin, pp 1147–1150.*) The bone marrow aspirate exhibits a proliferation of plasma cells that are characterized by well-defined perinuclear clear zones and by dense cytoplasmic basophilia due to increased RNA accumulations. Weakness, weight loss, recurrent infections, proteinuria, anemia, and abnormal proliferation of plasma cells in the bone marrow are findings that highly suggest the presence of multiple myeloma, a plasma cell dyscrasia. The more definitive diagnostic criteria are findings of M component in the results of serum electrophoresis and plasma cell levels of above 20% in the bone marrow. Multiple myeloma, which occurs more commonly in males than in females, shows an increasing incidence with increasing age, and most patients are in their seventies. Osteolytic, punched-out bone lesions are characteristic, especially in the skull. Because the process is lytic, alkaline phosphatase is usually not elevated. These osteolytic lesions result from the production of osteoclast-activating factor (OAF) by the myeloma cells. This results in increased serum calcium levels (hypercalcemia). OAF is in fact IL-6, and increased amounts of IL-6 are associated with a worse prognosis because the survival of the myeloma cells is dependent on IL-6. Myeloma is not associated with lymphadenopathy, but recurrent infections are frequent because of the severe suppression of normal immunoglobulins. In fact, infection is the most common cause of death in these patients and is usually due to encapsulated bacteria. There is no increase in viral infections in these patients because their cell-mediated immunity is normal.

Finally, note that glycogen accumulating abnormally in histiocytes (macrophages) is characteristic of the glycogen storage diseases (GSD), such as von Gierke's disease, type I GSD, which is due to a deficiency of glucose-6-phosphatase. Gaucher disease is a type of lysosomal storage disease that is due to a deficiency of beta-glucocerebrosidase. Excess glucocerebrosides accumulate within phagocytic cells.

232. The answer is e. (*Kumar, pp 681–682. Hoffman, pp 1410–1411.*) Waldenström's macroglobulinemia (WM), associated with a monoclonal production of IgM, is clinically distinct from multiple myeloma. It is somewhat like a cross between multiple myeloma (MM) and small lymphocytic lymphoma (SLL). As with myeloma, there is a monoclonal production of immunoglobulin (IgM) that produces an M spike. Unlike the case with myeloma, however, there are no lytic bone lesions and no hypercalcemia, and the bone marrow shows proliferation of plasma cells, lymphocytes, and plasmacytoid lymphocytes. Like SLL, WM is associated with infiltration of organs outside of the bone marrow by neoplastic cells. These include the lymph nodes and the spleen. (Involvement of these organs is unusual in patients with MM.) Because IgM is a large molecule (a pentamer), patients with WM are prone to developing the hyperviscosity syndrome, which consists of visual abnormalities, neurologic signs (headaches and confusion), bleeding, and cryoglobulinemia.

Other monoclonal proliferations of immunoglobulin include monoclonal gammopathy of undetermined significance (MGUS) and heavy-chain disease. MGUS may be associated with an M spike and increased marrow plasma cells, but the number of plasma cells will be less than 20%. Note that M proteins are found in 1 to 3% of asymptomatic persons over the age of 50. Heavy chain disease refers to types of plasma cell dyscrasia that are associated with the monoclonal production of immunoglobulin heavy chains only (not light chains). There are basically three types of heavy-chain disease: α heavy-chain disease, γ heavy-chain disease, and μ heavy-chain disease. α heavy-chain disease is seen primarily in the Mediterranean region, hence its other name, Mediterranean lymphoma. It is characterized by numerous plasma cells infiltrating the lamina propria of the small intestines. This disease is preceded by an abnormality called immunoproliferative small intestinal disease (IPSID), which is characterized by villous atrophy of the small intestines with steatorrhea. Unique patients with this disease are treated with antibiotics. γ heavy-chain disease is rare and is similar to non-Hodgkin's lymphoma. μ heavy-chain disease is found rarely in some patients with CLL.

233. The answer is b. (*Kumar, pp 701–702. Rubin, pp 1364–1365.*) Langerhans cell histiocytosis, previously known as histiocytosis X, refers to a spectrum of clinical diseases that are associated with the proliferation of Langerhans cells. These cells, not to be confused with the Langerhans-type giant cells found in caseating granulomas of tuberculosis, have Fc receptors and HLA-D/DR antigens and react with CD1 antibodies. These cells contain distinctive granules, seen by electron microscopy, that are rod-shaped organelles resembling tennis rackets. They are called LC (Langerhans cell) granules, pentilaminar bodies, or Birbeck granules. There are three general ·clinical forms of Langerhans histiocytosis. Acute disseminated LC histiocytosis (Letterer-Siwe disease) affects children before the age of 3 years. These children have cutaneous lesions that resemble seborrhea, hepatosplenomegaly, and lymphadenopathy. The LCs infiltrate the marrow, which leads to anemia, thrombocytopenia, and recurrent infections. The clinical course is usually rapidly fatal; however, with intensive chemotherapy 50% of patients may survive 5 years. Multifocal LC histiocytosis (Hand-Schüller-Christian disease) usually begins between the second and sixth years of life. The characteristic triad consists of bone lesions, particularly in the calvarium and the base of the skull; diabetes insipidus; and exophthalmos. These lesions are the result of proliferations of LCs. Lesions around the hypothalamus lead to decreased ADH production and signs of diabetes insipidus. Unifocal LC histiocytosis (eosinophilic granuloma), seen in older patients, is usually a unifocal disease, most often affecting the skeletal system. The lesions are granulomas that contain a mixture of lipid-laden Langerhans cells, macrophages, lymphocytes, and eosinophils.

In contrast, sarcoidosis is characterized by a proliferation of activated macrophages that form granulomas. It is not a proliferation of LCs. Dermatopathic lymphadenitis refers to a chronic lymphadenitis that affects the lymph nodes draining the sites of chronic dermatologic diseases. The lymph nodes undergo hyperplasia of the germinal follicles and accumulation of melanin and hemosiderin pigment by the phagocytic cells.

234. The answer is d. (*Kumar, pp 326, 369–371. Rubin, pp 370–372, 1094.*) Infectious mononucleosis is a benign lymphoproliferative disorder caused by infection with the Epstein-Barr virus (EBV). It typically occurs in young adults and presents with systemic symptoms, lymphadenopathy, and pharyngitis. Hepatosplenomegaly may be present. Peripheral blood shows an absolute lymphocytosis, and many lymphocytes are atypical with irregular nuclei and abundant basophilic vacuolated cytoplasm. These represent CD8+ T killer cells induced by EBV-transformed B lymphocytes. These atypical lymphocytes are usually adequate for diagnosis, along with a positive heterophil or monospot test (increased sheep red cell agglutinin). Administration of ampicillin for a mistaken diagnosis of streptococcal pharyngitis results in a rash in many patients.

Respiratory System

Questions

DIRECTIONS: Each item below contains a question or incomplete statement followed by suggested responses. Select the **one best** response to each question.

235. Histologic sections (routine H&E stain) of lung reveal the alveoli to be filled with pale, nongranular pink fluid. Neither leukocytes nor erythrocytes are present within this fluid. Which of the following is the most common cause of this abnormality?

a. Bacterial pneumonia
b. Congestive heart failure
c. Lymphatic obstruction by tumor
d. Pulmonary embolus
e. Viral pneumonia

236. A 7-year-old boy accidentally inhales a small peanut, which lodges in one of his bronchi. A chest x-ray reveals the mediastinum to be shifted toward the side of the obstruction. Which of the following pulmonary abnormalities is most likely present in this boy?

a. Absorptive atelectasis
b. Compression atelectasis
c. Contraction atelectasis
d. Patchy atelectasis
e. Hyaline membrane disease

237. A 26-year-old man barely survives a house fire. He is taken unconscious to the hospital where over the next several days he develops worsening signs of respiratory failure. A chest x-ray on the third hospital day reveals a complete "white-out" of both lungs. Laboratory evaluation finds severe hypoxemia that does not improve with 100% oxygen. Which of the following histologic changes is most likely to be seen in a biopsy specimen taken from his lungs?

a. Angioinvasive infiltrates of pleomorphic lymphoid cells
b. Deposits of needle-like crystals from the membranes of eosinophils
c. Infiltrating groups of malignant cells having intercellular bridges
d. Irregular membranes composed of edema, fibrin, and dead cells lining alveoli
e. Plexiform lesions within pulmonary arterioles

238. While recovering in bed 1 week after an abdominal hysterectomy, a 42-year-old woman develops acute shortness of breath with hemoptysis. Physical examination finds the patient to be afebrile with moderate respiratory distress, calf tenderness, and a widely split S_2. Which of the following is the most likely diagnosis?

a. Atelectasis
b. Bacterial pneumonia
c. Pulmonary embolus
d. Pulmonary hypertension
e. Viral pneumonia

239. A 25-year-old woman presents with a 6-month history of increasing fatigue and dyspnea. Physical examination finds that she is in moderate respiratory distress and cyanosis is present. An echocardiogram of her heart finds the thickness of the right ventricle to be increased, but the thickness of the left ventricle is within normal limits. Histologic sections from a lung biopsy reveal plexiform lesions within the pulmonary arterioles. Hyaline membranes are not found nor are areas of lung collapse present. Which of the following is the most important cause of the primary form of this disorder?

a. A congenital heart defect that produces a left-to-right shunt
b. Mutations involving the apical epithelial sodium ion channel
c. Mutations involving the bone morphogenetic protein receptor type 2
d. The presence of c-ANCA antibodies
e. The presence of p-ANCA antibodies

240. A 19-year-old woman presents with urticaria that developed after she took aspirin for a headache. She has a history of chronic rhinitis, and physical examination reveals the presence of nasal polyps. This patient is at an increased risk of developing which one of the following pulmonary abnormalities following the ingestion of aspirin?

a. Contraction atelectasis of the lower lung lobes
b. Destruction of the alveolar walls
c. Fibrosis of the alveolar interstitium
d. Mucus plugging of the bronchioles
e. Sclerosis of the small blood vessels

241. A 63-year-old man who is a long-term smoker presents with increasing shortness of breath and dyspnea. He has smoked more than two packs of cigarettes per day for more than 40 years. He denies having a productive cough or any recent infections. Physical examination reveals a thin elderly-appearing man in moderate respiratory distress. While sitting he leans forward slightly and breathes quickly through pursed lips. He is afebrile and his blood pressure is within normal limits. Examination of his chest reveals an increased anteroposterior diameter and his lungs are hyper-resonant to percussion. His respiratory rate is increased, but no clubbing or cyanosis is present. Chest x-ray reveals his heart to be of normal size, but there is hyperinflation of his lungs. Laboratory examination reveals that while breathing room air, his arterial Po_2 is decreased but his arterial Pco_2 is normal. Which of the following statements is a correct association concerning the pathogenesis of this man's pulmonary disease?

a. Destruction of entire acinus caused panlobular emphysema
b. Destruction of the cilia on the respiratory epithelial cells resulted in bronchiectasis
c. Destruction of the proximal acinus caused centrilobular emphysema
d. Hyperplasia of the respiratory smooth-muscle cells resulted in intrinsic asthma
e. Hyperplasia on the respiratory mucus glands caused chronic bronchitis

242. A 27-year-old man presents with a chronic productive cough. Pertinent medical history is that he has had recurrent sinusitis and numerous lower respiratory tract infections since childhood. He has been married for 6 years and has no children, although he and his wife do not use any form of birth control. His chest x-ray reveals the apex of the heart to be directed toward the right (the cardiac apical impulse is felt best in the sixth intercostal space), and a CBC reveals a normocytic normochromic anemia. Semen analysis reveals his spermatozoa to be immotile and lack the normal ATPase-containing dynein arms. Without treatment, which of the following changes is most likely to result from his disease?

a. Abnormal permanent dilation of the bronchi in the lungs
b. Destruction of the walls of the alveoli in the base of the lungs
c. Fatty metamorphosis of the hepatocytes in the liver
d. Hyperplasia of the smooth-muscle cells of the bronchioles in the lungs
e. Irreversible deposition of collagen in the subendothelial spaces in the liver

243. A 37-year-old woman presents with the acute onset of a productive cough, fever, chills, and pleuritic chest pain. A chest x-ray reveals consolidation of the entire lower lobe of her right lung. She unexpectedly dies before treatment due to a cardiac arrhythmia. Histologic examination of lung tissue taken at the time of autopsy reveals multiple suppurative, neutrophil-rich exudates filling the bronchi, bronchioles, and alveolar spaces. The majority of lung tissue from her right lower lung is involved in this inflammatory process. Hyaline membranes are not found. Which of the following is the most likely diagnosis?

a. Bronchiectasis
b. Bronchopneumonia
c. Interstitial pneumonitis
d. Lobar pneumonia
e. Pulmonary abscess

244. A 44-year-old alcoholic man presents with fever and a productive cough with copious amounts of foul-smelling purulent sputum. Physical examination finds that changing the position of this individual produces paroxysms of coughing. Which of the following is the most likely cause of this patient's signs and symptoms?

a. Esophageal cancer
b. Esophageal reflux
c. Myocardial infarction
d. Pulmonary abscess
e. Pulmonary infarction

245. A 25-year-old woman presents with fever, malaise, headaches, and muscle pain (myalgia). A chest x-ray reveals bilateral infiltrates. You draw a tube of blood from the patient (the tube contains anticoagulant) and place the tube in a cup of ice. After the blood has cooled, you notice that the red cells have agglutinated (not clotted). This agglutination goes away after you warm up the tube of blood. This patient's illness is most likely due to infection with which one of the following organisms?

a. Influenza A virus
b. *Mycoplasma pneumoniae*
c. *Streptococcus pneumoniae*
d. *Pneumocystis pneumoniae*
e. *Mycobacterium tuberculosis*

246. A 23-year-old HIV-positive man presents with a cough and increasing shortness of breath. A histologic section from a transbronchial biopsy stained with Gomori's methenamine-silver stain is shown in the photomicrograph. Which of the following is the most likely diagnosis?

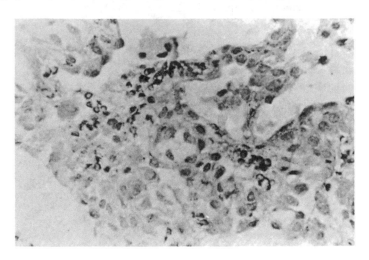

a. *Pseudomonas* pneumonia
b. *Aspergillus* pneumonia
c. *Pneumocystis carinii* pneumonia
d. Cytomegalovirus pneumonia
e. Influenza pneumonia

247. A routine chest x-ray performed on an asymptomatic 31-year-old man who works at sandblasting reveals a fine nodularity in the upper zones of the lungs and "eggshell" calcification of the hilar lymph nodes. The patient's serum calcium level is 9.8 mg/dL, while his total protein is 7.2 g/dL. He denies any history of drug use or cigarette smoking. A biopsy from his lung reveals birefringent particles within macrophages. This individual has an increased risk for developing which one of the listed disorders?

a. Anthracosis
b. Berylliosis
c. Myxomatosis
d. Sarcoidosis
e. Tuberculosis

248. A 65-year-old man who just retired after having worked for many years as a shipyard worker presents with increasing shortness of breath. Pertinent medical history is that he has been a long time smoker. A CT scan of his chest reveals thick, pleural plaques on the surface of his lungs. The associated picture is from a bronchial washing specimen from this patient. The dumbbell-shaped structures in this picture were found to stain blue with a Prussian blue stain. What are these structures?

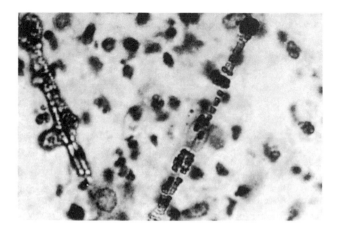

a. *Candida* species
b. Cholesterol crystals
c. Ferruginous bodies
d. Schaumann bodies
e. Silica particles

249. A 24-year-old African American woman presents with nonspecific symptoms including fever and malaise. A chest x-ray reveals enlarged hilar lymph nodes ("potato nodes"), while her serum calcium level is found to be elevated. Which of the following histologic abnormalities is most likely to be seen in biopsy specimens from these enlarged hilar lymph nodes?

a. Caseating granulomas
b. Dense, granular, PAS-positive, eosinophilic material
c. Markedly enlarged epithelial cells with intranuclear inclusions
d. Noncaseating granulomas
e. Numerous neutrophils with fibrin deposition

250. A 61-year-old man presents with increasing shortness of breath. A chest x-ray reveals a diffuse pulmonary infiltrate, while a transbronchial lung biopsy reveals variable patchy interstitial fibrosis with multiple fibroblastic foci. Sheets of "desquamated" cells within alveoli are not seen. What is the best diagnosis?

   a. Bronchiolitis obliterans-organizing pneumonia (BOOP)
   b. Cryptogenic organizing pneumonia (COP)
   c. Desquamative interstitial pneumonia (DIP)
   d. Idiopathic pulmonary fibrosis (IPF)
   e. Nonspecific interstitial pneumonia(NSIP)

251. A 44-year-old woman presents with hemoptysis and hematuria. Pertinent medical history includes repeated infections involving her sinuses. Physical examination finds a small perforation of her nasal septum with several surrounding mucosal ulcers, and a small amount of purulent material is seen leaking from her sinuses. Serum studies are positive for the presence of antineutrophil cytoplasmic antibodies, mainly against proteinase 3. Which of the following histologic abnormalities is most likely to be seen in a lung biopsy from this individual?

   a. Atypical lymphocytes invading blood vessels
   b. Granulomatous inflammation of blood vessels with numerous eosinophils
   c. Granulomatous inflammation of bronchi with Aspergillus species
   d. Large, serpiginous necrosis with peripheral, palisading macrophages
   e. Necrotizing hemorrhagic interstitial pneumonitis

252. A 45-year-old man presents with shortness of breath, cough with mucoid sputum, and some weight loss, and has diffuse, bilateral alveolar infiltrates on chest x-ray. Pulmonary function tests reveal decreased diffusing capacity and hypoxia. The patient had worked for several years at grinding aluminum. The photomicrograph below is from a lung biopsy. This granular material within the alveoli is intensely eosinophilic. The acquired form of this disorder is associated with the development of which one of the listed types of antibodies?

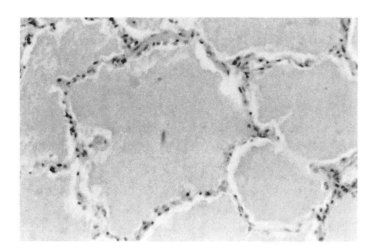

   a. Anti-centromere antibodies
   b. Anti-GM-CSF antibodies
   c. Anti-mitochondria antibodies
   d. Anti-*Pneumocystis carinii* antibodies
   e. Anti-smooth muscle antibodies

253. A 54-year-old man presents with several problems involving his face and pain in his shoulder. He states that he has smoked 2 packs of cigarettes a day for almost 40 years. Physical examination reveals ptosis of his left upper eyelid, constriction of his left pupil, and lack of sweating (anhidrosis) on the left side of his face. No other neurologic abnormalities are found. Which of the following tumors is most likely to be present in this individual?

a. A bronchioloalveolar carcinoma involving the left upper lobe
b. A small-cell carcinoma involving the hilum of his left lung
c. A squamous cell carcinoma involving the left mainstem bronchus
d. An adenocarcinoma involving the apex of his left lung
e. An endobronchial carcinoid tumor involving the right mainstem bronchus

254. During a routine physical examination, a 43-year-old man is found to have a 2.5-cm "coin" in the peripheral portion of his right upper lobe (RUL). Several sputum samples sent for cytology are unremarkable, and a bronchoscopic examination is also unremarkable. Surgery is performed and the mass is resected. Histologic examination reveals lobules of connective tissue that contain mature hyaline cartilage. These lobules are separated by clefts that are lined by respiratory epithelium. Which of the following is the most likely diagnosis?

a. Adenocarcinoma
b. Bronchioloalveolar carcinoma
c. Carcinoid
d. Fibroma
e. Hamartoma

255. A 67-year-old man who is a long-term smoker presents with weight loss, a persistent cough, fever, chest pain, and hemoptysis. Physical examination reveals a cachectic man with clubbing of his fingers and dullness to percussion over his right lower lobe. A chest x-ray reveals a 3.5-cm hilar mass on the right and postobstructive pneumonia of the right lower lobe. Sputum cytology is suspicious for malignant cells. Histologic examination of a transbronchial biopsy specimen reveals infiltrating groups of cells with scant cytoplasm. No glandular structures or keratin production are seen. The nuclei of these cells are about twice the size of normal lymphocytes and do not appear to have nucleoli. Which of the following is the most likely diagnosis?

a. Adenocarcinoma
b. Hamartoma
c. Large-cell undifferentiated carcinoma
d. Small-cell undifferentiated carcinoma
e. Squamous cell carcinoma

256. A 39-year-old woman presents with a cough and increasing shortness of breath. A chest x-ray is interpreted by the radiologist as showing a right lower lobe (RLL) pneumonia. No mass lesions are seen. The woman is treated with antibiotics, but her symptoms do not improve. On her return visit, the area of consolidation appears to be increased. Bronchoscopy is performed. No bronchial masses are seen, but a transbronchial biopsy is obtained in an area of mucosal erythema in the RLL. After the diagnosis is made, the RLL is removed and a section from this specimen reveals well-differentiated mucus-secreting columnar epithelial cells that infiltrate from alveolus to alveolus. Which of the following is the most likely diagnosis?

a. Bronchioloalveolar carcinoma
b. Carcinoid
c. Large cell carcinoma
d. Small cell carcinoma
e. Squamous cell carcinoma

257. A 49-year-old man presents with shaking chills and fever, pleuritic chest pain, and increasing shortness of breath. A chest x-ray reveals a right-sided pleural effusion. The lung in this area appears to be consolidated. The pleural fluid is tapped, and laboratory examination reveals numerous acute inflammatory cells. Which of the following is the basic defect that caused the accumulation of this pleural fluid?

a. Collagen-vascular disease involving the pleura
b. Obstruction of lymphatics by tumor
c. Right-sided congestive heart failure
d. Rupture of an aortic aneurysm
e. Suppurative infection of adjacent lung tissue

258. A 19-year-old woman presents with sudden, severe right-sided chest pain that developed shortly after she had been placing heavy boxes on shelves in her garage. Physical examination reveals an afebrile woman in mild respiratory distress. Breath sounds are markedly decreased on the right, and the right lung is hyperresonant to percussion. Which of the following is most likely present in this individual?

a. Pneumoconiosis
b. *Pneumocystis* infection
c. Bacterial pneumonia
d. Viral pneumonia
e. Pneumothorax

259. A 68-year-old man who worked for many years in the asbestos indus-try presents with weight loss and increasing chest pain. Examination of his sputum finds very rare asbestos bodies, while a CT scan shows a large mass involving the apical surface of his left lung. Surgery is performed and gross examination finds a lesion similar in appearance to that seen in the associated gross photograph of a sagittal section of the lung. Sections from this mass examined by electron microscopy reveal tumor cells with long microvilli on their surface. Which of the following is the most likely diagnosis?

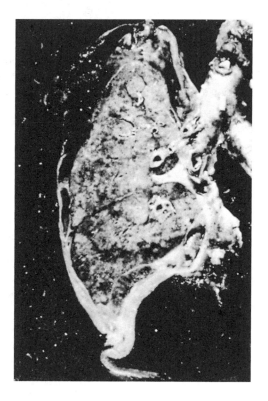

a. Malignant mesothelioma
b. Malignant thymoma
c. Metastatic malignant melanoma
d. Poorly differentiated adenocarcinoma
e. Small-cell carcinoma

Respiratory System

Answers

235. The answer is b. (*Kumar, pp 122, 562, 714–715.*) Pulmonary edema refers to excess accumulation of fluid in the extravascular spaces of the lung. Pulmonary edema can be classified based on the etiology into cardiogenic pulmonary edema and noncardiogenic pulmonary edema. Cardiogenic pulmonary edema results from abnormalities of hemodynamic (Starling) forces, while noncardiogenic pulmonary edema results from cellular injury. Causes of cardiogenic pulmonary edema include increased hydrostatic forces, as seen with congestive heart failure (the most common cause of pulmonary edema); decreased oncotic pressure, such as resulting from decreased albumin levels; and lymphatic obstruction. Noncardiogenic edema may be the result of either endothelial injury (infections, disseminated intravascular coagulopathy, or trauma) or alveolar injury (from inhaled toxins, aspiration, drowning, or near drowning). Microscopically, pulmonary edema reveals the alveoli to be filled with pale pink fluid. Cardiogenic edema may lead to alveolar hemorrhages and hemosiderin-laden macrophages (heart failure cells). Where cardiogenic edema is present, chest x-rays show an increase in the caliber of the blood vessels in the upper lobes, perivascular and peribronchial fluid ("cuffing"), and Kerley B lines (fluid in the interlobular septa). Noncardiogenic edema produces a "whiteout" of the lungs.

236. The answer is a. (*Kumar, pp 713–714. Rubin, p 600.*) Atelectasis refers to lung collapse. It is divided into four types. Absorptive (obstructive) atelectasis results from airway obstruction, such as occurs with mucus, tumors, or foreign bodies. The air within the lungs distal to the obstruction is absorbed, the lung collapses, and the mediastinum then shifts toward the collapsed lung. With compression, atelectasis fluid within the pleural cavity, such as seen with congestive heart failure (CHF), causes increased pleural pressure, which collapses lung tissue. In this instance, the mediastinum shifts away from the collapsed lung. In contraction, atelectasis fibrosis causes collapse of lung tissue. Patchy atelectasis may result from loss of pulmonary surfactant, which is seen in hyaline membrane disease of the newborn.

237. The answer is d. (*Damjanov, pp 1503–1505. Kumar, pp 715–716. Rubin, pp 615–617.*) Adult respiratory distress syndrome (ARDS) is a syndrome characterized clinically by the rapid onset of severe, life-threatening respiratory insufficiency. ARDS has also been called adult respiratory failure, shock lung, traumatic wet lung, pump lung, and diffuse alveolar damage (DAD). The initial and basic lesion in ARDS is diffuse damage to the alveolar wall. Protein-rich edema fluid then leaks into the alveolar spaces and combines with fibrin and dead cells to produce hyaline membranes that line the alveoli and are the characteristic histologic feature of ARDS. In the acute edematous stage, the lungs are congested (pulmonary congestion) and show pulmonary edema with interstitial inflammation. Collapsed, airless pulmonary parenchyma is called atelectasis and can also be seen in ARDS. These other changes, although present in ARDS, are not pathognomonic.

In contrast, angioinvasive infiltrates of pleomorphic lymphoid cells are seen with lymphomatoid granulomatosis, a disease of middle-aged individuals that is characterized by an angiocentric and angioinvasive infiltrate of atypical lymphoid cells. Deposits of needle-like crystals from the membranes of eosinophils, called Charcot-Leyden crystals, can be seen in patients with asthma, while infiltrating groups of malignant cells having intercellular bridges characterize squamous cell carcinoma. Plexiform lesions within pulmonary arterioles are diagnostic of pulmonary hypertension.

238. The answer is c. (*Kumar, pp 136, 742–743. Braunwald, pp 634–635.*) Pulmonary emboli may be caused by thrombi, air (after surgery), amniotic fluid (complications of labor), fat (associated with trauma causing fractures of long bones), or tumors (renal cell carcinomas invading the vena cava). Pulmonary emboli are common and are found in about 10 to 20% of hospital autopsies. Occlusions of the pulmonary arteries by blood clots are almost always embolic, arising from thrombi in the deep veins of the leg [deep vein thromboses (DVTs)]. Typical settings for the development of deep vein thrombosis include increased venous stasis and hypercoagulable states, such as after surgery. Calf tenderness, associated with DVTs, is a useful clinical sign that points toward pulmonary emboli as the cause of breathing problems after surgery. Pulmonary emboli may produce other clinical symptoms, such as anxiety, pleuritic chest pain, dyspnea, fever, cough, hemoptysis, or sudden death. Hypoxemia results from increased A-a gradients, the result of increased alveolar dead space. The majority of pulmonary thromboemboli do no harm and eventually organize or lyse;

however, depending on the size of the embolus and the hemodynamic status of the patient, a pulmonary infarct may be produced. Pulmonary infarcts grossly have an apex pointing toward the occluded vessel and a pyramidal base extending toward the pleural surface. The histologic hallmark is ischemic necrosis of the lung.

239. The answer is c. (*Kumar, pp 528–529, 541, 743–744. Rubin, pp 652–654.*) Pulmonary vascular sclerosis refers to the vascular changes associated with pulmonary hypertension. Elevation of the mean pulmonary arterial pressure is the result of endothelial dysfunction and vascular changes. The vascular changes vary with the size of the vessel. The main arteries have atheromas that are similar to systemic atherosclerosis, but are not as severe. Medium-sized arteries show intimal thickening and neomuscularization. Smaller arteries and arterioles show intimal thickening, medial hypertrophy, and reduplication of the internal and external elastic membranes. A distinctive arteriolar change, a plexiform lesion, consists of intraluminal angiomatous tufts that form webs. This pattern is thought to be diagnostic of primary hypertension.

The changes of pulmonary vascular sclerosis may be primary or secondary. Primary pulmonary vascular sclerosis almost always occurs in young women, who develop fatigue, syncope (with exercise), dyspnea on exertion (DOE), and chest pain. Recent studies have found that primary pulmonary hypertension is caused by mutations involving the bone morphogenetic protein receptor type 2 (BMPR2) signaling pathway. BMPR2 is an important cell-surface protein for various cytokines including transforming growth factor-β (TGF-β), bone morphogenetic protein (BMP), activin, and inhibin. BMPR2 normally inhibits vascular smooth muscle cell proliferation and stimulates apoptosis of these cells. Therefore defects involving BMPR2 can lead to uncontrolled vascular smooth muscle proliferation.

Secondary pulmonary vascular sclerosis may occur at any age, and symptoms depend on the underlying cause. Possible causes of secondary pulmonary hypertension include certain types of heart disease, such as mitral valve disease, left ventricular failure, and congenital valvular disease with left-to-right shunt as well as certain types of pulmonary disease, such as chronic obstructive or interstitial lung disease and recurrent pulmonary emboli. Pulmonary hypertension is also associated with diet pills (Redux and Fen-Phen), while "exotic" causes include *Crotalaria spectabilis* ("bush tea") and adulterated olive oil.

In contrast to the histologic changes seen with pulmonary hypertension, biopsies of the lung from individuals with the Churg-Strauss syndrome (allergic vasculitis) show necrotizing vasculitis with granulomas. This syndrome is associated with the presence of p-ANCA. The lung from patients with Wegener's granulomatosis, which is associated with c-ANCA, has areas of necrosis that are characteristically large and serpiginous with peripheral palisading of macrophages. Finally, the rare Liddle syndrome, which is characterized by salt-sensitive hypertension, results from mutations involving the apical epithelial sodium ion channel of renal tubules.

240. The answer is d. (*Kumar, pp 714, 716–732. Schneider, p 201. Rubin, pp 630–633.*) Asthma is a pulmonary disease that is caused by excessive bronchoconstriction secondary to airways that are hyperreactive to numerous stimuli. Because of the obstruction to airflow along the airways asthma is classified as a type of chronic obstructive pulmonary disease (COPD). This group of disorders also includes bronchiectasis (abnormal dilation of the bronchi), chronic bronchitis (hyperplasia of the bronchial submucosal glands) and emphysema (destruction of the alveolar walls).

Asthma has been divided into extrinsic and intrinsic forms. Extrinsic asthma includes atopic (allergic) asthma, occupational asthma, and allergic bronchopulmonary aspergillosis. The intrinsic category includes nonreaginic asthma and pharmacologic asthma. The former is related to respiratory tract infections, while the latter is often related to aspirin sensitivity. These aspirin-sensitive patients often have recurrent rhinitis and nasal polyps. In these patients, the aspirin initiates an asthmatic attack by inhibiting the cyclooxygenase pathway of arachidonic acid metabolism without affecting the lipoxygenase pathway. This causes the relative excess production of the leukotrienes, which are bronchoconstrictors.

Pathologic findings in patients with asthma include hyperplasia of the bronchial goblet cells and hypertrophy of the bronchial smooth muscle cells. Excess secretions from the goblet cells leads to mucus plugging of bronchioles. These mucus plugs can be seen in sputum specimens as Curschmann's spirals and may contain fragments of eosinophil membranes called Charcot-Leyden crystals. Excess numbers of eosinophils is also characteristic of asthma.

In contrast to the histologic findings seen with asthma, fibrosis of the alveolar interstitium is seen with interstitial pneumonia, while sclerosis of the small blood vessels is characteristic of pulmonary hypertension. Finally, atelectasis refers to the collapse of lung tissue and contraction atelectasis can result from any disorder that causes fibrosis of the lung.

241. The answer is c. (*Kumar, pp 717–722. Rubin, pp 625–630.*) An individual who has trouble breathing, and while sitting leans forward slightly and breathes quickly through pursed-lips, and is also found to have an increased anteroposterior diameter to their chest ("barrel chest") most likely has emphysema. This abnormality, which results from abnormal dilation of the air spaces distal to the terminal bronchioles, may be classified based on the anatomic location of the abnormal dilation within the respiratory lobule. The normal respiratory lobule is composed of three to five terminal bronchioles and their acini, which in turn are composed of a respiratory bronchiole, alveolar ducts, alveolar sacs, and alveoli. Emphysema may affect the proximal acinus (centrilobular emphysema), the distal acinus (paraseptal emphysema), or the entire acinus (panlobular emphysema). It is postulated that emphysema results from an imbalance between elastase, which is produced by neutrophils and macrophages and destroys the walls of airways, and antielastase, which inactivates elastase. Cigarette smoking, which is associated with the production of centrilobular emphysema, increases elastase activity and decreases α_1 antitrypsin activity. In contrast, there is a well-established association between panacinar emphysema and a hereditary deficiency of α_1 antitrypsin, an enzyme that functions as an anti-elastase. This enzyme is coded for by proteinase-inhibitor (Pi) genes on chromosome 14. The normal Pi allele is M, and the normal homozygote is MM. The Z allele yields the lowest level of antiproteinase, and the Pi ZZ homozygote is the most deficient in α_1 antitrypsin.

242. The answer is a. (*Kumar, pp 727–728. Rubin, pp 600–601.*) Patients with bronchiectasis have a persistent, productive cough due to abnormally dilated bronchi, which are the result of a chronic necrotizing infection. Patients with Kartagener's syndrome have the triad of bronchiectasis, recurrent sinusitis, and situs inversus. The respiratory problems associated with this syndrome are caused by abnormal motility of the cilia, which is due to abnormalities of the ATPase-containing dynein arms. Abnormal cilia inhibit the normal functioning of the respiratory epithelium, which is to clear microorganisms and foreign particles within the respiratory mucus. This results in repeated respiratory infections. Males with this condition tend to be sterile because of the ineffective motility of the tails of the sperm.

In contrast, patients with asthma develop episodic wheezing due to bronchial smooth-muscle hyperplasia and excess production of mucus. Extrinsic (allergic) asthma may be related to IgE (type I) immune reactions; intrinsic (nonallergic) asthma may be triggered by infections or drugs. Clinically there is an elevated eosinophil count in the peripheral blood, and Curschmann's spirals and Charcot-Leyden crystals may be found in the sputum. Emphysema is abnormal dilation of the alveoli due to destruction of the alveolar walls. Steatosis refers to the accumulation of triglyceride within the cytoplasm of hepatocytes, while cirrhosis results from the irreversible deposition of collagen in the subendothelial spaces in the liver.

243. The answer is d. (*Kumar, pp 747–756. Rubin, pp 601–606. Chandrasoma, pp 488, 794, 882–883.*) Pulmonary infections may be caused by bacteria, fungi, viruses, or mycoplasma. Classically the onset of bacterial pneumonia is sudden, with malaise, shaking chills, fever, peripheral leukocytosis, and a cough with sputum production. Bacterial infections generally result in a polymorphonuclear (neutrophil) response. Bacterial infection of the lung (pneumonia) results in consolidation of the lung, which may be patchy or diffuse. Patchy consolidation of the lung is seen in bronchopneumonia (lobular pneumonia), while diffuse involvement of an entire lobe is seen in lobar pneumonia. Histologically, bronchopneumonia is characterized by multiple, suppurative neutrophil-rich exudates that fill the bronchi and bronchioles and spill over into the adjacent alveolar spaces. In contrast, lobar pneumonia is characterized by four distinct stages: congestion, red hepatization, gray hepatization, and resolution. Finally, inflammation of the interstitium of the lung (e.g., the alveolar walls or septae) can be seen with viral infections, while bronchiectasis results from abnormal permanent dilation of the bronchi.

244. The answer is d. (*Kumar, p 753. Rubin, pp 614–615.*) A pulmonary abscess is a localized suppurative process within the pulmonary parenchyma that is characterized by tissue necrosis and marked acute inflammation. Possible causes of a lung abscess include aerobic and anaerobic streptococci, *Staphylococcus aureus*, and many gram-negative organisms. Aspiration more often gives a right-sided single abscess, because the airways on the right side are more vertical. Antecedent pneumonia gives rise to multiple diffuse abscesses. The abscess cavity is filled with necrotic suppurative debris unless it communicates with an air passage. Clinically an individual with a lung abscess will have a prominent cough producing copious amounts of foul-smelling, purulent sputum. Changes in position evoke paroxysms of coughing. There is also fever, malaise, and clubbing of the fingers and toes. With antibiotic therapy 75% of lung abscesses resolve. Complications of a lung abscess include pleural involvement (empyema) and bacteremia, which could result in brain abscesses or meningitis.

245. The answer is b. (*Kumar, p 751. Rubin, pp 613–614.*) Acute interstitial pneumonia refers to inflammation of the interstitium of the lung that is the result of infection, typically with either M. *pneumoniae* or viruses such as influenza A and B. This type of pneumonia is called primary atypical pneumonia because it is atypical when compared to the "typical" bacterial pneumonia, such as produced by S. *pneumoniae*. These bacterial pneumonias are characterized by acute inflammation (neutrophils) within the alveoli. In contrast, acute interstitial pneumonia is characterized by lymphocytes and plasma cells within the interstitium, that is, the alveolar septal walls. Viral cytopathic effects, such as inclusion bodies or multinucleated giant cells, may be seen histologically with certain viral infections. Certain viruses produce pneumonia in certain patient groups, for example, respiratory syncytial virus in infants and adenovirus in military recruits. Infection with M. *pneumoniae* results in the production of a nonspecific cold IgM antibody, which characteristically reacts with red cells having the I antigen. Because most adult red cells have I antigens, blood from a patient with mycoplasma pneumonia will hemagglutinate when cooled. This type of reaction is not seen with infection by either P. *pneumoniae* or *Mycobacterium tuberculosis*.

246. The answer is c. (*Damjanov, pp 1006–1008. Kumar, pp 753–756.*) Infection by the protozoan P. *carinii* is characterized by the presence of oval and helmet-shaped organisms whose capsules are made more visible by use of Gomori's methenamine-silver staining technique. This organism, although it has low virulence, is opportunistic; it is often seen to attack severely ill, immunologically depressed patients. It is frequently the first opportunistic infection to be diagnosed in HIV-1-positive patients, and it is a leading cause of death in patients with AIDS.

247. The answer is e. (*Kumar, pp 732–737. Rubin, pp 633–636.*) Tuberculosis is more common in individuals with silicosis, a type of pneumoconiosis seen in sandblasters and mine workers, which is perhaps the most common chronic occupational disease in the world. The pneumoconioses are pulmonary diseases that are caused by nonneoplastic lung reactions to several types of environmental dusts. The characteristic pathology of silicosis is pulmonary fibrosis. Early in the disease there are multiple, very small nodules in the upper zones of the lung, which produces a fine nodularity on x-ray. These areas histologically show fibrosis and birefringent particles. The fibrotic lesions may also be found in the hilar lymph nodes, which can become calcified and have an "eggshell" pattern on x-ray examination. Silica depresses cell-mediated immunity, and crystalline silica may inhibit pulmonary macrophages, which may be why individuals with silicosis are at a high risk for developing tuberculosis. There is no clear relationship between silicosis and the development of cancer. This is in contrast to asbestosis, which is associated with the development of lung cancer and mesothelioma. Asbestos also results in larger areas of fibrosis, and histologically asbestos (ferruginous) bodies are found.

Reactions to coal (carbon) may result in anthracosis; simple coal worker's pneumoconiosis, which is composed of multiple small nodules; or complicated coal worker's pneumoconiosis, which is composed of fibrotic nodules that are larger than 2 cm (progressive massive fibrosis). In the chronic state, beryllium elicits a cell-mediated immunity response, seen histologically as noncaseating granulomas. Noncaseating granulomas are also seen in patients with sarcoidosis, a disease of unknown etiology that may cause enlargement of the hilar lymph nodes ("potato nodes"). Neither berylliosis nor sarcoidosis is associated with exposure to silica. Finally, myxomatosis is a disease of rabbits that is caused by a myxoma virus. It is not a disease of humans.

248. The answer is c. (*Damjanov, pp 1536–1541. Kumar, pp 735–737. Rubin, pp 637–639.*) The segmented or beaded, often dumbbell-shaped bodies are ferruginous bodies that are probably asbestos fibers coated with iron and protein. The term ferruginous body is applied to other inhaled fibers that become iron-coated; however, in a patient with interstitial lung fibrosis or pleural plaques, ferruginous bodies are probably asbestos bodies. The type of asbestos mainly used in America is chrysotile, mined in Canada, and it is much less likely to cause mesothelioma or lung cancer than is crocidolite (blue asbestos), which has limited use and is mined in South Africa. Cigarette smoking potentiates the relatively mild carcinogenic effect of asbestos. In contrast, laminated spherical (Schaumann's) bodies are found in granulomas of sarcoid and chronic berylliosis, while *Candida* species histologically may show elongated chains of yeast without hyphae (pseudohyphae), and silica particles are very small and are birefringent.

249. The answer is d. (*Henry, pp 291, 1040. Lever, pp 322–326. Braunwald, pp 759–760. Kumar, pp 737–739.*) Sarcoidosis is a systemic disease characterized by noncaseating granulomas in multiple organs. The diagnosis of sarcoidosis depends on finding these noncaseating granulomas in commonly affected sites. In 90% of cases, bilateral hilar lymphadenopathy ("potato nodes") or lung involvement is present and can be revealed by chest x-ray or transbronchial biopsy. The eye and skin are the next most commonly affected organs, so that both conjunctival and skin biopsies are clinical possibilities. Noncaseating granulomas may be found in multiple infectious diseases, such as fungal infections, but sarcoidosis is not caused by any known organism. Therefore, before the diagnosis of sarcoidosis can be made, cultures must be taken from affected tissues, and there must be no growth of any organism that may produce granulomas. In patients with sarcoidosis, blood levels of angiotensin-converting enzyme are increased, and this may also be used as a clinical test. In the past, the Kveim skin test was used to assist in the diagnosis of sarcoidosis, but because it involves injecting into patients extracts of material from humans, it is no longer used.

250. The answer is d. (*Kumar, pp 729–732. Rubin, pp 643–648.*) Interstitial or idiopathic pulmonary fibrosis (IPF) is a slowly progressive disease with no recognizable etiology. This disease entity has many names, such as chronic interstitial pneumonitis and cryptogenic fibrosing alveolitis. Another common name is usual interstitial pneumonitis (UIP), which refers to the histologic pattern of fibrosis with IPF. The term Hamman-Rich syndrome used to refer to a rapidly aggressive form of IPF, but this term now is used for acute lung injury due to acute interstitial pneumonia.

The pathogenesis of IPF involves damage to type I pneumocytes with the subsequent proliferation of type II pneumocytes and secretion of factors by macrophages that cause fibrosis. IPF is thought to occur secondary to repeated cycles of acute lung injury (alveolitis) that damages different portions of the lung with time. That is, IPF is a process that is variable over "space and time." Exuberant wound healing is associated with excess fibroblastic proliferation and fibroblastic foci that are characteristic of IPF. The end-stage form of IPF is characterized by large cysts with intervening fibrosis, which imparts the gross appearance of a "honeycomb lung." There are several subtypes of IPF, which are characterized by their histologic appearance. Lymphocytic interstitial pneumonitis (LIP) has numerous lymphocytes, Giant cell interstitial pneumonitis (GIP) has giant cells, and plasma cell interstitial pneumonitis (PIP) has numerous plasma cells. LIP is seen in patients with Sjögren syndrome or AIDS and is associated with an increased risk of developing lymphoma.

Desquamative interstitial pneumonitis (DIP), which is characterized histologically by sheets of cells within the alveoli, used to be thought of as a subtype of IPF, but now DIP is known to be a smoking-related disease. Cryptogenic organizing pneumonia (COP) describes a characteristic histologic appearance of polypoid plugs of loose organizing connective tissue within alveolar ducts and alveoli. COP used to be called bronchiolitis obliterans-organizing pneumonia (BOOP). Patients usually present with cough and dyspnea. Finally nonspecific interstitial pneumonia (NSIP) is a "wastebasket" diagnosis for lung biopsies having interstitial inflammation and fibrosis that does not have any diagnostic features of the other interstitial lung diseases. Patients with NSIP have a better prognosis than patients with IPF.

251. The answer is d. (*Kumar, pp 541–542, 746–747. Rubin, pp 650–652.*) The pulmonary hemorrhagic syndromes are characterized by hemorrhage within the alveoli, which may be severe enough to produce hemoptysis. Several of these diseases are associated with blood vessel abnormalities, namely, inflammation of the vessels (angiitis). Necrotizing granulomatous arteritis affecting the upper and lower respiratory tracts and the kidneys is seen in patients with Wegener's granulomatosis. These areas of necrosis are characteristically large and serpiginous, and exhibit peripheral palisading of macrophages. In patients with Wegener's granulomatosis, the nose, sinus, antrum, and trachea often exhibit ulcerations. Originally the disease was lethal, but the prognosis is now much improved by immunosuppressive drugs. Laboratory findings reveal a positive ANCA (if kidney involved), mainly c-ANCA. Involvement of the kidneys may produce hematuria.

Goodpasture's syndrome is another pulmonary hemorrhagic syndrome that may produce hematuria. This syndrome is characterized by the development of a necrotizing hemorrhagic interstitial pneumonitis and rapidly progressing glomerulonephritis because of antibodies directed against the capillary basement membrane in alveolar septa and glomeruli. A linear IgG immunofluorescence pattern is present, which is characteristic of a type II hypersensitivity reaction. The prognosis for Goodpasture's syndrome has been markedly improved by intensive plasma exchange to remove circulating anti-basement membrane antibodies and by immunosuppressive therapy to inhibit further antibody production.

Finally, eosinophilic granulomatous arteritis occurs in some patients with asthma who have eosinophilic pulmonary infiltrates; this abnormality is called Churg-Strauss syndrome. The areas of necrosis are not large and serpiginous as in Wegener's. Granulomatous inflammation centered around bronchi (bronchocentric granulomatosis) is often related to allergic pulmonary aspergillosis (histologically aspergillus species appear as thin septate hyphae with acute angle-branching). Lymphomatoid granulomatosis is a disease of middle-aged people that is characterized by an angiocentric and angioinvasive infiltrate of atypical lymphoid cells.

252. The answer is b. (*Kumar, pp 238, 741, 903. Rubin, pp 618–619.*) Pulmonary alveolar proteinosis (PAP) is a rare disease that is characterized histologically by the accumulation of intensely eosinophilic, proteinaceous, granular substance in the intra-alveolar and bronchiolar spaces. The alveolar walls are relatively normal, without inflammatory exudate or fibrosis, although type II pneumocytes may be hyperplastic. The process is often patchy, with groups of normal alveoli alternating with groups of affected alveoli. Acicular (cholesterol) clefts and densely eosinophilic bodies (necrotic cells) are found within the granular material. Distinction from edema fluid may be difficult, but PAP alveolar material stains with periodic acid–Schiff (PAS). At low power, alveolar material seen in *P. carinii* pneumonia may also mimic PAP, but with high power the foamy material seen with *Pneumocystis* is not present in PAP. In PAP, the material is surfactant accumulation due either to overproduction or to failure of macrophage clearance.

There are three distinct clinical classes of this disease: acquired, congenital, and secondary PAP. Currently it is postulated that acquired PAP is associated with the development of anti-GM-CSF antibodies. Congenital PAP is quite rare and is associated with mutations of genes coding for either surfactant protein B, GM-CSF, and GM receptor β chain. Secondary PAP is associated with occupational exposure to silica or aluminum dusts. It also occurs in immunosuppressed patients and toxic drug reactions and is often associated with infections by organisms such as nocardia, fungi, and TB (possible impaired macrophage killing). The treatment of choice is bronchoalveolar lavage to remove the proteinaceous debris.

In contrast, anti-centromere antibodies are seen with limited systemic sclerosis (specifically the CREST syndrome), anti-mitochondria antibodies with primary biliary cirrhosis, and anti-smooth muscle antibodies with autoimmune (lupoid) hepatitis.

253. The answer is d. (*Kumar, pp 757–764. Rubin, p 657.*) Horner syndrome occurs with apical (superior sulcus) tumors of any type (Pancoast tumor), but because most peripheral cancers of the lung are adenocarcinomas, most tumors of the apex of the lung are adenocarcinomas. Horner syndrome is characterized by enophthalmos, ptosis, miosis, and anhidrosis on the same side as the lesion due to invasion of the cervical sympathetic nerves. Involvement of the brachial plexus causes pain and paralysis in the ulnar nerve distribution.

254. The answer is e. (*Damjanov, pp 1541–1545. Kumar, p 765.*) Pulmonary hamartomas, although infrequent, are still the most common of all benign lung tumors. Hamartomas consist of various tissues normally found in the organ where they develop, but in abnormal amounts and arrangements. In the lung they consist of lobules of connective tissue often containing mature cartilage, fat, or fibrous tissue and separated by clefts lined by entrapped respiratory epithelium. The peak incidence is at age 60, and the tumor is usually found as a well-circumscribed, peripheral "coin" lesion on routine chest x-ray. Unless the radiographic findings are pathognomonic of hamartoma with "popcorn ball" calcifications, the lesion should be excised or at least carefully followed. Conservative excision is curative.

255. The answer is d. (*Kumar, pp 759–762. Rubin, pp 657–659.*) Lung cancers are classified according to their histologic appearance. First, they are divided into two groups based on the size of the tumor cells, namely, small-cell carcinomas and non–small-cell carcinomas. Small-cell carcinomas, also called "oat cell" carcinomas, contain scant amounts of cytoplasm, and their nuclei are small and round and rarely have nucleoli. These malignancies, which are of neuroendocrine origin and display neurosecretory granules on electron microscopy, may cause a variety of paraneoplastic syndromes, such as from the synthesis and secretion of hormones such as ACTH and serotonin. Other effects not well understood on the neuromuscular system include central encephalopathy and Eaton-Lambert syndrome, a myasthenic syndrome resulting from impaired release of acetylcholine and usually associated with pulmonary oat cell carcinoma. Oat cell carcinomas form 20 to 25% of primary lung tumors, occur most frequently in men of middle age or older, have a strong association with cigarette smoking, and carry a poor prognosis, as they metastasize early (e.g., bone marrow metastases). The non–small-cell carcinomas are classified as to the differentiation of the tumor cells. Squamous cell carcinomas are characterized by keratin pearl formation, intracytoplasmic keratin, or the formation of intercellular bridges. Adenocarcinomas are characterized by the formation of glandular structures. They are typically found at the periphery of the lung (peripheral carcinomas) and sometimes may be found in an area of previous scar (scar carcinoma). Non–small-cell carcinomas of the lung that do not form glands or show squamous differentiation are called undifferentiated large-cell carcinomas.

256. The answer is a. (*Damjanov, pp 1541–1545. Kumar, pp 759–762.*) One type of bronchogenic carcinoma that has unique characteristics is bronchioloalveolar carcinoma (BAC). This tumor is characterized by well-differentiated, mucus-secreting columnar epithelial cells that infiltrate along the alveolar walls and spread from alveolus to alveolus through the pores of Kohn. This pneumonic spread can be mistaken for pneumonia on chest x-ray. These tumors, which make up about 2 to 5% of bronchogenic carcinomas, do not arise from the major bronchi. Instead they are thought to arise in terminal bronchioles from Clara cells. Even though these tumors may be multiple, they are well differentiated and have a good prognosis.

257. The answer is e. (*Kumar, pp 766–767. Rubin, pp 299, 664.*) The causes of pleural effusions may be classified as being inflammatory or non-inflammatory. Inflammatory edema may be caused by increased vascular permeability. Inflammation in the adjacent lung, such as with collagen vascular diseases, produces a serofibrinous exudate. Suppurative inflammation in the adjacent lung, such as with a bacterial pneumonia, may produce a suppurative pleuritis, which is called an empyema.

In contrast, the formation of noninflammatory edema is related to abnormalities involving the Starling forces and may result in the formation of noninflammatory pleural effusions. Increased hydrostatic pressure, such as is seen with congestive heart failure, causes hydrothorax, which is a transudate. Decreased oncotic pressure, such as is seen with renal disease associated with albuminuria, also causes hydrothorax. Increased intra-pleural negative pressure produced by atelectasis causes hydrothorax, while decreased lymphatic drainage, which can be caused by a tumor obstructing lymphatics, produces chylothorax. Chylothorax is characterized by milky fluid that contains finely emulsified fats. An additional type of noninflammatory pleural effusion is hemothorax, which may be caused by trauma or ruptured aortic aneurysm.

258. The answer is e. (*Kumar, pp 767–768. Rubin, pp 663–664.*) Pneumothorax refers to the accumulation of air in the pleural cavity. Types of pneumothorax include spontaneous pneumothorax, traumatic pneumothorax, and therapeutic pneumothorax. Spontaneous pneumothorax is most commonly associated with emphysema, asthma, and tuberculosis. One special type, however, is idiopathic spontaneous pneumothorax, which occurs primarily in young people. This disorder results from rupture of subpleural blebs. These blebs are most often located in the apex of the lung, and rupture is usually related to stretching or raising the arms. Recurrence of idiopathic spontaneous pneumothorax is common.

259. The answer is a. (*Kumar, pp 768–770. Rubin, p 666.*) Malignant mesothelioma and adenocarcinoma are two neoplasms that may involve the pleural surfaces, as seen in the gross photograph. Malignant mesothelioma arises from the pleural surfaces and develops with significant and chronic exposure to asbestos (usually occupationally incurred). As the malignant mesothelioma spreads, it lines the pleural surfaces, including the fissures through the lobes of the lungs, and results in a tight and constricting encasement. This restricts the excursions of the lungs during ventilation. Adenocarcinoma of the lung also may invade the pleural surfaces and spread in an advancing manner throughout the pleural lining. The differential diagnosis histologically between an epithelial type of malignant mesothelioma and an adenocarcinoma may be difficult and sometimes impossible without special techniques. A characteristic feature seen by electron microscopy is numerous long microvilli on the surface of cells from mesotheliomas. Other histologic characteristics that favor the diagnosis of malignant mesothelioma over adenocarcinoma include positive acid mucopolysaccharide staining that is inhibited by hyaluronidase, perinuclear keratin staining (not peripheral), and negative staining with CEA and Leu-M_1.

Head and Neck

Questions

DIRECTIONS: Each item below contains a question or incomplete statement followed by suggested responses. Select the **one best** response to each question.

260. A 48-year-old man living in an underdeveloped country presents with pain in the left side of his face. Physical examination reveals a large, indurated area involving the left side of his jaw with multiple sinuses draining pus. This draining material contains a few scattered small yellow granules. This lesion was most likely caused by an infection with which one of the following organisms?

a. *Streptococcus pyogenes*
b. *Borrelia vincentii*
c. *Corynebacterium diphtheriae*
d. *Klebsiella rhinoscleromatis*
e. *Actinomyces israelii*

261. A 4-year-old boy presents with multiple laryngeal squamous papillomas. Obtaining a history, you discover this boy has had the same types of lesions removed in the past, but they have now recurred. Which of the following viruses is most closely associated with this boy's condition?

a. Cytomegalovirus (CMV)
b. Epstein-Barr virus (EBV)
c. Herpes simplex virus (HSV)
d. Human immunodeficiency virus (HIV)
e. Human papillomavirus (HPV)

262. A 61-year-old man presents because of recent problems he has had trying to read the newspaper. Physical examination finds mild blurring of his central vision along with drusen within Bruch's membrane beneath the retinal pigment epithelium. What is the correct diagnosis?

a. Closed-angle glaucoma
b. Fuchs dystrophy
c. Macular degeneration
d. Retinitis pigmentosa
e. Retrolental fibroplasia

263. Histologic sections from a 3-cm mass found in the mandible of a 55-year-old woman reveal a tumor consisting of nests of tumor cells that appear dark and crowded at the periphery of the nests and loose in the center (similar to the stellate reticulum of a developing tooth). Grossly, the lesions consist of multiple cysts filled with a thick, "motor oil"–like fluid. Which of the following is the most likely diagnosis?

a. Pleomorphic adenoma
b. Ameloblastoma
c. Mucoepidermoid carcinoma
d. Adenoid cystic carcinoma
e. Acinic cell carcinoma

264. A 24-year-old woman presents after having several "attacks" that last for about 24 h. She states that during these attacks she develops nausea, vomiting, vertigo, and ringing in her ears. Physical examination reveals a sensorineural hearing loss. Which of the following is the most likely cause of this woman's signs and symptoms?

a. Acute suppurative inflammation of the middle ear
b. Dilation of the cochlear duct and saccule
c. Obstruction of the middle ear by a cyst filled with keratin
d. Destruction of the tympanic membrane by a benign neoplasm
e. New bone formation around the stapes and the oval window

265. A 2-month-old male infant, who was born at term without any prenatal abnormalities, is being evaluated for possible visual problems. He is noted to have an abnormal white light reflex involving his right eye, and examination finds a large mass that has almost completely filled the posterior chamber of this eye. Which of the following cells are most likely to be seen proliferating in histologic sections from this mass?

a. Benign fibroblasts and endothelial cells
b. Foamy macrophages with cytoplasmic clear vacuoles
c. Plasmacytoid cells within a dense Congo red–positive stroma
d. Small cells forming occasional rosette structures
e. Spindle-shaped cells with cytoplasmic melanin

266. A 37-year-old woman presents with a recurrent swelling in her left upper eyelid. The lesion is biopsied by an ophthalmologist, and a section from that specimen is seen in the photomicrograph. Which of the following is the most likely diagnosis?

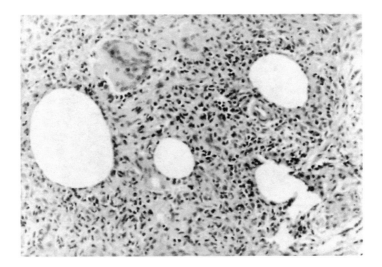

a. Chalazion
b. Hordeolum
c. Xanthelasma
d. Hydrocystoma
e. Sebaceous carcinoma

267. A 28-year-old man presents with a small, painless swelling in his neck. Physical examination finds a 7-mm, smooth, nontender, fluctuant mass located in the anterior midline, near the central portion of the hyoid bone. The mass moves up and down as this patient swallows. The mass is excised and histologic sections reveal a cystic lesion lined by pseudostratified columnar epithelium. Lymphoid tissue is not present in the wall of the cyst. Which of the following is the most likely diagnosis?

a. Branchial cleft cyst
b. Dentigerous cyst
c. Odontogenic keratocyst
d. Radicular cyst
e. Thyroglossal duct cyst

268. A 41-year-old man presents with a slowly enlarging mass on the right side of his face. Physical examination finds a 2.5-cm mass involving the superficial lobe of his right parotid gland. Histologic sections reveal a papillary tumor with cleftlike spaces lined by oncocytic cells as seen in the associated picture. Which of the following is the most likely diagnosis?

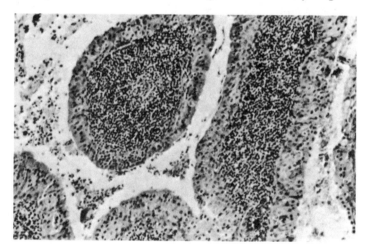

a. Adenoid cystic carcinoma
b. Lymphoepithelioma
c. Sebaceous lymphadenoma
d. Thyroglossal duct neoplasm
e. Warthin's tumor

269. A 35-year-old woman presents with slowly progressive weakness involving the left side of her face. She says she cannot completely close her left eye. Physical examination finds facial asymmetry characterized by flattening of the entire left side of her face, but no abnormalities are seen on the right side. A 1.5-cm mass is found involving the deep portion of the left parotid gland. At the time of surgery the mass is found to be infiltrating along the facial nerve. Which of the following histologic changes is most likely to be seen in a biopsy specimen taken from this mass?

a. A mixture of epithelial structures and mesenchyme-like stroma
b. A mixture of squamous epithelial cells and mucus-secreting cells
c. Atypical cells forming tubular and cribriform patterns
d. Infiltrating groups of vacuolated epithelial cells
e. Papillary folds composed of a double layer of oncocytic cells

Head and Neck

Answers

260. The answer is e. (*Kumar, pp 349, 776–778. Rubin, pp 361, 380, 406–407, 1303, 1320.*) Numerous diseases result from bacterial infections of the oral cavity. *A. israelii,* a normal inhabitant of the mouth, is a branched, filamentous gram-positive bacteria that may produce an indurated (lumpy) jaw with multiple draining fistulas or abscesses. Small yellow colonies, called sulfur granules, may be seen in the draining material. Scarlet fever, a disease of children, is caused by several strains of β-hemolytic group A streptococci (*S. pyogenes*). An erythrogenic toxin damages vascular endothelium and produces a rash on the skin and oral mucosa. The tongue in a patient with scarlet fever may be fiery red with prominent papillae (raspberry tongue) or white-coated with hyperemic papillae (strawberry tongue). Acute necrotizing ulcerative gingivitis (Vincent's angina or trench mouth) is caused by two symbiotic organisms, a fusiform bacillus and a spirochete (*B. vincentii*), the combination being termed fusospirochetosis. *C. diphtheriae* causes diphtheria, which is characterized by oral and pharyngeal pseudomembranes and a peripheral lymphocytosis. Rhinoscleroma, a chronic inflammation of the nose, is caused by *K. rhinoscleromatis* and histologically is characterized by numerous foamy macrophages, called Mikulicz cells.

261. The answer is e. (*Kumar, pp 371, 784–785. Rubin, pp 594–596.*) Tumors of the larynx may be reactive proliferations or neoplastic growths. The laryngeal nodule is a common abnormality formed as a reactive process to excessive use; as such it may be found in singers and is called a "singer's nodule." These nodules are solitary, produce hoarseness, and histologically reveal a polyp consisting of fibrosis, dilated vascular spaces, and myxomatous degeneration of the stroma. Laryngeal neoplasms may be either benign or malignant. Squamous papillomas are benign neoplasms that occur in two clinical forms. One form is typically solitary and occurs in adults (solitary squamous papilloma), while the other form is multiple and occurs in children (juvenile papillomatosis). The latter form is associated with human papillomavirus (HPV) and may recur locally after excision. Malignant neoplasms of the larynx are most often squamous cell carcinomas.

262. The answer is c. (*Kumar, pp 1422, 1428–1429, 1431–1432, 1439, 1441–1442.*) Age-related macular degeneration (ARMD) is the most common cause of irreversible vision loss in the United States and in the entire industrial world. There are two basic types of ARMD: exudative (wet) and nonexudative (dry). Exudative ARMD is characterized by choroidal neovascular (CNV) membranes located under the retina. The nonexudative (atrophic) form of ARMD has atrophic and hypertrophic changes in the retinal pigment epithelium (RPE) along with deposits in Bruch's membrane (drusen) beneath the RPE. Between 10 and 20% of the cases of dry ARMD will progress to wet ARMD. Symptoms of dry ARMD tend to be milder and include blurred central vision and problems with contrast. Wet ARMD have painless progressive blurring of their central vision that is more severe.

The clinical term glaucoma refers to visual loss and changes in the optic disk that usually result from increased intraocular pressure. There are two basic types of glaucoma: open angle glaucoma and closed angle glaucoma. Open angle glaucoma is more common, while closed angle glaucoma results from obstruction to aqueous flow, usually at the angle between the iris and cornea. Acute angle closure may cause sudden eye pain and loss of vision when leaving a dark room (or with the use of mydriatics).

Fuchs endothelial dystrophy is a type of corneal dystrophy that results from loss of endothelial cells on the inner portion of the cornea. Early in the disease process these endothelial cells produce basement membrane material, called guttata, which can be seen with slit-lamp examination. Eventual loss of endothelial cells leads to stromal edema of the cornea and loss of vision. In contrast, retinitis pigmentosa is a disease caused by the loss of cones and rods (begins at periphery) and leads to night blindness and loss of peripheral vision. Finally, retrolental fibroplasia refers to the formation of a fibrovascular mass behind lens. This abnormality, also called retinitis of prematurity (ROP), is seen in premature infants who received high-dose oxygen.

263. The answer is b. (*Kumar, p 782. Rubin, pp 1310–1311.*) A rare tumor of the oral cavity (found most commonly in the mandible) that is similar to the enamel organ of the tooth is the ameloblastoma. This locally aggressive tumor consists of nests of cells that at their periphery are similar to ameloblasts and centrally are similar to the stellate reticulum of the developing tooth. A similar lesion occurs in the sella turcica and is called a craniopharyngioma. In contrast, pleomorphic adenomas, mucoepidermoid carcinomas, adenoid cystic carcinomas, and acinic cell carcinomas are all tumors that originate in salivary glands.

264. The answer is b. (*Kumar, pp 787–788. Rubin, pp 1331–1333.*) Ménière's disease is an abnormality that is characterized by periodic episodes of vertigo that are often accompanied by nausea and vomiting, sensorineural hearing loss, and tinnitus (ringing in the ears). These symptoms are related to hydropic dilation of the endolymphatic system of the cochlea. Inflammation of the middle ear (otitis media), which occurs most often in children, may be acute or chronic. If otitis media is caused by viruses, there may be a serous exudate, but if it is produced by bacteria, there may be a suppurative exudate. Acute suppurative otitis media is characterized by acute suppurative inflammation (neutrophils), while chronic otitis media involves chronic inflammation with granulation tissue. Chronic otitis media may cause perforation of the eardrum or may lead to the formation of a cyst within the middle ear that is filled with keratin, called a cholesteatoma. The name is somewhat of a misnomer, as cholesterol deposits are not present. Otosclerosis, a common hereditary cause of bilateral conduction hearing loss, is associated with formation of new spongy bone around the stapes and the oval window. Patients present with progressive deafness. Tumors of the middle ear are quite rare, but a neoplasm that arises from the paraganglia of the middle ear (the glomus jugulare or glomus tympanicum) is called a chemodectoma. Other names for this tumor include nonchromaffin paraganglioma and glomus jugulare tumor. This lesion is characterized histologically by lobules of cells in a highly vascular stroma (zellballen). A similar tumor that occurs in the neck is called a carotid body tumor.

265. The answer is d. (*Kumar, pp 299–302, 1442–1443. Rubin, pp 1563–1565.*) Retinoblastoma is the most common malignant tumor of the eye in children. Clinically, retinoblastoma may produce a white pupil (leucoria). This is seen most often in young children in the familial form of retinoblastoma, which is due to a deletion involving chromosome 13. These familial cases of retinoblastoma are frequently multiple and bilateral, although like all the sporadic, nonheritable tumors they can also be unifocal and unilateral. Histologically, rosettes of various types are frequent (similar to neuroblastoma and medulloblastoma). There is a good prognosis with early detection and treatment; spontaneous regression can occur but is rare. Retinoblastoma belongs to a group of cancers (osteosarcoma, Wilms' tumor, meningioma, rhabdomyosarcoma, uveal melanoma) in which the normal cancer suppressor gene (antioncogene) is inactivated or lost, with resultant malignant change. Retinoblastoma and osteosarcoma arise after loss of the same genetic locus— hereditary mutation in the q14 band of chromosome 13.

In contrast to the histologic appearance of retinoblastoma, a proliferation of benign fibroblasts and endothelial cells, which can form a retrolental mass, is seen with retinopathy of prematurity (ROP), a cause of blindness in premature infants that is related to the therapeutic use of high concentrations of oxygen. The presence of foamy macrophages with cytoplasmic clear vacuoles is not a specific histologic finding and can be seen with several disorders. Congo red–positive stroma, however, is characteristic of medullary carcinoma of the thyroid, while spindle-shaped cells with cytoplasmic melanin is characteristic of malignant melanoma, the most common primary intraocular malignancy of adults.

266. The answer is a. (*Kumar, pp 1424–1426. Rubin, p 1538. Goldman, p 228. Weidner, p 2174.*) Many lesions of the eyelid are submitted for pathologic examination. One of the most common eyelid lesions is the chalazion, a chronic inflammatory reaction to lipid released into the tissue from the eyelid's sebaceous glands of Meibom or Zeis. Characteristic histologic features of this lesion include a chronic inflammatory reaction with giant cells that surround empty spaces where the lipid vacuoles from the sebaceous glands had been located. Because the major clinical disorder to be differentiated from chalazia is sebaceous carcinoma, ophthalmologists biopsy recurrent lesions suspected of being chalazia to rule out sebaceous carcinoma. In contrast hordeolums (styes) are acute staphylococcal infections of the eyelash follicles (external hordeolum) or the Meibomian glands (internal hordeolum). Xanthelasmas (yellow plaques on the skin) histologically reveal aggregates of foamy macrophages within the dermis. Hydrocystomas are one type of cyst that may affect the eyelid and may be lined by apocrine or eccrine cells.

267. The answer is e. (*Kumar, pp 782, 788–790. Weidner, pp 306, 332–333.*) Two cysts that occur in the neck are the branchial cleft cyst (usually located in the anterolateral part of the neck) and the thyroglossal duct cyst (usually located in the anterior part of the neck). Each of these cysts may histologically reveal a lining composed of squamous epithelium or pseudostratified columnar epithelium. Branchial cleft cysts, which arise from remnants of the branchial (pharyngeal) apparatus, may contain lymphoid tissue, while thyroglossal duct cysts may move up and down as the patient swallows.

There are several other types of cysts that occur in and around the oral cavity. The most common type is the radicular cyst. These cysts result from chronic inflammation of the tooth apex. Histologic sections reveal chronic inflammation of the tooth apex with epithelialization of periapical granulation tissue. Other types of oral cysts include follicular cysts (which arise from the epithelium of the tooth follicle), odontogenic keratocysts (which consist of keratinized squamous epithelium), and inclusion (fissural) cysts (which are fluid-filled cysts lined by squamous or respiratory epithelial cells). Follicular cysts are called dentigerous cysts because the associated tooth is unerupted, while odontogenic keratocysts are important because they may recur and act aggressively. These keratocysts may also be associated with basal cell carcinomas of the skin. Mucoceles, which typically occur on or near the lips due to a ruptured minor salivary gland, consist of a cyst filled with mucous material. They lack an epithelial lining.

268. The answer is e. (*Kumar, pp 791–794. Rubin, pp 1314–1315.*) The salivary glands give rise to a wide variety of tumors, the majority of which are of epithelial origin and benign. Most tumors occur in adults and have a slight female predominance. Approximately 75 to 85% occur in the parotids, 10 to 20% in the submandibular glands, and the remainder in the minor glands. In the parotid the vast majority are benign, whereas in the minor glands 35 to 50% are malignant. Clinically, most tumors of the salivary glands present as palpable masses, regardless of histologic type. The most common neoplasm of the parotid gland is the pleomorphic adenoma (mixed tumor), which histologically reveals epithelial structures embedded within a mesenchyme-like stroma consisting of mucoid, myxoid, or chondroid tissue. A malignant tumor may develop from a pleomorphic adenoma, in which case it is called a carcinoma ex pleomorphic adenoma.

The second most common tumor is Warthin's tumor (papillary cystadenoma lymphomatosum), which histologically reveals cleftlike spaces lined by oncocytic epithelial cells overlying a stroma with a dense lymphocytic infiltrate. The epithelial cells are oncocytic because their pink cytoplasm is packed with mitochondria. This epithelial portion probably arises from early duct cells that become entrapped within developing parotid lymph nodes during embryogenesis. Warthin's tumors occur mainly in the lower regions of the parotid gland, especially near the angle of the mandible and on rare occasion may be bilateral. They are completely benign neoplasms, although they carry some undesirable synonyms: adenolymphoma, which is a misnomer, and papillary cystadenoma lymphomatosum, a term undesirable both for the lymphomatosum part as well as its length. For these reasons most prefer the term Warthin's tumor.

In contrast to these two benign tumors, adenoid cystic carcinomas of the salivary glands histologically have tubular or cribriform patterns. This malignancy has a characteristic tendency to invade along perineural spaces. Lymphoepithelioma is a tumor that is recognized by hyperplastic duct epithelium surrounded by lymphoid tissue, while sebaceous lymphadenomas contain sebaceous cells within the lymphoid tissue. Finally, thyroglossal duct cysts are located in the midline of the neck but may be found extending up to the base of the tongue, and there is a similarity between the lymphoid islands seen in thyroglossal duct cysts and in Warthin's tumors; however, thyroid follicles may lead to the correct diagnosis in the former.

269. The answer is c. (*Kumar, pp 791–794. Rubin, pp 1315–1316.*) Three malignant tumors of the salivary glands are adenoid cystic carcinoma, mucoepidermoid carcinoma, and acinic cell carcinoma. Adenoid cystic carcinomas form tubular or cribriform patterns histologically and have a tendency to invade along perineural spaces, especially the facial nerve. This involvement can produce Bell's palsy, which is characterized by flattening of one side of the face. Mucoepidermoid carcinomas consist of a mixture of squamous epithelial cells and mucus-secreting cells. The mucus-secreting cells of a mucoepidermoid carcinoma can demonstrate intracellular mucin with a special mucicarmine stain. Acinic cell carcinomas contain glands with cleared or vacuolated epithelial cells. Finally, a mixture of epithelial structures and mesenchyme-like stroma is seen with pleomorphic adenomas, while papillary folds composed of a double layer of oncocytic cells is characteristic of Warthin's tumors.

Gastrointestinal System

Questions

DIRECTIONS: Each item below contains a question or incomplete statement followed by suggested responses. Select the **one best** response to each question.

270. A newborn infant is noted to have coughing and cyanosis during feeding. This infant is also noted to have marked gastric dilation due to "swallowed" air. Workup reveals that this infant has the most common type of esophageal atresia. Which one of the following statements correctly describes this type of congenital abnormality?

a. Atresia of the esophagus with fistula between both segments and the trachea
b. Atresia of the esophagus with fistula between the trachea and the blind upper segment
c. Atresia of the esophagus with fistula between the trachea and the distal esophageal segment
d. Atresia of the esophagus without tracheoesophageal fistula
e. Fistula between a normal esophagus and the trachea

271. A 49-year-old woman presents with increasing problems swallowing food (progressive dysphagia). X-ray studies with contrast reveal that she has a markedly dilated esophagus above the level of the lower esophageal sphincter (LES). No lesions are seen within the lumen of the esophagus. Which of the following is the most likely cause of this disorder?

a. Decreased LES resting pressure
b. Absence of myenteric plexus in the body of esophagus
c. Absence of myenteric plexus at the LES
d. Absence of submucosal plexus in the body of esophagus
e. Absence of submucosal plexus at the LES

272. A 45-year-old male alcoholic with a history of portal hypertension presents with vomiting of blood (hematemesis) and hypotension. He denies any history of vomiting nonblood material or retching prior to vomiting blood. During workup he dies suddenly. Which of the following histologic changes is most likely to be seen in a biopsy specimen taken from his esophagus?

a. Metaplastic columnar epithelium
b. Decreased ganglion cells in the myenteric plexus
c. Dilated blood vessels in the submucosa
d. Mucosal outpouchings
e. Numerous intraepithelial neutrophils

273. A 45-year-old man presents with increasing "heartburn," especially after eating or when lying down. Endoscopic examination finds a red velvety plaque located at the distal esophagus. Biopsies from this area, taken approximately 4 cm proximal to the gastroesophageal junction reveal metaplastic columnar epithelium as seen in the associated picture. Which of the following is the most likely diagnosis?

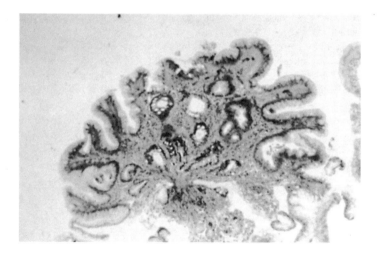

a. Acquired achalasia
b. Barrett's esophagus
c. Hamartomatous polyp
d. Metastatic adenocarcinoma
e. Reflux esophagitis

274. A 71-year-old man presents with dysphagia and is found to have a 5-cm mass that is located in the middle third of the esophagus and extends into adjacent lung tissue. Which of the following statements best describes the expected microscopic appearance of this lesion?

a. A mass composed of benign cartilage
b. A mass composed of benign smooth-muscle cells
c. Infiltrating groups of cells forming glandular structures
d. Infiltrating sheets of cells forming keratin
e. Infiltrating single cells having intracellular mucin

275. A 2-week-old neonate presents with regurgitation and persistent, severe projectile vomiting. An olive-like epigastric mass is felt during physical examination. A chest x-ray does not reveal the presence of bowel gas in the chest cavity. This infant's mother did not have polyhydramnios during this pregnancy. Which of the following is the most appropriate treatment for this infant's condition?

a. Oral medication with omeprazole and clarithromycin
b. Oral medication with vancomycin or metronidazole
c. Surgery to cut a hypertrophied stenotic band at the pylorus
d. Surgery to remove a mass of the adrenal gland
e. Surgery to resect an aganglionic section of the intestines

276. A 49-year-old woman taking ibuprofen for increasing joint pain in her hands presents with increasing pain in her midsternal area. Gastroscopy reveals multiple, scattered, punctate hemorrhagic areas in her gastric mucosa. Biopsies from one of these hemorrhagic lesions reveal mucosal erosions with edema and hemorrhage. No mucosal ulceration is seen. Which of the following is the most likely diagnosis?

a. Active chronic gastritis
b. Acute gastritis
c. Autoimmune gastritis
d. Chronic gastritis
e. Peptic ulcer disease

277. A biopsy of the antrum of the stomach of an adult who presents with epigastric pain reveals numerous lymphocytes and plasma cells within the lamina propria, which is of normal thickness. There are also scattered neutrophils within the glandular epithelial cells. A Steiner silver stain from this specimen is positive for a small, curved organism. These histologic changes are most consistent with infection by which one of the following organisms?

a. Enteroinvasive *Escherichia coli*
b. Enterotoxigenic *E. coli*
c. *Helicobacter pylori*
d. *Salmonella typhi*
e. *Shigella* species

278. A 51-year-old man presents with epigastric pain that is lessened whenever he eats. A gastroscopy is performed to evaluate these gastric symptoms and a solitary gastric ulcer is seen. Which one of the listed gross findings if present would be most suspicious for the lesion being a malignant ulcer?

a. Diameter greater than 2 cm
b. Location on the lesser curvature
c. Outward radiating rugae
d. Perforation into the peritoneal cavity
e. Raised peripheral margins

279. A 56-year-old woman presents with a small mass overlying her left clavicle. She states that she has lost about 15 pounds over the past several months and has had trouble falling asleep at night because of "heartburn." She states that her last menstrual period was 10 years ago, and she denies any vaginal bleeding. Physical examination finds a solitary enlarged lymph node over her left clavicle. The lymph node measures 1.5 cm in greatest dimension, and a biopsy from this enlarged node reveals numerous malignant cells that are similar in appearance to those seen in the picture below. These cells stain positively for mucin. Which of the following abnormalities is most likely to be present in this individual?

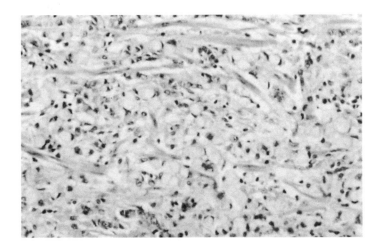

a. Adenocarcinoma of the esophagus
b. Clear cell carcinoma of the kidney
c. Colloid carcinoma of the breast
d. Mucoepidermoid carcinoma of the parotid
e. Signet cell carcinoma of the stomach

280. A 53-year-old man presents with increasing gastric pain and is found to have a 3-cm mass located in the anterior wall of his stomach. This mass is resected and histologic examination reveals a tumor composed of cells having elongated, spindle-shaped nuclei. The tumor does not connect to the overlying gastric epithelium and is instead found only in the wall of the stomach. The tumor cells stain positively with CD117, but negatively with both desmin and S-100. Special studies find that these tumor cells have abnormalities of the KIT gene. Which of the following is the most likely diagnosis?

a. Ectopic islet cell adenoma (VIPoma)
b. Gastrointestinal stromal tumor (GIST)
c. Submucosal leiomyoma ("fibroid tumor")
d. Lymphoma of mucosa-associated lymphoid tissue (MALToma)
e. Nonchromaffin paraganglioma (chemodectoma)

281. A 2-year-old boy presents with painless rectal bleeding. His stools are found to be brick-colored, and after further workup, the bleeding is thought to be secondary to the abnormality seen in the picture below. Which of the following is the basic defect that caused this developmental abnormality of the small intestines?

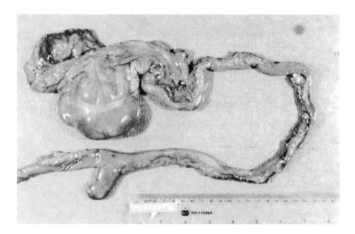

a. Failure of the hepatic duct to close
b. Failure of the intestinal loop to retract
c. Failure of the midgut to rotate
d. Failure of the urachus to close
e. Failure of the vitelline duct to close

282. A 3-year-old girl presents with the abrupt onset of colicky abdominal pain, abdominal distention, and stool with blood and mucus ("currant jelly" stools). Physical examination finds a slightly tender, sausage-shaped mass in the right upper quadrant of her abdomen. Which of the following is the most likely diagnosis?

a. Acute appendicitis with abscess formation
b. Acute diverticulitis with perforation
c. Aneurysm of the mesenteric artery
d. Intussusception of the cecum
e. Volvulus of the sigmoid colon

283. A 10-month-old, previously healthy male infant develops a severe, watery diarrhea 2 days after visiting the pediatrician for a routine checkup. Which of the following complications is this infant most at risk of developing?

a. Aplastic anemia
b. Intestinal obstruction
c. Iron deficiency
d. Megaloblastic anemia
e. Severe dehydration

284. A 2-year-old girl is being evaluated for vomiting, diarrhea, and failure to thrive. A small intestinal biopsy reveals changes that are similar in appearance to those changes seen in the picture. Additionally, laboratory studies find the presence of antiendomysial autoantibodies. Which of the following is the most appropriate therapy for this infant?

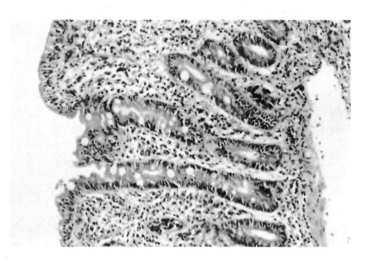

a. Daily skin exposure to light of 470 nm
b. Dietary restriction of the water-insoluble wheat protein gluten
c. Dietary supplementation with megadoses of vitamin C
d. Surgical resection of the aganglionic segment
e. Triple antibiotic therapy with metronidazole, bismuth salicylate, and tetracycline

285. A 45-year-old man presents with fever, chronic diarrhea, and weight loss. He is found to have multiple pain and swelling of his joints (migratory polyarthritis) and generalized lymphadenopathy. Physical examination reveals skin hyperpigmentation. A biopsy from his small intestines reveals the presence of macrophages in the lamina propria that contain PAS-positive cytoplasm. Which of the following is the most likely diagnosis?

a. Abetalipoproteinemia
b. Crohn's disease
c. Hartnup disease
d. Nontropical sprue
e. Whipple's disease

286. A 29-year-old woman presents with colicky lower abdominal pain and frequent bloody diarrhea with mucus. Physical examination finds fever and peripheral leukocytosis, while multiple stool examinations fail to reveal any ova or parasites. A colonoscopy reveals the rectum and sigmoid portions of her colon to have superficial mucosal ulcers with hemorrhage, but regions more proximal are within normal limits. Which of the following histologic changes is most likely to be seen in a biopsy specimen taken from her rectum?

a. Crypt abscesses with crypt distortion
b. Dilated submucosal blood vessels with focal thrombosis
c. Increased thickness of the subepithelial collagen layer
d. Noncaseating granulomas with scattered giant cells
e. Numerous eosinophils within the lamina propria

287. A 39-year-old man presents with bloody diarrhea. Multiple stool examinations fail to reveal any ova or parasites. A barium examination of the patient's colon reveals a characteristic "string sign." A colonoscopy reveals the rectum and sigmoid portions of the colon to be unremarkable. A biopsy from the terminal ileum reveals numerous acute and chronic inflammatory cells within the lamina propria. Worsening of the patient's symptoms results in emergency resection of the distal small intestines. Gross examination of this resected bowel reveals deep, long mucosal fissures extending deep into the muscle wall. Several transmural fistulas are also found. Which of the following is the most likely diagnosis?

a. Ulcerative colitis
b. Lymphocytic colitis
c. Infectious colitis
d. Eosinophilic colitis
e. Crohn's disease

288. A 62-year-old man presents after fainting at home approximately 1 h ago. He says that for the past day he has had increasing left-sided abdominal pain, and also he has noted bright red blood in his stool. He denies any history of vomiting or diarrhea. Physical examination finds a low-grade fever and gross blood on rectal examination. Further workup finds abnormalities in his colon that are similar in appearance to the abnormalities seen in the gross picture of his colon. Which of the following is the most likely cause of his GI bleeding?

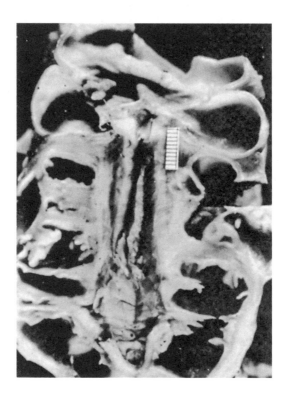

a. Angiodysplasia
b. Appendicitis
c. Diverticulosis
d. Hemorrhoids
e. Intussusception

289. A 39-year-old woman presents with chronic abdominal cramps, watery diarrhea, and periodic facial flushing. Physical examination reveals wheezing and a slightly enlarged liver. Workup reveals several masses within the liver and a large mass in the small intestine. Which of the following substances is likely to be elevated in her urine?

a. 5-hydroxyindoleacetic acid (5-HIAA)
b. Aminolevulinic acid (ALA)
c. N-formiminoglutamate (FIGlu)
d. Normetanephrine
e. Vanillylmandelic acid (VMA)

290. During routine colonoscopy of a 65-year-old man, a 2-mm "dewdrop"-like polyp is found in the sigmoid colon. A biopsy of this lesion is seen in the picture below. Which of the following is the most likely diagnosis?

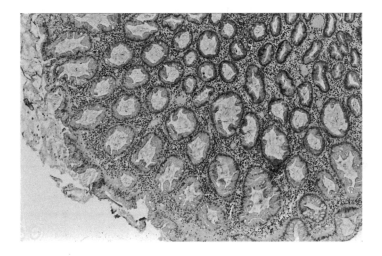

a. Hyperplastic polyp
b. Hamartomatous polyp
c. Inflammatory polyp
d. Adenomatous polyp
e. Lymphoid polyp

291. A 26-year-old man presents because of the development of multiple lesions on his face and within his oral cavity. Physical examination finds multiple flesh-colored facial papules along with multiple papillomas of the oral cavity and multiple keratoses that are located on the dorsal surface of his hands. A biopsy from one of the facial lesions is diagnosed by the pathologist as being a trichilemmoma. Further workup finds a small nodule in the thyroid gland and multiple polyps of the small and large intestines. A biopsy from one of the intestinal polyps is diagnosed as being a hamartoma. Which of the following is the most likely diagnosis?

a. Cowden disease
b. Familial adenomatous polyposis
c. Gardner's syndrome
d. Peutz-Jeghers syndrome
e. Turcot's syndrome

292. A 38-year-old woman presents with increasing fatigue. Her past medical history is remarkable for the development of endometrial adenocarcinoma 3 years prior. Physical examination at this time is unremarkable except for heme-positive stool. Laboratory examination finds her hematocrit to be slightly decreased and hypochromic microcytic red cells are present in her peripheral smear. An upper GI is unremarkable, but a barium enema study finds a 4-cm mass in the left side of his colon having an "apple core" appearance and a 2-cm mass in the right colon. Biopsies of these masses find multiple adenocarcinomas. She has no previous history of colon polyps. Further workup finds that several of her relatives have a history of colon cancer and it is thought that she may have the hereditary nonpolyposis colon carcinoma (HNPCC) syndrome. Germ line mutations of which one of the following genes is often present in this syndrome?

a. APC
b. K-RAS
c. MSH2
d. p53
e. SMAD

293. An 18-year-old woman presents with abdominal pain localized to the right lower quadrant, nausea and vomiting, mild fever, and an elevation of the peripheral leukocyte count to 17,000/μL. An appendectomy is performed. Which of the following statements best describes the expected microscopic appearance of her appendix?

a. An appendix with a normal appearance
b. Neutrophils within the muscular wall
c. Lymphoid hyperplasia and multinucleated giant cells within the muscular wall
d. A dilated lumen filled with mucus
e. A yellow tumor nodule at the tip of the appendix

294. An autopsy is performed on a 19-year-old woman who died from an overdose of acetaminophen. Which of the following histologic changes is most likely to be seen in a biopsy specimen taken from her liver?

a. Centrilobular necrosis
b. Focal scattered necrosis
c. Geographic necrosis
d. Midzonal necrosis
e. Periportal necrosis

295. A 2-year-old girl is being evaluated for strikingly yellow skin and is found to have elevated serum levels of indirect bilirubin. After appropriate workup the diagnosis of type II Crigler-Najjar syndrome is made. She is then treated with phenobarbital, which causes hyperplasia of the smooth endoplasmic reticulum in hepatocytes and decreases her serum indirect bilirubin levels. What is the basic defect that caused this child's illness?

a. Acute intravascular hemolysis of red blood cells
b. Decreased activity of bilirubin-UDP-glucuronyl transferase
c. Defective metabolism of the urea cycle
d. Reduced uptake of unconjugated bilirubin by hepatocytes
e. Formation of mercaptans in the gut

296. A full-term normal male breast-fed infant develops a slight yellow color to his skin on his sixth day of life. Laboratory examination finds his serum bilirubin levels to be slightly elevated (due to increased indirect bilirubin), but the levels are less than 6 mg/dL. Additionally, serum hemoglobin levels are within normal limits. The elevated bilirubin levels last for about 5 weeks. Which of the following is the most likely cause of these signs and symptoms?

a. Breastfeeding jaundice
b. Breast milk jaundice
c. Hemolytic disease of the newborn
d. Inspissated bile syndrome
e. Physiologic jaundice of the newborn

297. A 21-year-old woman notices her urine suddenly turned dark soon after she started taking oral contraceptives. She is otherwise asymptomatic. Physical examination finds a slight yellow color to her skin, and laboratory tests find mildly elevated serum direct bilirubin levels. A liver biopsy, which grossly is a black color, shows pigmented cytoplasmic globules in hepatocytes. Further workup documents mutations involving the gene that codes for the multidrug resistance protein 2 (MRP2). Which one of the following is most likely to result from mutations of this gene?

a. Decreased synthesis of albumin
b. Decreased synthesis of gamma-glutamyl transpeptidase
c. Increased excretion of copper into bile
d. Increased metabolism of carnitine by the liver
e. Impaired canalicular transport of bilirubin glucuronide

298. A 44-year-old man presents with the sudden onset of severe right upper quadrant (RUQ) abdominal pain, ascites, tender hepatomegaly, and hematemesis. These symptoms are suggestive of Budd-Chiari syndrome. Which of the following is the most likely cause of this disorder?

a. Obstruction of the common bile duct
b. Obstruction of the intrahepatic sinusoids
c. Thrombosis of the hepatic artery
d. Thrombosis of the hepatic vein
e. Thrombosis of the portal vein

299. A 27-year-old woman presents with headaches, muscle pain (myalgia), anorexia, nausea, and vomiting. She denies any history of drug or alcohol use, but upon further questioning she states that recently she has lost her taste for coffee and cigarettes. Physical examination reveals a slight yellow discoloration of her scleras, while laboratory results indicate a serum bilirubin level of 1.8 mg/dL, and aminotransferases (AST and ALT) levels are increased. Which of the following is the most likely diagnosis?

a. Gilbert's syndrome
b. Chronic hepatitis
c. Amebic liver abscess
d. Acute viral hepatitis
e. Acute hepatic failure

300. A 4-year-old boy presents with mild fatigue and malaise. Several other children in the day-care center he attends 5 days a week have developed similar illnesses. Physical examination finds mild liver tenderness, but no lymphadenopathy is noted. Laboratory examination finds mildly elevated serum levels of liver enzymes and bilirubin. The boy recovers from his mild illness without incident. Which of the following organisms is the most likely cause of this child's illness?

a. Cytomegalovirus (CMV)
b. Epstein-Barr virus (EBV)
c. Group A β-hemolytic streptococcus
d. Hepatitis A virus
e. Hepatitis B virus

301. Which of the following hepatitis profile patterns is most consistent with an asymptomatic hepatitis B carrier?

	Hepatitis B Surface Antigen (HBsAg)	Hepatitis B e Antigen (HBeAg)	Antibody to Surface Antigen (anti-HBs)	Antibody to Core Antigen (anti-HBc)
a.	Positive	Negative	Negative	Negative
b.	Positive	Positive	Negative	Negative
c.	Positive	Positive	Negative	Positive
d.	Positive	Negative	Negative	Positive
e.	Negative	Negative	Positive	Positive

302. A 48-year-old man with fatigue is being evaluated for a 1-year history of elevated serum liver enzymes. A liver biopsy is taken and the pathology report of this specimen states there is grade 2 inflammatory activity with piecemeal necrosis and stage 1 fibrosis. The term "piecemeal necrosis" refers to which one of the following pathologic abnormalities?

a. Congo red–positive extracellular deposits surrounding necrotic hepatocytes in acinar zone 1
b. Destruction of the limiting plate with necrosis of hepatocytes surrounding the portal triad
c. Fibrosis around the central hepatic veins with apoptosis of adjacent hepatocytes
d. Necrosis of hepatocytes extending from the portal area of one hepatic lobule to the central vein of an adjacent lobule
e. Random necrosis of individual or small clusters of hepatocytes in acinar zone 3

303. A 48-year-old man presents with fatigue and slight malaise. Physical examination is unremarkable except for slight tenderness in the upper right quadrant of his abdomen. Laboratory examination reveals mild elevation of the liver enzymes. He is followed over the next year and is found to have intermittent hyperbilirubinemia along with episodic elevations in his serum transaminase levels (AST and ALT). During these episodes the AST/ALT ratio is less than 1. A liver biopsy reveals chronic inflammation of the portal triads that spills over into the hepatocytes and moderate fatty change of the hepatocytes. No hepatocytes with ground-glass cytoplasm are found. Which of the following viral proteins is thought to be in part responsible for the persistent infection in this individual?

a. The VP1 capsid protein of hepatitis A virus
b. The nucleocapsid core protein of hepatitis B virus
c. The E2 protein of hepatitis C virus
d. The delta antigen of hepatitis D virus
e. The ORF3 protein of hepatitis E virus

304. A 49-year-old woman presents with increasing fatigue and is found to have elevated liver enzymes (AST and ALT). You follow her in your clinic and find over the next 9 months that her liver enzymes have remained elevated. All serologic tests for viral markers are within normal limits. A liver biopsy reveals chronic inflammation in the portal triads that focally destroys the limiting plate and "spills over" into the adjacent hepatocytes. There are no granulomas present, and there is no evidence of fibrosis surrounding any of the bile ducts within the portal triads. Anti-smooth-muscle antibodies and antinuclear antibodies are found in the patient's serum. An LE cell test is positive. Which of the following is the most likely diagnosis?

a. Autoimmune hepatitis
b. Chronic persistent hepatitis
c. Primary biliary cirrhosis
d. Primary sclerosing cholangitis
e. Systemic lupus erythematosus

305. Dilated sinusoids and irregular cystic spaces filled with blood within the liver, which may rupture and lead to massive intraabdominal hemorrhage, are most closely associated with which one of the following substances?

a. Salicylates
b. Estrogens
c. Anabolic steroids
d. Acetaminophen
e. Vinyl chloride

306. A 49-year-old man presents with symptoms that developed following a long weekend of binge drinking. His serum reveals a gamma-glutamyl transferase (GGT) level of 65 IU/L. A liver biopsy reveals fatty change (steatosis) of numerous hepatocytes. Which of the following biochemical abnormalities is most likely responsible for this patient's liver abnormality?

a. Decreased free fatty acid delivery to the liver
b. Decreased production of triglycerides
c. Increased mitochondrial oxidation of fatty acids
d. Increased NADH production
e. Increased release of lipoproteins

307. A 55-year-old man presents with increasing fatigue, weakness, anorexia, and jaundice over the past several months. Physical examination finds mild ascites and gynecomastia. A liver biopsy reveals regenerative nodules of hepatocytes surrounded by fibrosis, as seen in the picture below. Which of the following is the source of the excess collagen deposited in these fibrotic bands?

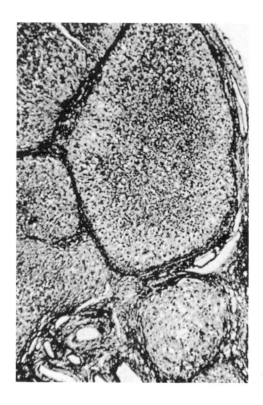

a. Hepatocytes
b. Kupffer cells
c. Ito cells
d. Endothelial cells
e. Bile duct epithelial cells

308. A 45-year-old obese woman presents with increasing fatigue, malaise, and fullness in the right upper quadrant of her abdomen. Pertinent clinical history includes type II diabetes mellitus and hyperlipidemia. Laboratory test finds elevated liver enzymes along with increased serum cholesterol. Which one of the following clinical procedures or tests should be used to confirm a diagnosis of nonalcoholic steatohepatitis?

a. Abdominal magnetic resonance imaging
b. Liver biopsy
c. Liver ultrasonography
d. Oral cholecystogram
e. Quantitative serum ferritin

309. A 36-year-old man presents because his skin has been darkening recently. Physical examination finds his skin to have a dark, somewhat bronze color. Workup reveals signs of diabetes mellitus. His serum iron is found to be 1150 mg/dL, and his transferrin saturation is 98%. A liver biopsy is performed and reveals extensive deposits of hemosiderin in the hepatocytes and Kupffer cells. Which one of the listed genes is mutated in the familial form of this man's disease?

a. ATP7B gene
b. CFTR gene
c. FIC1 gene
d. HFE gene
e. MDR3 gene

310. A 5-year-old girl is brought in with severe vomiting that developed suddenly 5 days after she had a viral infection. Upon questioning, her parents indicate that she was given aspirin for several days to treat a fever that occurred with the viral illness. She is hospitalized and quickly develops signs of cerebral edema. Microscopic examination of a liver biopsy from this young girl would most likely reveal what abnormality?

a. Increased intracellular copper
b. Marked microvesicular steatosis
c. Numerous Mallory bodies
d. PAS-positive intracytoplasmic inclusions
e. PAS-negative intracytoplasmic inclusions

311. A 36-year-old man presents with jaundice and pruritus. Physical examination finds a diffuse yellow discoloration to his skin. Laboratory examination reveals markedly elevated serum levels of alkaline phosphatase, but neither antinuclear nor antimitochondrial antibodies are present. A liver biopsy revealed reactive hepatocytes and fibrosis in the sinusoids. The portal tracts showed marked fibrosis around the bile ducts, but no granulomas were seen. While waiting for a liver transplant he developed a malignancy and died. Which of the following tumors is most closely associated with his liver disease?

a. Cholangiocarcinoma
b. Gallbladder carcinoma
c. Gastric carcinoma
d. Hepatoblastoma
e. Pancreatic carcinoma

312. A 26-year-old presents with right upper quadrant abdominal pain and is found to have a large cyst in the right lobe of his liver. X-rays reveal the cyst to have a calcified wall. The cyst is then surgically excised. Examination of this tissue histologically reveals a thick, acellular, laminated eosinophilic wall. The fluid within the cyst is found to be granular and contain numerous small larval capsules with scoleces ("brood capsules"). Which of the following is the most likely diagnosis?

a. Pyogenic liver abscess
b. Amebic liver abscess
c. Hydatid cyst
d. Schistosomiasis
e. Oriental cholangiohepatitis

313. An oval lesion is found in the right lobe of the liver in an otherwise asymptomatic 24-year-old woman. Surgical resection finds a single well-demarcated lesion that has a prominent, central, stellate white scar. Which of the following diagnoses is most consistent with this gross appearance?

a. Metastatic adenocarcinoma
b. Focal nodular hyperplasia
c. Hemangioma
d. Hepatocellular carcinoma
e. Nodular regenerative hyperplasia

314. A 51-year-old male alcoholic with a history of chronic liver disease presents with increasing weight loss and ascites. Physical examination reveals a slightly enlarged, soft, nontender prostate. Examination of the scrotum is unremarkable, and fecal occult blood tests are negative. A chest x-ray is unremarkable, but a CT scan of the abdomen reveals a single mass in the left lobe of the liver. Workup reveals elevated levels of α-fetoprotein in this patient's blood. Which of the following is the most likely diagnosis?

a. Angiosarcoma
b. Cholangiocarcinoma
c. Hepatoblastoma
d. Hepatocellular carcinoma
e. Metastatic colon cancer

315. A 12-year-old boy with sickle cell anemia presents with recurrent severe right upper quadrant colicky abdominal pain. At the time of surgery, multiple dark black stones are found within the gallbladder. These stones are composed of which one of the following substances?

a. Bilirubin
b. Carbon
c. Cholesterol
d. Struvite
e. Urate

316. A 54-year-old man presents with a high fever, jaundice, and colicky abdominal pain in the right upper quadrant. The gallbladder cannot be palpated on physical examination. Workup reveals hemoglobin level of 15.3 g/dL, unconjugated bilirubin level of 0.9 mg/dL, conjugated bilirubin level of 1.1 mg/dL, and alkaline phosphatase level of 180 IU/L. Which of the following is the most likely diagnosis?

a. Acute cholecystitis
b. Chronic cholecystitis
c. Bile duct obstruction by a stone
d. Carcinoma of the gallbladder
e. Carcinoma of the head of the pancreas

317. An infant is brought in by his mother, who says that his skin tastes salty. With time this patient's pancreas is expected to undergo progressive fibrosis with atrophy of the exocrine glands and cystic dilation of the ducts. Which of the following is the basic abnormality in this infant?

a. Decreased synthesis of surface receptor
b. Decreased intracellular cAMP
c. Decreased glycosylated chloride channel
d. Increased phosphorylation of chloride channel
e. Increased ductal secretion of water

318. Germ line mutations in the cationic trypsinogen (PRSS1) gene can produce an autosomal dominant disorder that usually begins in childhood and is characterized by recurrent bouts of severe inflammation that produces which one of the listed disorders?

a. Acute cholecystitis
b. Acute colitis
c. Acute pancreatitis
d. Chronic gastritis
e. Chronic hepatitis

319. A 45-year-old man presents with weight loss, steatorrhea, and malabsorption. A CT scan of the abdomen reveals a questionable mass in the head of the pancreas. A biopsy specimen microscopically reveals chronic inflammation and atrophy of the pancreatic acini with marked fibrosis. No malignancy is identified. Which of the following is the most common cause of this disorder in adults in the United States?

a. Abdominal trauma
b. Chronic alcoholism
c. Cystic fibrosis
d. Gallstones
e. Hyperlipidemia

320. A 48-year-old male alcoholic presents with malaise, fever, and mid-abdominal pain that radiates to his back. Pertinent medical history includes repeated bouts of pancreatitis that mainly occur after times of binge drinking. Physical examination finds a low-grade fever, and a mass is palpated in the epigastric area. An abdominal CT scan finds a fluid-filled mass in the pancreas. This mass is removed at celiotomy and has a similar appearance to the cystic mass shown in the photograph. It is filled with clear fluid, and histologic sections reveal a large cystic structure that lacks an epithelial lining. Which of the following is the most likely diagnosis?

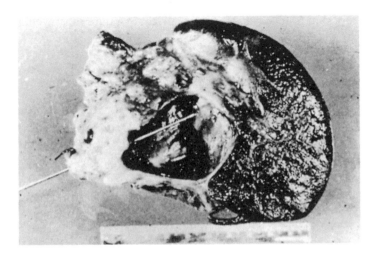

a. Cylindroma
b. Hydrocystoma
c. Pseudocyst
d. Pseudomyxoma
e. Syringoma

321. According to Courvoisier's law, a pancreatic cancer located in the head of the pancreas should be suspected in an individual with which one of the following clinical signs?

a. Migratory thrombophlebitis
b. Obstructive jaundice and a dilated gallbladder
c. Obstructive jaundice and a nonpalpable gallbladder
d. Steatorrhea and a nontender gallbladder
e. Steatorrhea and a tender gallbladder

322. A 45-year-old man with a 2 year history of a mild, non-ketotic diabetes mellitus and anemia presents with the new onset of a necrolytic migratory skin rash. What is the cell of origin of a tumor that would most likely produce this set of clinical signs?

a. A cell of the pancreas
b. B cell of the pancreas
c. C cell of the thyroid
d. D cell of the stomach
e. G cell of the stomach

323. A 44-year-old woman presents with repeated episodes of feeling "light-headed" that are associated with sweating and a feeling like she is about to faint. She says that she feels better if she drinks some orange juice and eats a candy bar during one of these episodes. Physical examination is unremarkable, but laboratory examination finds decreased serum levels of glucose along with elevated levels of insulin. The combination of hypoglycemia, symptoms of hypoglycemia, and symptoms of hypoglycemia relieved by glucose is the definition of which of the following clinical triads?

a. Beck's triad
b. Charcot's triad
c. Marchiafava's triad
d. Virchow's triad
e. Whipple's triad

324. A 20-year-old woman is found to have elevated blood glucose levels on several occasions. She is otherwise asymptomatic and is of normal height and normal weight. Laboratory evaluation does not detect the presence of islet cell autoantibodies in this young woman. Several members in successive generations of her family, however, have been diagnosed as having diabetes mellitus. Further tests find that her mother also has mildly elevated blood glucose levels but is not obese and is otherwise asymptomatic. Which of the following is the most likely diagnosis?

a. Insulin-dependent diabetes mellitus
b. Mature-onset diabetes of the young
c. Non–insulin-dependent diabetes mellitus
d. Type 1 diabetes mellitus
e. Type 2 diabetes mellitus

325. A 12-year-old nonobese boy presents for evaluation after becoming sick at school. Pertinent recent medical history includes weight loss with polyphagia, polydipsia, and polyuria. Laboratory examination finds hyperglycemia, while urinary examination reveals increased glucose and trace ketones. Which of the following abnormalities is most likely to be present in this boy?

a. Amyloid deposition in the pancreatic islets
b. Atrophy and destruction of the pancreatic acini
c. Decreased numbers of insulin receptors on adipocytes
d. Lymphocytic infiltration in the pancreatic islets
e. Mutations in the gene that codes for hexokinase

326. A 35-year-old obese woman of normal height is found to have hyperglycemia that lasts for several hours following a meal. Further workup reveals normal fasting serum glucose levels. Physical examination is otherwise unremarkable. A decreased amount of which one of the following is most closely associated with insulin resistance and the development of postprandial hyperglycemia?

a. Adiponectin
b. Free fatty acids
c. Pramlintide
d. Gamma-peroxisome proliferator-activator receptor
e. Tumor necrosis factor-alpha

327. A 57-year-old woman with a long history of type 2 diabetes mellitus is being evaluated for progressive renal failure. A kidney biopsy reveals nodular glomerulosclerosis and hyaline arteriolosclerosis. Electron microscopic examination finds a diffuse thickening of the basement membrane of the glomerular capillaries. Which of the following is the primary defect responsible for the thickening of the renal basement membrane in this individual?

a. Deposition of immune complexes in the subendothelial space
b. Increased intracellular production of sorbitol
c. Loss of glomerular polyanions
d. Nonenzymatic glycosylation of proteins
e. Production of antibodies to type IV collagen

Gastrointestinal System

Answers

270. The answer is c. (*Kumar, pp 799–800. Rubin, pp 670–671.*) The most common congenital anomaly of the esophagus is tracheal-esophageal fistula (TEF). Congenital anomalies of the esophagus are classified into five types, but only four types are associated with esophageal atresia. Type A abnormalities consist of atresia of the esophagus without a connection to the trachea (no fistula). Type B consists of atresia of the esophagus with a fistula between the trachea and the blind upper segment, while type C (the most common type) is characterized by atresia of the esophagus with a fistula between the trachea and the distal esophageal segment. Type D involves esophageal atresia with a fistula between both segments and the trachea, while type E is characterized by a fistula between a normal esophagus and the trachea. This abnormality involves no atresia. To summarize, type A has no fistula, type B connects to the upper segment, type C to the lower segment, and type D to both segments. These defects are dangerous because material that is swallowed may pass into the trachea (aspiration) either directly (types B, D, and E) or indirectly through reflux in that there is a blind upper pouch present (types A and C). Additionally, gastric dilation can occur due to "swallowed" air in those anomalies in which the trachea communicates with the lower esophagus (types C, D, and E). Also important is the fact that any defect that interferes with fetal swallowing in utero will produce polyhydramnios during pregnancy.

271. The answer is b. (*Kumar, pp 800–801. Rubin, pp 672–673.*) Achalasia, which means "un-relaxation," is a term that describes the absence of normal lower esophageal sphincter (LES) relaxation. This condition results from decreased or absent ganglion cells in the myenteric plexus in the body of the esophagus. The etiology of this neuronal loss is unknown in many cases; however, some cases are secondary to other diseases, such as diabetes mellitus, amyloidosis, sarcoidosis, and Chagas' disease, which is caused by *Trypanosoma cruzi*. Because of the increased LES pressure and the absence of peristaltic waves in the lower esophagus, the esophagus in these patients is dilated and tortuous above the level of the LES. Barium x-ray studies reveal this dilation. The distal esophagus has a characteristic "beaklike" appearance.

Patients with achalasia have an increased risk of developing aspiration pneumonia and squamous cell carcinoma.

272. The answer is c. (*Kumar, pp 802–803.*) Most lesions of the esophagus present with similar symptoms, such as heartburn and dysphagia, but the most serious disease, which carries the risk of exsanguination, is bleeding esophageal varices. Varices occur in about two-thirds of all patients with cirrhosis, and in the majority of patients the etiology is alcoholic cirrhosis. The cirrhosis causes portal hypertension, which shunts blood into connecting channels between the portal and caval systems, such as the subepithelial plexus of veins in the lower esophagus. Varices produce no symptoms until they rupture and cause massive bleeding (hematemesis), which may lead to death. Other diseases, such as gastritis, esophageal laceration (Mallory-Weiss tears), or peptic ulcer disease, may cause hematemesis.

In contrast, columnar epithelium in the distal esophagus is seen with Barrett's esophagus; decreased ganglion cells in the myenteric plexus are seen with achalasia, a disorder that is characterized by aperistalsis, incomplete relaxation of the lower esophageal sphincter (LES) with swallowing, and increased resting tone of the LES, all of which lead to esophageal dilation and symptoms of progressive dysphagia.

273. The answer is b. (*Kumar, pp 803–805. Rubin, pp 673–676.*) The presence of columnar epithelium lining part or all of the distal esophagus is known as Barrett's esophagus. It is considered an acquired change resulting from reflux of acidic gastric contents with ulceration of the esophageal squamous epithelium and replacement by metaplastic, acid-resistant, columnar epithelium. Endoscopically it has a velvety-red appearance. Microscopically, intestinal-type epithelium is most common, but gastric-type epithelium is also seen. Varying degrees of dysplasia may be present. The risk of carcinoma is increased 30- to 40-fold. Virtually all of these tumors are of the adenocarcinoma type and they account for up to 10% of all esophageal cancers.

274. The answer is d. (*Kumar, pp 806–809. Rubin, pp 679–680.*) Carcinoma of the esophagus accounts for about 10% of malignancies of the GI tract, but for a disproportionate number of cancer deaths. Predisposing factors include smoking, esophagitis, and achalasia. Of these carcinomas, 60 to 70% are squamous cell carcinomas that characteristically begin as lesions in situ. Adenocarcinoma occurs mainly in the lower esophagus and may arise in up to

10% of cases of Barrett's esophagus. Anaplastic and small cell variants also occur. Polypoid lesions are most common, followed by malignant ulceration and diffusely infiltrative forms. Tumors tend to spread by direct invasion of adjacent structures, but lymphatic and hematogenous spread may occur. Distant metastases are, however, a late feature. Five-year survival is less than 10%.

275. The answer is c. (*Kumar, pp 799–800, 812.*) Several congenital abnormalities of the gastrointestinal tract present with specific symptoms. Infants with congenital hypertrophic pyloric stenosis present in the second or third week of life with symptoms of regurgitation and persistent severe vomiting. Physical examination reveals a firm mass in the region of the pylorus. Surgical splitting of the muscle in the stenotic region is curative. Diaphragmatic hernias, if large enough, may allow abdominal contents— including portions of the stomach, intestines, or liver—to herniate into the thoracic cavity and cause respiratory compromise. Congenital aganglionic megacolon (Hirschsprung's disease) is caused by failure of the neural crest cells to migrate all the way to the anus, resulting in a portion of distal colon that lacks ganglion cells and both Meissner's submucosal and Auerbach's myenteric plexuses. This results in a functional obstruction and dilation proximal to the affected portion of colon. Symptoms of Hirschsprung's disease include failure to pass meconium soon after birth followed by constipation and possible abdominal distention.

276. The answer is b. (*Kumar, pp 812–813. Rubin, pp 682–684.*) Gastritis is a nonspecific term that describes any inflammation of the gastric mucosa. Acute gastritis refers to the clinical situation of gastric mucosal erosions (not mucosal ulcers). Acute gastritis is also known as hemorrhagic gastritis or acute erosive gastritis. Acute gastritis is associated with the use of nonsteroidal anti-inflammatory drugs, such as aspirin, ibuprofen, and corticosteroids, and also with alcohol, chemotherapy, ischemia, shock, and even severe stress. Two types of stress ulcers are Curling's ulcers, seen in patients with severe burns, and Cushing's ulcers, seen in patients with intracranial lesions. Grossly acute gastritis appears as multiple, scattered, punctate (less than 1 cm) hemorrhagic areas in the gastric mucosa. This is helpful in differentiating acute gastritis from peptic ulcers, which tend to be solitary and larger. Microscopically the gastric mucosa from a patient with acute gastritis is likely to reveal mucosal erosions, scattered neutrophils, edema, and possibly hemorrhage.

277. The answer is c. (*Kumar, pp 813–816. Rubin, pp 684–687.*) Chronic gastritis is histologically characterized by the presence of lymphocytes and plasma cells. It is important to realize that the presence of neutrophils within the glandular epithelium indicates active inflammation and may be the main type of inflammation present (acute gastritis) or may be combined with more numerous chronic inflammations (active chronic gastritis). Chronic gastritis is divided into subgroups based either on etiology (immunologic or infectious), location (antrum or body), histopathology, or clinical features. *H. pylori* gastritis is associated with infection by *H. pylori*, a small, curved, gram-negative rod that is found in approximately 20% of the general population. The organisms are found in the mucus overlying the surface/foveolar epithelium. These changes tend to affect primarily the antral or antral-body-fundic mucosa. This is the type of gastritis normally associated with active chronic gastritis. The therapy for *Helicobacter* is either triple therapy (metronidazole, bismuth salicylate, and either amoxicillin or tetracycline) or double therapy (omeprazole and clarithromycin).

In contrast, autoimmune gastritis, also known as diffuse corporal atrophic gastritis or type A atrophic gastritis, is characterized by the presence of autoimmune antibodies including parietal cell antibodies and intrinsic factor antibodies. This type of gastritis is associated with pernicious anemia and achlorhydria. Pernicious anemia is the result of decreased intrinsic factor, which in turn produces a vitamin B_{12} deficiency. This vitamin deficiency causes megaloblastic anemia and subacute combined disease of the spinal cord. Histologically there is diffuse atrophy (reduced mucosal thickness), gland loss, widespread intestinal metaplasia, and variable chronic and acute inflammation. These changes are found predominantly in the body-fundus mucosa (usually absent in the antrum). There is an increased risk for gastric cancer, but these patients do not develop peptic ulcers.

278. The answer is e. (*Kumar, pp 816–820. Rubin, pp 688–694.*) Benign peptic ulcers are associated with the effects of acid and may occur anywhere in the gastrointestinal tract exposed to acid-peptic activity. Over 98% of cases occur in the stomach or duodenum, with duodenal cases outnumbering gastric cases 4 to 1. Peptic ulcers tend to be solitary lesions, but ulcers associated with Zollinger-Ellison syndrome are typically multiple and frequently involve distal duodenum and jejunum. Duodenal ulceration appears to be related to hypersecretion of acid. Gastric ulceration typically occurs in a setting of normo- or hypochlorhydria with abnormality of mucosal defense mechanisms, back-diffusion of acid, and possibly local ischemia. *H. pylori* is present in up to 100% of patients with duodenal ulcers and about 75% of patients with gastric ulcers.

Note that gastric ulcers can be either benign peptic ulcers or malignant ulcers associated with gastric cancers. Certain gross and microscopic characteristics help to differentiate benign peptic ulcers from malignant ulcers. Benign peptic ulcers tend to be round and regular with punched-out straight walls. The margins are only slightly elevated and rugae radiate outward from the ulcer. Raised peripheral margins are quite characteristic of malignant lesions, which are also irregular in appearance. Most benign peptic ulcers are located in the first portion of the duodenum or the stomach. The anterior wall of the duodenum is a more common location than the posterior wall, while benign gastric ulcers are most commonly located on the lesser curvature. The location of the ulcer, however, does not differentiate a benign ulcer from a malignant ulcer. Most benign ulcers are less than 2 cm in diameter, but they can be large. Most malignant ulcers are large, but they too can be less than 2 cm in diameter. Therefore, size can not be used to tell a benign ulcer from a malignant ulcer. Also both benign and malignant ulcers can erode through the wall of the stomach and perforate into the peritoneal cavity.

Histologically the surface of a benign ulcer shows acute inflammation and necrotic fibrinoid debris, while the base has active granulation tissue overlying a fibrous scar. Grossly, the floor of the ulcer is smooth. The gastric epithelium adjacent to the benign ulcer is reactive and is characterized by numerous mitoses and epithelial cells with prominent nucleoli. Malignant ulcers obviously have malignant cells infiltrating at the margins of the ulcer. Additionally, *H. pylori* may be seen with either type of ulcer, and its presence is not diagnostic for the type of ulcer. It is also found in 20% of the general population.

279. The answer is e. (*Kumar, pp 793, 822–826, 1017–1018, 1145–1146. Rubin, pp 696–699.*) "Signet ring cell" carcinoma is a morphologic variant of adenocarcinoma that most often originate from the stomach. In these tumors, intracellular mucin vacuoles (which stain positively with a mucin stain) coalesce and distend the cytoplasm of tumor cells. This compresses the nucleus toward the edge of the cell and creates a signet ring appearance. Tumors of this type are usually deeply invasive and fall into the category of advanced gastric carcinoma. There is often a striking desmoplasia with thickening and rigidity of the gastric wall, which may result in the so-called linitis plastica ("leather bottle") appearance. Advanced gastric carcinoma is usually located in the pyloroantrum, and the prognosis is poor, with 5-year survival of only 5 to 15%.

Colloid (mucinous) carcinoma of the breast also has malignant cells that secrete mucin, but the mucin is found extracellular and not within the cytoplasm. A mucoepidermoid carcinoma of the parotid gland may have intracytoplasmic mucus-filled vacuoles, but they do not have a "signet ring cell" appearance, and additionally there are areas within the tumor that have squamous features. Finally, the cytoplasm of the clear cell carcinoma of the kidney is clear because of cytoplasmic glycogen and lipids and not mucin.

280. The answer is b. (*Feldman, pp 666, 847. Berman, 578–582.*) Gastrointestinal stromal tumors (GIST) are mesenchymal tumors of the GI tract that are lumped together because of a common histologic finding of spindle-shaped tumor cells. Seventy percent of GIST occur in the stomach, most of these behaving in a benign fashion, and 30% occur in the small intestines, most of these behaving in a malignant fashion. GIST have abnormalities of KIT gene. Therapy for this type of tumor is with the tyrosine kinase inhibitor Glivec (formerly known as STI571), which is also used to treat chronic myelocytic leukemia (CML). GIST stain positively with CD117 (the KIT protein) and negatively with desmin and S-100. Spindle cell tumors that are negative for CD117 and positive for desmin are leiomyomas, which are also found in the wall of the stomach.

In contrast, MALTomas, lymphomas of mucosa-associated lymphoid tissue, are indolent B-cell lymphomas that are forms of marginal zone lymphomas. They typically involve sites outside of lymph nodes, such as the gastrointestinal tract, thyroid gland, breast, skin, or lungs. Finally, chemodectomas are benign, chromaffin-negative tumors of the chemoreceptor system. Common locations are the neck (carotid body tumor) and the inner ear (glomus jugulare tumor).

281. The answer is e. (*Cotran, pp 804–805. Rubin, pp 703–704.*) The presence of a Meckel's diverticulum should be suspected in an infant or child who presents with significant painless rectal bleeding. This type of diverticulum occurs in the ileum, usually within 30 cm of the ileocecal valve, and is present in approximately 2% of normal persons. It results from failure of the vitelline duct to close and is found on the antimesenteric border of the intestine. Heterotopic gastric or pancreatic tissue may be present in about one-half of cases. Peptic ulceration, which occurs as a result of acid secretion by heterotopic gastric mucosa, may occur in the adjacent ileum. Complications include perforation, ulceration, intestinal obstruction, intussusception, and neoplasms, including carcinoid tumors.

In contrast, failure of the intestinal loop to retract back into the abdomen can be seen with gastroschisis, which is a disorder that results from a congenital defect in the anterior abdominal wall. There is protrusion of the intestines outside of the abdomen. Failure of the midgut to rotate during embryogenesis can lead to intestinal malrotation, which can lead to abnormal twisting of the intestines. This can obstruct the intestinal blood supply and can cause gangrene. Finally, incomplete attenuation of the urachus (which normally forms the median umbilical ligament in the adult) can lead to formation of a urachal cyst, urachal sinus, or urachal fistula. Urachal sinuses and fistulas can leak urine at the site of the umbilicus.

282. The answer is d. (*Cotran, pp 825–826. Rubin, p 717.*) Intussusception refers to a condition in which one portion of the GI tract is pulled into the lumen of an adjoining portion of the GI tract. The most common location for this is the terminal ileum, and there are two types of patients who are most at risk, namely weaning infants and adults with a polypoid mass. It is thought that in weaning infants, exposure to new antigens causes hypertrophy of the lymphoid follicles in the terminal ileum and this may result in intussusception. Intussusception produces a classic triad of signs that includes sudden colicky abdominal pain, abdominal distention, and a "currant jelly" stool due to the vascular compromise produced by pulling of the mesentery.

In contrast, the combination of fever, leukocytosis, and right lower quadrant abdominal pain is suggestive of acute appendicitis, while fever, leukocytosis, and left lower quadrant abdominal pain is suggestive of acute diverticulitis. Finally, a volvulus, which is a "twisting" of the intestines, also produces acute abdominal pain, inability to pass flatus, and a markedly distended abdomen, but it usually occurs in the sigmoid colon of the elderly due to redundant mesentery. A barium study may show a "bird beak" sign.

283. The answer is e. (*Kumar, pp 832–833. Behrman, pp 1081–1083. Rubin, p 365.*) Rotavirus is a major cause of diarrhea in children between the ages of 6 and 24 months. Clinical symptoms consisting of vomiting and watery (secretory) diarrhea begin about 2 days after exposure. Usually rotavirus infection is self-limited, but fluid loss from the secretory diarrhea can be dramatic, and severe dehydration is the most common complication. Indeed, death from dehydration can occur, particularly in developing countries. Still, rotavirus may cause as many as 100 deaths annually in the United States.

In contrast to rotavirus, aplastic anemia in children with chronic hemolytic anemias can result from infection with parvovirus. Intestinal obstruction can result from infection by ascariasis (human roundworm), while iron deficiency can result from blood loss by infection with hookworms, and megaloblastic anemia from infection with the fish tapeworm D. latum.

284. The answer is b. (Kumar, pp 843–844. Rubin, pp 712–714.) Celiac disease, or gluten-sensitive enteropathy, is an inflammatory condition of the small intestinal mucosa related to dietary gluten. It is more common in females and shows familial clustering. It is associated with the presence of antigliadin (IgG or IgA) antibodies and endomysial (IgA) antibodies, the latter being a very good predictive laboratory test. Histologically it is characterized by villus atrophy with hyperplasia of underlying crypts and increased mitotic activity. The surface epithelium shows disarray of the columnar epithelial cells and increased intraepithelial lymphocytes. There is a chronic inflammatory infiltrate in the lamina propria. Definitive diagnosis in patients with these features on biopsy depends on response to a gluten-free diet and subsequent gluten challenge.

In contrast, daily skin exposure to light of 440 to 470 nm is used to treat infants with elevated serum bilirubin levels, while surgical resection of an aganglionic segment of colon is the treatment for Hirschsprung's disease, and triple antibiotic therapy with metronidazole, bismuth salicylate, and tetracycline is one antibiotic treatment for infection with H. pylori. Finally, dietary supplementation with megadoses of vitamin C has uncertain medical benefit.

285. The answer is e. (Kumar, pp 844–845. Rubin, pp 711–717.) The causes of malabsorption are vast, but in a few cases biopsy specimens of the small intestine may provide clues to a specific diagnosis. Whipple's disease is a systemic disease associated with malabsorption, fever, skin pigmentation, lymphadenopathy, and arthritis. Biopsy of the small intestine typically reveals the lamina propria to be infiltrated by numerous PAS-positive macrophages that contain glycoprotein and rod-shaped bacteria. The organism, Tropheryma whippelii, is a gram-positive actinomycete. The disease responds promptly to broad-spectrum antibiotic therapy. Abetalipo-proteinemia is a genetic defect in the synthesis of apolipoprotein B that leads to an inability to synthesize prebetalipoproteins (VLDLs), beta-lipoproteins (LDLs), and chylomicrons. These individuals have no chylomicrons, VLDLs, or LDLs in their blood. A biopsy of the small intestine reveals the mucosal absorptive cells to be vacuolated by lipid (triglyceride) inclusions, and peripheral smear reveals numerous acanthocytes, which are red blood cells that have numerous irregular spikes on their cell surface. The symptoms of malabsorption may be partially reversed by ingestion of medium-chain triglycerides rather than long-chain triglycerides because these medium-chain triglycerides are absorbed directly into the portal system and are not incorporated into lipoproteins. Tropical and nontropical (celiac) sprue are both characterized by shortened to absent villi in the small intestines (atrophy). Celiac sprue is a disease of malabsorption related to a sensitivity to gluten, which is found in wheat, oats, barley, and rye. This disease is related to HLA-B8 and to previous infection with type 12 adenovirus. These patients respond to removal of gluten from their diet. Tropical sprue is an acquired disease found in tropical areas, such as the Caribbean, the Far East, and India. It is the result of a chronic bacterial infection. Granulomas in mucosa and submucosa of an intestinal biopsy, if infectious causes have been excluded, are highly suggestive of Crohn's disease. Fibrosis of the lamina propria and submucosa may be seen in patients with systemic sclerosis. Bacterial overgrowth, a result of numerous causes such as the blind loop syndrome, strictures, achlorhydria, or immune deficiencies, may also cause malabsorption. Treatment is with appropriate antibiotics.

286. The answer is a. (*Kumar, pp 846–851. Rubin, pp 727–734.*) The term inflammatory bowel disease (IBD) is used to describe two idiopathic disorders that have many similar features, Crohn's disease and ulcerative colitis. Histologically, both of these diseases produce distorted crypt architecture with crypt destruction and loss. These abnormalities of the colonic crypts help to differentiate IBD from infectious colitis. Both Crohn's disease and ulcerative colitis produce acute and chronic inflammation of the colonic mucosa. Lymphocytes and plasma cells are increased in number in the lamina propria. Neutrophils may be seen within the colonic epithelium and, if present within the lumens of the crypts, may produce crypt abscesses. This latter change, however, is more commonly associated with ulcerative colitis.

One important way to differentiate between these two inflammatory bowel diseases is the location of involved colon. Crohn's disease may affect any portion of the GI tract, but most commonly there is involvement of the terminal ileum (regional enteritis) or the proximal portion (right side) of the colon. GI involvement is segmental with skip areas. In contrast, almost all cases of ulcerative colitis involve the rectum, and involvement extends proximally (left side) without skip lesions (diffuse involvement). This involvement causes the mucosa to bleed and forms large areas of mucosal ulceration.

In contrast to IBD, dilated submucosal blood vessels with focal thrombosis describes the histologic appearance of thrombosed hemorrhoids, while increased thickness of the subepithelial collagen layer is characteristic of collagenous colitis. Patients with collagenous colitis are usually middle-aged women who present with a chronic watery diarrhea. Related to collagenous colitis is the additional histologic finding of numerous lymphocytes, this condition being called lymphocytic colitis. Eosinophilic colitis refers to the histologic finding of numerous eosinophils in the mucosa of the colon. Some of these cases are idiopathic and the patients may be asymptomatic, but some cases are associated with diseases which cause eosinophilia, such as parasites.

287. The answer is e. (*Kumar, pp 846–851. Rubin, pp 727–734.*) The two inflammatory bowel diseases (IBDs), Crohn's disease (CD) and ulcerative colitis (UC), are both chronic, relapsing inflammatory disorders of unknown etiology. They both may show very similar morphologic features and associations, such as mucosal inflammation, malignant transformation, and extragastrointestinal manifestations that include erythema nodosum (especially ulcerative colitis), arthritis, uveitis, pericholangitis (especially with ulcerative colitis, in which sclerosing pericholangitis may produce obstructive jaundice), and ankylosing spondylitis. CD is classically described as being a granulomatous disease, but granulomas are present in only 25 to 75% of cases. Therefore, the absence of granulomas does not rule out the diagnosis of CD. CD may involve any portion of the gastrointestinal tract and is characterized by focal (segmental) involvement with "skip lesions." Involvement of the intestines by CD is typically transmural inflammation, which leads to the formation of fistulas and sinuses. The deep inflammation produces deep longitudinal, serpiginous ulcers, which impart a "cobblestone" appearance to the mucosal surface of the colon. Additionally in Crohn's disease, the mesenteric fat wraps around the bowel surface, producing what is called "creeping fat," and the thickened wall narrows the lumen, producing a characteristic "string sign" on x-ray. This narrowing of the colon, which may produce intestinal obstruction, is grossly described as a "lead pipe" or "garden hose" colon. In contrast to CD, UC affects only the colon, and the disease involvement is continuous. The rectum is involved in all cases, and the inflammation extends proximally. Because UC involves the mucosa and submucosa, but not the wall, fistula formation and wall thickening are absent (but toxic megacolon may occur). Grossly, the mucosa displays diffuse hyperemia with numerous superficial ulcerations. The regenerating, nonulcerated mucosa appears as "pseudopolyps."

288. The answer is c. (*Kumar, pp 854–855. Rubin, pp 725–727.*) One of the most common abnormalities of the colon seen in older patients is diverticulosis (multiple outpouchings of the mucosa into and through the muscular wall). Sometimes GI diverticula are classified as being either true diverticula or false diverticula. True diverticula have all layers of the intestine in the diverticulum, an example being Meckel's diverticulum, while false diverticulum lack the muscle layer, an example being the usual type of colonic diverticula seen in older patients. These false colonic diverticula are found in the sigmoid region (the left side) in a double vertical row along the antimesenteric taenia coli. They are thought to be the result of decreased dietary fiber that increases intraluminal pressure. Most diverticula are asymptomatic, but they may cause rectal bleeding or they may become inflamed, somewhat analogously to inflammation of the appendix (associated with fever, leukocytosis, and right-sided abdominal pain). Patients with inflamed diverticula (diverticulitis) present with fever, peripheral leukocytosis, and left-sided abdominal pain (left-sided appendicitis).

In contrast, angiodysplasia refers to dilated tortuous vessels (vascular ectasia) usually of the right side of the colon in elderly individuals. Angiodysplasia may produce lower GI bleeding (and hence iron-deficiency anemia) and may be seen with radiographic examination. Hemorrhoids are dilations of the anal and perianal venous plexi. External hemorrhoids involve the inferior hemorrhoidal plexus, internal hemorrhoids the superior hemorrhoidal plexus. Thrombosis of external hemorrhoid can produce acute constant anal pain that is worse with defecation with a tense purple mass in anal verge. Finally intussusception refers to "telescoping" of one portion of the GI tract into the lumen of an adjoining portion of the GI tract.

289. The answer is a. (*Kumar, pp 856–857, 866–868. Rubin, pp 720–721.*) The patient shows signs of the carcinoid syndrome, which include flushing, diarrhea, and bronchoconstriction. The syndrome results from elaboration of serotonin (5-hydroxytryptamine) by a primary carcinoid tumor in the lungs or ovary or from hepatic metastases from a primary carcinoid tumor in the gastrointestinal tract. However, primary appendiceal carcinoid tumors, the most common gastrointestinal carcinoid tumors, very rarely metastasize and are virtually always asymptomatic. Carcinoid tumors arise from cells of the neuroendocrine system, which, as part of the amine precursor uptake and decarboxylation (APUD) system, are capable of secreting many products. Grossly, carcinoid tumors, which tend to be multiple when they occur in the stomach or intestines, are characteristically solid and firm and have a yellow-tan appearance on sectioning. Histologically they are composed of nests of relatively bland-appearing monotonous cells. Diagnosis is based on finding increased urinary 5-hydroxyindoleacetic acid (5-HIAA) excretion from metabolism of excess serotonin. In contrast, increased urinary levels of aminolevulinic acid (ALA) are seen with lead toxicity, increased N-formiminoglutamate (FIGlu) with folate deficiency, and increased normetanephrine or vanillylmandelic acid (VMA) with tumors of the adrenal medulla (pheochromocytoma in adults and neuroblastoma in children).

290. The answer is a. (*Kumar, pp 857–861. Rubin, pp 736–742.*) Colonic polyps are either nonneoplastic, which have no malignant potential, or neoplastic, which are precursors of cancer. Most colon polyps are nonneoplastic and are the result of abnormal maturation or inflammation. Hyperplastic polyps histologically have a serrated "saw tooth" appearance, while grossly they tend to be small and have a "dewdrop" appearance. These polyps are thought to be an aging change and are not associated with malignant transformation. Inflammatory polyps or pseudopolyps may be formed by inflamed regenerating epithelium, as seen with Crohn's disease or ulcerative colitis. Juvenile (retention) polyps contain abundant stroma and dilated glands filled with mucus, while lymphoid polyps contain intramucosal lymphoid tissue. Hamartomatous polyps are similar to juvenile polyps, but they also contain smooth muscle. An interesting fact about juvenile polyps, which are typically found in children or young adults, is that they are prone to self-amputation, and patients may find them floating in the toilet (which can be disturbing for the patient).

In contrast to the nonneoplastic polyps, neoplastic polyps arise from proliferative, dysplastic epithelium, which is characterized by stratification of cells having plump, elongated nuclei. As a group these dysplastic polyps are called adenomatous polyps. Based on their architecture, they are further classified as either tubular adenomas, villous adenomas, or mixed tubulovillous adenomas. The risk for malignancy is dependent on the size of the polyp and the type and the amount of dysplasia present. The risk for developing a malignancy is greater for large villous polyps that have severe dysplasia.

291. The answer is a. (*Kumar, pp 859, 861–862. Rubin, pp 740–741.*) Although most colonic polyps occur sporadically, there are several conditions in which colonic polyposis is familial and sometimes associated with extraintestinal abnormalities. Cowden (multiple hamartoma) syndrome is an autosomal dominant disorder that results from a germ line mutation of the PTEN (phosphatase and tensin homolog) gene and is characterized by the formation of intestinal hamartomas, facial trichilemmomas, acral keratoses, and oral papillomas. Although the intestinal hamartomas are not premalignant, this syndrome is associated with an increased risk for the development of thyroid and breast cancers.

Gardner's syndrome is an autosomal recessive disorder characterized by the association of colonic polyposis with multiple osteomas, fibromatosis, and cutaneous cysts. Some people think that Gardner's syndrome is a variant of familial polyposis coli (FAP). This disorder, which is usually transmitted as an autosomal dominant condition, results from a genetic defect involving the APC gene on chromosome 5q21. FAP is characterized by the formation of multiple adenomatous colonic polyps, with a minimum of 100 polyps necessary for diagnosis. As with sporadic adenomatous polyps, there is a risk of malignancy, and this increases to 100% within 30 years of diagnosis. Panproctocolectomy is therefore usually recommended.

The Peutz-Jeghers syndrome is characterized by hamartomatous polyps of the small intestine, oral pigmentation, and a slightly increased risk for carcinoma especially of extracolonic sites, such as the ovary, while Turcot's syndrome refers to the association of colonic polyposis with central nervous system tumors.

292. The answer is c. (*Kumar, pp 862–868. Rubin, pp 742–746.*) Colon cancer is a frequent type of cancer in adults of the United States. It may be found in the left side of the colon (producing a "napkin ring" or "apple core" appearance) or the right side of the colon (producing a polypoid mass). In either location, chronic bleeding may produce heme-positive stools and an iron-deficiency (hypochromic-microcytic) anemia. Histologically, the vast majority of colon cancers are adenocarcinomas.

It is now thought that there are two pathways that lead to the development of colon cancer: the APC/beta-caterin pathway and the microsatellite instability pathway. The former pathway involves the development of cancer from pre-existing adenomas and is called the adenoma-carcinoma sequence, while the latter pathway is not associated with pre-existing adenomas and instead is characterized by genetic lesions in DNA mismatch repair genes. This second pathway is associated with the hereditary nonpolyposis colon carcinoma (HNPCC) syndrome, which is an autosomal dominant familial syndrome (Lynch syndrome) that is characterized by an increased risk of colorectal cancer (often multiple). Lynch syndrome type I is associated with colorectal carcinoma only (predominately of the right side), while Lynch syndrome type II is associated with extraintestinal cancer, particularly of the endometrium. The HNPCC syndrome is associated with germ-line mutations involving any of the five genes that are involved in DNA repair, but the majority of mutations involve either the MSH2 or MLH1 genes. In contrast, the APC/beta-caterin pathway involves the following genes: APC (adenomatous polyposis coli) gene, which regulates levels of beta-catenin, K-RAS, SMAD, p53, and many other genes.

293. The answer is b. (*Kumar, pp 870–872. Rubin, pp 748–749.*) Acute appendicitis, a disease found predominantly in adolescents and young adults, is characterized histologically by acute inflammatory cells (neutrophils) within the mucosa and muscular wall. Clinically, acute appendicitis causes right lower quadrant pain, nausea, vomiting, a mild fever, and a leukocytosis in the peripheral blood. These symptoms may not occur in the very young or the elderly. The inflamed appendiceal wall may become gangrenous and perforate in 24 to 48 h. Even with classic symptoms, the appendix may be histologically unremarkable in up to 20% of the cases. False-positive diagnoses are to be preferred to the possible severe or fatal complications of a false-negative diagnosis of acute appendicitis that results in rupture. Lymphoid hyperplasia with multinucleated giant cells (Warthin-Finkeldey giant cells) is characteristic of measles (rubeola). These changes can be found in the appendix, but this is quite rare. Dilation of the lumen of the appendix, called a mucocele, may be caused by mucosal hyperplasia, a benign cystadenoma, or a malignant mucinous cystadenocarcinoma. If the latter tumor ruptures, it may seed the entire peritoneal cavity, causing the condition called pseudomyxoma peritonei. The most common tumor of the appendix is the carcinoid tumor. Grossly it is yellow in color and is typically located at the tip of the appendix. Histologically, carcinoids are composed of nests or islands of monotonous cells. Appendiceal carcinoids rarely metastasize.

294. The answer is a. (*Kumar, pp 25–26, 880–881.*) The type and distribution of necrotic hepatocytes is often a clue as to the cause of the hepatic injury. Focal scattered necrosis is characteristic of viral hepatitis, but may also be seen with bacterial infections or other toxic insults. In focal necrosis, there is necrosis of single hepatocytes, or small clusters of hepatocytes, that is randomly located in some, but not all, of the liver lobules. In contrast, zonal necrosis refers to the finding of hepatocellular necrosis in identical areas in all of the liver lobules. There are basically three types of zonal necrosis. Centrilobular (acinar zone 3) necrosis is characteristic of ischemic injury (heart failure or shock), toxic effects (acetaminophen toxicity), carbon tetrachloride exposure, or chloroform ingestion. Drugs such as acetaminophen may be metabolized in zone 1 to toxic compounds that cause necrosis of zone 3 hepatocytes because they receive the blood from zone 1. Midzonal (zone 2) necrosis is quite rare, but may be seen in yellow fever, while periportal (zone 1) necrosis is seen in phosphorus poisoning or eclampsia. Submassive necrosis refers to liver cell necrosis that crosses the normal lobular boundaries. Classically the necrosis goes from portal areas to central veins (or vice versa) and is called bridging necrosis. If the hepatocellular necrosis is severe, it is called massive necrosis. This type of extensive necrosis is described as acute yellow atrophy, because grossly the liver appears soft, yellow, flabby, and decreased in size with a wrinkled capsule. It may be produced by hepatitis viruses (usually B or C), drugs, or chemicals.

295. The answer is b. (*Kumar, pp 881–882, 885–888. Kumar, pp 848–851. Henry, pp 264–266.*) Jaundice is caused by increased blood levels of bilirubin, which results from abnormalities in bilirubin metabolism. Bilirubin, the end product of heme breakdown, is taken up by the liver, where it is conjugated with glucuronic acid by the enzyme bilirubin UDP-glucuronosyl transferase (UGT) and then secreted into the bile. Unconjugated bilirubin is not soluble in an aqueous solution, is complexed to albumin, and cannot be excreted in the urine. Unconjugated hyperbilirubinemia may result from excessive production of bilirubin, which occurs with hemolytic anemias (acute intravascular hemolysis also produces hemoglobinemia, hemoglobinuria and decreased levels of haptoglobin.). Unconjugated hyperbilirubinemia can also result from reduced hepatic uptake of bilirubin, as occurs in Gilbert's syndrome, a mild disease associated with a subclinical hyperbilirubinemia. Unconjugated hyperbilirubinemia may result from impaired conjugation of bilirubin. Examples of diseases resulting from impaired conjugation include physiologic jaundice of the newborn and Crigler-Najjar syndrome, which result from either decreased UGT activity (type II) or absent UGT activity (type I). Individuals with type II Crigler-Najjar syndrome may not need any therapy, or their condition may be managed with phenobarbital, which is metabolized in the smooth endoplasmic reticulum in hepatocytes. Therapy with this drug causes hyperplasia of the smooth endoplasmic reticulum in hepatocytes and indirectly increases the levels of bilirubin-UDP-glucuronyl transferase.

In contrast, a defective urea cycle, which results in hyperammonemia, and a foul-smelling breath (fetor hepaticus) are both signs of liver failure. Fetor hepaticus is thought to occur due to volatile, sulfur-containing mercaptans being produced in the gut. Despite various underlying causes, the clinical features of all types of liver failure are similar. If liver cell necrosis is present, serum hepatic enzymes, such as LDH, ALT, and AST, will be increased. Additionally, deranged bilirubin metabolism results in jaundice (mainly conjugated hyperbilirubinemia), while a decreased synthesis of albumin (hypoalbuminemia) results in ascites. Symptoms of hepatic encephalopathy, a metabolic disorder of the neuromuscular system, include stupor, hyperreflexia, and asterixis (a peculiar flapping tremor of the hands). Finally, impaired estrogen metabolism in males can result in gynecomastia, testicular atrophy, palmar erythema, and spider angiomas of the skin.

296. The answer is b. (*Goldman, p 899. Kumar, pp 887–888. Rubin, p 766.*) Breast milk jaundice is a cause of neonatal jaundice that begins between days 4 and 7 of life. In contrast, physiologic jaundice of the newborn refers to mild elevation of the serum bilirubin levels that begins on days 2 to 4 of life. This abnormality is generally the result of decreased levels of bilirubin UDP-glucuronosyl transferase (UGT), while breast milk jaundice may be due to hormones in breast milk (possibly beta-glucuronidases) that inhibit UGT. It is important to clinically differentiate breast milk jaundice from physiologic jaundice of the newborn in order to predict the length of the hyperbilirubinemia. The elevated indirect bilirubin with breast milk jaundice persists longer (up to 6 weeks) than physiologic jaundice (usually less than 2 weeks). Also note that breast milk jaundice is different from breast-feeding jaundice, which occurs before first 4 to 7 days of life and is caused by insufficient breast milk (decreased plasma volume).

With these abnormalities the increased serum bilirubin is mainly unconjugated (indirect) bilirubin. In full-term infants, the maximum bilirubin levels are less than 6 mg/dL (normal is less than 2 mg/dL). It is important to realize that in newborns the blood-brain barrier is not fully developed and unconjugated bilirubin may be deposited in the brain, particularly in the lipid-rich basal ganglia, producing severe neurologic abnormalities. Grossly the brain has a bright yellow pigmentation that is called kernicterus. Note that kernicterus does not result unless serum bilirubin levels are greater than 20 mg/dL. Treatment, if needed, consists of exposing the skin to light (440 to 470 nm), which activates oxygen and converts bilirubin to photobilirubin. This substance is hydrophilic and can be excreted in the urine.

Finally, with hemolytic disease of the newborn serum hemoglobin levels are decreased, while inspissated bile syndrome, which can contribute to jaundice, is seen in neonates with sepsis in which thick bile can cause obstruction.

297. The answer is e. (*Kumar, pp 885–890, 910–911. Chandrasoma, pp 636–637.*) In contrast to unconjugated bilirubin, conjugated bilirubin is water-soluble, nontoxic, and readily excreted in the urine. Conjugated hyperbilirubinemia may result from either decreased hepatic excretion of conjugates of bilirubin, such as in Dubin-Johnson syndrome (DJS), or impaired extrahepatic bile excretion, as occurs with extrahepatic biliary obstruction. DJS is an autosomal recessive disorder that results from mutations involving the multidrug resistance protein 2 (MRP2), which is also called the human canalicular organic anion transporter (cMOAT) protein. This results in defective excretion of bilirubin glucuronide and other organic anions from hepatocytes. The diagnosis of DJS can be made by finding the urine ratio of coproporphyrin I to coproporphyrin III to be increased. Normally coproporphyrin I is excreted in the bile, while coproporphyrin III is excreted in the urine, but with DJS coproporphyrin I is not excreted normally into the bile. With DJS the liver is grossly black and pigmented cytoplasmic globules are found in hepatocytes. Rotor's syndrome is similar to Dubin-Johnson syndrome but the liver is not black grossly; and the liver histology is normal.

In contrast, decreased synthesis of albumin and gamma-glutamyl transpeptidase can be seen with liver failure; DJS is not associated with liver failure. Decreased (not increased) excretion of copper into the bile is seen with Wilson's disease, while a deficiency of carnitine can be seen with inherited defects of fatty acid beta-oxidation.

298. The answer is d. (*Kumar, pp 917–920. Rubin, pp 809–810.*) Abnormalities of the hepatic blood flow occur in various disease states and result in characteristic symptoms. Because of their dual blood supply, arterial occlusion of either the hepatic artery or the portal vein rarely results in liver infarcts. However, thrombosis of branches of the hepatic artery may result in a pale (anemic) infarct, or possibly a hemorrhagic infarct due to blood flow from the portal vein. In contrast, occlusion of the portal vein, which may be caused by cirrhosis or malignancy, may result in a wedge-shaped red area called an infarct of Zahn. This is a misnomer, however, because it is not really an infarction but instead is the result of focal sinusoidal congestion. Hepatic vein thrombosis (Budd-Chiari syndrome) is associated with polycythemia vera, pregnancy, and oral contraceptives. Clinically, Budd-Chiari syndrome is characterized by the sudden onset of severe right upper quadrant abdominal pain, ascites, tender hepatomegaly, and hematemesis. Occlusion of the central veins, called veno-occlusive disease, may be rarely seen in Jamaican drinkers of alkaloid-containing bush tea, but is much more commonly found following bone marrow transplantation (up to 25% of allogenic marrow transplants).

299. The answer is d. (*Kumar, pp 897–898. Chandrasoma, pp 643–645.*) Several clinical syndromes may develop after exposure to any of the viruses that cause hepatitis, including asymptomatic hepatitis, acute hepatitis, fulminant hepatitis, chronic hepatitis, and the carrier state. Asymptomatic infection in individuals is documented by serologic abnormalities only. Liver biopsies in patients with acute hepatitis, either the anicteric phase or the icteric phase, reveal focal necrosis of hepatocytes (forming Councilman's bodies) and lobular disarray resulting from ballooning degeneration of the hepatocytes. These changes are nonspecific, but the additional finding of fatty change is suggestive of hepatitis C virus (HCV) infection. Clinically, acute viral hepatitis is classified into three phases. During the prodrome phase, patients may develop symptoms that include anorexia, nausea and vomiting, headaches, photophobia, and myalgia. An unusual symptom associated with acute viral hepatitis is altered olfaction and taste, especially the loss of taste for coffee and cigarettes. The next phase, the icteric phase, involves jaundice produced by increased bilirubin. Patients may also develop light stools and dark urine (due to disrupted bile flow) and ecchymoses (due to decreased vitamin K). The final phase is the convalescence phase. Fulminant hepatitis refers to massive necrosis and is seen in about 1% of patients with either hepatitis B or C, but very rarely with hepatitis A infection. The biggest risk for fulminant hepatitis is coinfection with both hepatitis B and D. Chronic hepatitis is defined as elevated serum liver enzymes for longer than 6 months. Patients may be either symptomatic or asymptomatic.

300. The answer is d. (*Kumar, pp 890–891. Chandrasoma, pp 641–643.*) Several types of viruses are implicated as being causative agents of viral hepatitis. Each of these has unique characteristics. Hepatitis A virus, an RNA picornavirus, is transmitted through the fecal-oral route (including shellfish) and is called infectious hepatitis. It is associated with small outbreaks of hepatitis in the United States, especially among young children at day care centers. Hepatitis B virus, which causes "serum hepatitis," is associated with the development of a serum sickness-like syndrome in about 10% of patients. Immune complexes of antibody and HBsAg are present in patients with vasculitis. Hepatitis C virus is characterized by episodic elevations in serum transaminases and also by fatty change in liver biopsy specimens. Hepatitis D virus is distinct in that it is a defective virus and needs HBsAg to be infective. Hepatitis E virus is characterized by waterborne transmission. It is found in underdeveloped countries and has an unusually high mortality in pregnant females. It is important to remember that the liver may be infected by other viruses, such as yellow fever virus, Epstein-Barr virus (EBV, the causative agent of infectious mononucleosis), CMV, and/or herpes virus. The latter is characterized histologically by intranuclear eosinophilic inclusions (Cowdry bodies) and nuclei that have a ground-glass appearance.

301. The answer is d. (*Kumar, pp 891–894. Rubin, pp 774–777.*) Hepatitis B virus (HBV) is a member of the DNA-containing hepadnaviruses. The mature HBV virion is called the Dane particle. Products of the HBV genome include the nucleocapsid [hepatitis B core antigen (HBcAg)], envelope glycoprotein [hepatitis B surface antigen (HBsAg)], and DNA polymerase. After exposure to HBV, there is a relatively long asymptomatic incubation period, averaging 6 to 8 weeks, followed by an acute disease lasting several weeks to months. HBsAg is the first antigen to appear in the blood. It appears before symptoms begin, peaks during overt disease, and declines to undetectable levels in 3 to 6 months. HBeAg, HBV-DNA, and DNA polymerase appear soon after HBsAg. HBeAg peaks during acute disease and disappears before HBsAg is cleared. The presence of either HBsAg or HBeAg without antibodies to either is seen early in hepatitis B infection. Anti-HBsAg appears at about the time of the disappearance of HBsAg and indicates complete recovery. Anti-HBc first appears much earlier, shortly after the appearance of HBsAg, and levels remain elevated for life. Its presence indicates previous HBV infection, but not necessarily that the hepatitis infection has been cleared. Persistence of HBeAg is an important indicator of continued viral replication with probable progression to chronic hepatitis. With normal recovery from hepatitis B, both HBsAg and HBeAg are absent from the blood, while anti-HBs and anti-HBc are present. If anti-HBs is never produced, then HBsAg may not be cleared. In this case, the patient may remove the HBeAg and be an asymptomatic carrier, or the HBeAg may persist and the patient could be a chronic carrier who has progressed to chronic active hepatitis. In both of these conditions, anti-HBc is still present.

302. The answer is b. (*Kumar, pp 898–899. Goldman, 791–793.*) Chronic hepatitis has been defined clinically as an inflammatory process of the liver that lasts longer than 6 months. The diagnosis and classification of chronic hepatitis has changed somewhat over the past several years. Previously chronic hepatitis was classified histologically into chronic active hepatitis and chronic persistent hepatitis. In chronic active hepatitis, an intense inflammatory reaction with numerous plasma cells spreads from portal tracts into periportal areas. The reaction destroys the limiting plate and causes necrosis of the hepatocytes surrounding the portal triad. This histologic change is called "piecemeal necrosis" or "interface hepatitis." Chronic persistent hepatitis was differentiated from chronic active hepatitis by the fact that the portal inflammation did not extend into the periportal areas; that is, there was no piecemeal necrosis.

Today chronic hepatitis is given a histologic grade, which is based on the inflammation activity present, and a histologic stage, which is based on the amount of fibrosis present. A histologic grade of 0 is characterized by minimal portal inflammation and no changes in the hepatic lobule, while a grade of 4 is characterized by severe limiting plate destruction with bridging necrosis. Mild to moderate piecemeal necrosis is seen with inflammatory activity grades 2 and 3. Stage 0 fibrosis is characterized by minimal to no fibrosis, while stage 4 fibrosis is characterized by cirrhosis.

In contrast to destruction of the limiting plate, Congo red–positive extracellular deposits surrounding hepatocytes are diagnostic for amyloidosis; fibrosis around central hepatic veins suggests alcoholic liver disease; and apoptosis of hepatocytes suggests viral hepatitis.

303. The answer is c. (*Kumar, pp 890–897. Rubin, pp 779–781.*) The hepatitis viruses are responsible for most cases of chronic hepatitis, but the chance of developing chronic hepatitis varies considerably depending on which type of hepatitis virus is the infecting agent. Neither hepatitis A nor hepatitis E virus infection is associated with the development of chronic hepatitis, but chronic hepatitis develops in about 50% of patients with hepatitis C. This high incidence of developing chronic hepatitis, along with episodic elevations in serum transaminases, which result from repeated bouts of hepatic damage, fatty change in liver biopsy specimens, and persistent infection are all characteristics of hepatitis C. These clinical hallmarks are thought to result from the fact that the hepatitis C RNA polymerase (NS5B) is quite unstable and gives rise to multiple genotypes and subtypes. That is, within a single individual there can be several dozen mutant strains that developed from the original strain that infected the person. In addition, the E2 protein of the envelope of hepatitis C is the most variable region of the entire viral genome. This variability allows the virus to escape from anti-HCV antibodies and allows the emergence of new mutated strains that can cause repeated bouts of hepatic damage and lead to chronic infection.

In contrast, about 5% of adults infected with hepatitis B develop chronic hepatitis, and about one-half of these patients progress to cirrhosis. Liver biopsies may reveal a characteristic "ground glass" appearance to the cytoplasm of the hepatocytes. Finally, chronic hepatitis can develop in 5% to more than 80% of individuals infected with hepatitis D. Infection with this virus occurs in one of two clinical settings. There might be acute coinfection by hepatitis D and hepatitis B, which results in chronic hepatitis in less than 5% of cases. If, instead, hepatitis D is superinfected on a chronic carrier of hepatitis B virus, then about 80% of cases progress to chronic hepatitis.

304. The answer is a. (*Kumar, p 903. Chandrasoma, pp 652–653.*) Chronic hepatitis is defined clinically by the presence of elevated serum liver enzymes for longer than 6 months. Liver biopsies in patients with chronic hepatitis may reveal inflammation that is limited to the portal areas (chronic persistent hepatitis), or the inflammation may extend into the adjacent hepatocytes. This inflammation causes necrosis of the hepatocytes (piecemeal necrosis) and is called chronic active hepatitis. These changes are nonspecific and can be seen with hepatitis B virus (HBV) or hepatitis C virus (HCV) infection. The finding of hepatocytes with ground-glass eosinophilic cytoplasm is highly suggestive of HBV infection, while fatty change (steatosis) is suggestive of HCV. A clinically distinct subtype of chronic hepatitis is called chronic autoimmune ("lupoid") hepatitis. This disease occurs in young females who have no serologic evidence of viral disease. These patients have increased IgG levels and high titers of autoantibodies, such as anti-smooth-muscle antibodies and antinuclear antibodies. They also have test positive for LE, which is the basis for the name lupoid hepatitis, but there is no relationship of this disease to systemic lupus erythematosus. The prognosis for these patients is poor, as many progress to cirrhosis.

In contrast to chronic hepatitis, two disorders that are classified as primary biliary diseases are primary biliary cirrhosis (PBC) and primary sclerosing cholangitis (PSC). Primary biliary cirrhosis is primarily a disease of middle-aged females and is characterized by pruritus, jaundice, and hypercholesterolemia. More than 90% of patients have antimitochondrial autoantibodies, particularly to mitochondrial pyruvate dehydrogenase. A characteristic lesion, called the florid duct lesion, is seen in portal areas and is composed of a marked lymphocytic infiltrate and occasional granulomas. Primary sclerosing cholangitis is characterized by fibrosing cholangitis that produces concentric "onion-skin fibrosis" in portal areas. It is associated with chronic ulcerative colitis, one type of inflammatory bowel disease.

305. The answer is c. (*Kumar, pp 903–904.*) Hepatic injury can result from a wide range of drugs, chemicals, and toxins. Peliosis hepatis is an abnormality of the hepatic blood flow that results in sinusoidal dilation and the formation of irregular blood-filled lakes, which may rupture and produce massive intraabdominal hemorrhage or hepatic failure. Peliosis hepatitis is most often associated with the use of anabolic steroids, but more rarely it may be associated with oral contraceptives. Reye's syndrome, characterized by microvesicular fatty change in the liver and encephalopathy, has been related to the use of salicylates in children with viral illnesses. Acetaminophen toxicity results in centrilobular liver necrosis, while estrogens may be related to thrombosis of the hepatic or portal veins. Several hepatic tumors are related to exposure to vinyl chloride, including angiosarcoma and hepatocellular carcinoma.

306. The answer is d. (*Kumar, pp 904–907. Chandrasoma, pp 8–10.*) Alcohol can produce hepatic steatosis via several mechanisms, such as increased fatty acid synthesis, decreased triglyceride utilization, decreased fatty acid oxidation, decreased lipoprotein excretion, and increased lipolysis. Ethanol is taken up by the liver and is converted into acetaldehyde by either alcohol dehydrogenase (the major pathway), microsomal P-450 oxidase, or peroxisomal catalase. These pathways also convert nicotinamide adenine dinucleotide (NAD) to NADH. This excess production of NADH changes the normal hepatic metabolism away from catabolism of fats and toward anabolism of fats (lipid synthesis), resulting in decreased mitochondrial oxidation of fatty acids and increased hepatic production of triglyceride. Ethanol also increases lipolysis and inhibits the release of lipoproteins. Increased lipolysis increases the amount of free fatty acids that reach the liver.

307. The answer is c. (*Fawcett, pp 657–660. Kumar, pp 882–883. Rubin, pp 796–798.*) Cirrhosis refers to fibrosis of the liver that involves both central veins and portal triads. This fibrosis is the result of liver cell necrosis and regenerative hepatic nodules. These nodules consist of hyperplastic hepatocytes with enlarged, atypical nuclei, irregular hepatic plates, and distorted vasculature. There is distortion of the normal lobular architecture. These changes diffusely involve the entire liver; they are not focal. It is thought that the fibrosis is the result of fibril-forming collagens that are released by Ito cells, which are fat-containing lipocytes found within the space of Disse of the liver. They normally participate in the metabolism and storage of vitamin A, but they can secrete collagen in the fibrotic (cirrhotic) liver. Normally types I and III collagens (interstitial types) are found in the portal areas and occasionally in the space of Disse or around central veins. In cirrhosis, types I and III collagens are deposited throughout the hepatic lobule. These Ito cells are initiated by unknown factors and then are further stimulated by such factors as platelet-derived growth factor and transforming growth factor-beta to secrete collagen.

In contrast to Ito cells, endothelial cells normally line the sinusoids and demarcate the extrasinusoidal space of Disse. Attached to the endothelial cells are the phagocytic Kupffer cells, which are part of the monocyte-phagocyte system. Bile ducts, and thus the epithelial cells that form them, are found in the portal triads of the liver.

308. The answer is b. (*Kumar, pp 907–908. Angulo, pp 1221–1231.*) Nonalcoholic fatty liver disease (NAFLD) is a type of chronic hepatitis characterized by liver damage similar to alcohol-induced liver damage except it occurs in individuals who do not abuse alcohol. Risk factors for NAFLD include diabetes mellitus, obesity, hyperlipidemia, and rapid weight loss. Patients are usually asymptomatic, but can develop fatigue, malaise, right upper quadrant abdominal discomfort, and hepatomegaly. Laboratory findings include elevated liver enzymes along with increased serum cholesterol, triglyceride, and glucose. Ultrasonography reveals a diffuse increased density that is similar in appearance to cirrhosis. Liver biopsy, which is the best diagnostic test for confirming the diagnosis, reveals macrovesicular steatosis, which refers to the accumulation of neutral lipid (triglyceride) in hepatocytes. Steatosis can be divided into two types: macrovesicular steatosis, with a single large vacuole, peripheral nucleus, and microvesicular steatosis, with many small vacuoles, central nucleus. Alcohol is the most common cause of macrovesicular steatosis, but it is also characteristic of NAFLD. Note that nonalcoholic steatohepatitis (NASH) is a subtype of NAFLD and is characterized by the combination of steatosis, inflammation, and hepatocyte ballooning and necrosis. The diagnosis of steatohepatitis can only be made with a liver biopsy.

309. The answer is d. (*Kumar, pp 889–890, 908–912. Chandrasoma, pp 655–658.*) Several quite different liver diseases result from abnormalities of metabolism. Hemochromatosis results from excessive accumulation of body iron. The disease may be primary or secondary. Primary (familial) hemochromatosis is a genetic disorder of iron metabolism that is inherited as an autosomal recessive disease. Excess iron is absorbed from the small intestines because of a mutation of the HFE gene, the product of which normally controls the small intestinal absorption of iron. The classic clinical triad for this disease consists of micronodular pigment cirrhosis, diabetes mellitus, and skin pigmentation. The combination of diabetes and skin pigmentation is called bronze diabetes. In the majority of patients, serum iron is above 250 mg/dL, serum ferritin is above 500 ng/dL, and iron (transferrin) saturation approaches 100%. In patients with primary hemochromatosis, the excess iron is deposited in the cytoplasm of parenchymal cells of many organs, including the liver and pancreas. Liver deposition of iron leads to cirrhosis, which in turn increases the risk of hepatocellular carcinoma. Iron deposition in the islets of the pancreas leads to diabetes mellitus. Iron deposition in the heart leads to congestive heart failure, which is the major cause of death in these patients. Deposition of iron in the joints leads to arthritis, while deposition in the testes leads to atrophy.

Secondary hemochromatosis, also called systemic hemosiderosis, is most common in patients with hemolytic anemias, such as thalassemia. Excess iron may also be due to an excessive number of transfusions or to increased absorption of dietary iron. In idiopathic (primary) hemochromatosis, iron accumulates in the cytoplasm of parenchymal cells, but in secondary hemochromatosis the iron is deposited in the mononuclear phagocytic system. In both conditions the iron is deposited as hemosiderin, which stains an intense blue color with Prussian blue stain. Because the iron deposition does not usually occur in the parenchymal cells in secondary hemochromatosis, there usually is no organ dysfunction or injury.

In contrast to the HFE gene, the ATP7B gene codes for a copper-transporting ATPase located on the canicular membrane of hepatocytes. The resultant defective excretion of copper into the bile is the basic abnormality of Wilson's disease, which is one of the inherited cholestatic disorders. Cystic fibrosis, which is caused by mutations of the CFTR gene, is another familial disease that can cause intrahepatic cholestasis. Finally, a group of disease referred to as progressive familial intrahepatic cholestasis (PFIC) result from mutations of genes coding for proteins located on the apical (canalicular) membrane of hepatocytes. PFIC-1, also called Byler syndrome, results from mutations involving the FIC1 gene, while PFIC-2 results from mutations involving the BSEP gene, and PFIC-3 from mutations of the MDR3 gene.

310. The answer is b. (*Kumar, pp 888, 904, 910–913. Chandrasoma, pp 655–658.*) Reye's syndrome (RS) is an acute postviral illness that is seen mainly in children. It is characterized by encephalopathy, microvesicular fatty change of the liver, and widespread mitochondrial injury. Electron microscopy (EM) reveals large budding or branching mitochondria. The mitochondrial injury results in decreased activity of the citric acid cycle and urea cycle and defective β-oxidation of fats, which then leads to the accumulation of serum fatty acids. The typical patient presents several days after a viral illness with pernicious vomiting. RS is associated with hyperammonemia, elevated serum free fatty acids, and salicylate (aspirin) ingestion.

In contrast, Wilson's disease, which is related to excess copper deposition within the liver and basal ganglia of the brain, is characterized by varying liver disease and neurologic symptoms. The liver changes vary from fatty change to jaundice to cirrhosis, while the neurologic symptoms consist of a Parkinson-like movement disorder and behavioral abnormalities. A liver biopsy may reveal steatosis, necrotic hepatocytes, or cholestasis. Increased copper can be demonstrated histologically using the rhodamine stain. Mallory's bodies, which are aggregates of cytokeratin intermediate filaments within hepatocytes, are characteristic of alcoholic liver disease, but they are not specific and can also be seen with Wilson's disease, primary biliary cirrhosis, and other disorders. Alpha1 antitrypsin deficiency causes both liver disease and lung disease, especially panacinar emphysema. Liver biopsies reveal red blobs within the cytoplasm of hepatocytes that are PAS-positive and diastase-resistant. Abundant intracytoplasmic inclusions are also present in Dubin-Johnson syndrome (DJS), but these inclusions are PAS-negative. DJS is associated with a conjugated hyperbilirubinemia that results from decreased hepatic excretion of conjugates of bilirubin.

311. The answer is a. (*Kumar, pp 926–927. Rubin, pp 795–796.*) Diseases of the biliary tract may lead to manifestations of jaundice, and, if prolonged and severe, may lead to cirrhosis. These diseases can be classified as either primary or secondary. Two primary causes of biliary cirrhosis are primary sclerosing cholangitis (PSC) and primary biliary cirrhosis (PBC). PSC is characterized histologically by fibrosing cholangitis that produces concentric "onion-skin" fibrosis in portal areas. It is highly associated with chronic ulcerative colitis. There is an increased risk of developing cholangiocarcinoma, a malignancy of bile ducts, in patients with PSC. In contrast, PBC is primarily a disease of middle-aged women and is characterized by pruritus, jaundice, and hypercholesterolemia. More than 90% of patients have antimitochondrial autoantibodies, particularly the M2 antibody to mitochondrial pyruvate dehydrogenase. A characteristic lesion, called the florid duct lesion, is seen in portal areas and is composed of a marked lymphocytic infiltrate and occasional granulomas. In contrast, causes of secondary biliary cirrhosis include biliary atresia, gallstones, and carcinoma of the head of the pancreas. Histologic examination of the liver may reveal bile stasis in the interlobular bile ducts and bile duct proliferation in the portal areas.

312. The answer is c. (*Kumar, pp 406–407.*) There are numerous organisms other than viruses that can cause infections of the liver and result in liver disease. Bacteria may cause nonsuppurative or suppurative infections. The latter can result in the formation of pyogenic liver abscesses, which clinically cause high fever, right upper quadrant abdominal pain, and hepatomegaly. There are several parasites that can cause hepatic disease. Infection with the ova of *Echinococcus granulosus* may produce a hydatid cyst within the liver, which is characterized by a thick, acellular, laminated eosinophilic wall (seen on x-ray as a calcified wall). The fluid within the cyst is granular and contains numerous small larval capsules with scoleces, called "brood capsules." Spillage of this cyst fluid at the time of surgery may produce anaphylactic shock and be deadly. Amebic trophozoites of *E. histolytica* reach the liver from the colonic submucosa and produce multiple, small amebic liver abscesses that coalesce to form large cysts with thick "anchovy paste" inside. Trophs of *Entamoeba* can be found within the wall of the cyst. Schistosomiasis (*Schistosoma mansoni* in the Middle East and *S. japonicum* in the Far East) can cause liver disease, as the adult worm lives in the intestinal venous plexus and eggs may reach the liver via the portal vein. Acute disease results in granulomas, while chronic infection produces a characteristic "pipe stem" fibrosis. Oriental cholangiohepatitis, seen in eastern Asia, is characterized by infection of bile ducts with *Clonorchis sinensis*.

313. The answer is b. (*Kumar, pp 922–923. Rubin, pp 823–825.*) Neoplasms of the liver, either benign or malignant, have characteristic microscopic or gross appearances. Benign tumors of the liver include hemangiomas (the most common), focal nodular hyperplasias, nodular regenerative hyperplasias, and adenomas. Hemangiomas are characterized by numerous small endothelial-lined spaces filled with blood. The lack of erythrocytes or blood would raise the possibility of the lesion being a lymphangioma, while pleomorphic or atypical endothelial cells would suggest the possibility of an angiosarcoma. Focal nodular hyperplasia, which has a characteristic gross appearance of a central stellate scar within the tumor, microscopically reveals hepatic nodules surrounded by fibrous bands having numerous proliferating bile ducts. This type of tumor is related to birth-control pills, but has no association with malignancy. In contrast, nodular regenerative hyperplasia involves the entire liver and forms multiple spherical nodules. Histologic sections reveal plump hepatocytes surrounded by rims of atrophic cells. Nodular regenerative hyperplasia is clinically important because it is associated with the subsequent development of portal hypertension. Two types of hepatic adenomas are the liver cell adenoma and the bile duct adenoma. Liver cell adenomas are seen in female patients taking birth-control pills. These adenomas may bleed, but are not associated with malignancy. Histologically, cords of hepatocytes are present, but there is no lobular architecture.

314. The answer is d. (*Kumar, pp 923–926. Chandrasoma, pp 659–662.*) The most common primary malignancy of the liver is the hepatocellular carcinoma (hepatoma). These tumors are associated with certain viral infections (hepatitis B and hepatitis C viruses), aflatoxin (produced by *Aspergillus flavus*), and cirrhosis. Microscopic sections of these tumors reveal pleomorphic tumor cells that form trabecular patterns, which are similar to the normal architecture of the liver. Hepatomas may secrete α–fetoprotein (AFP), but this tumor marker may also be seen in yolk sac tumors or fetal neural tube defects. Clinically, hepatocellular carcinomas have a tendency to grow into the portal vein or the inferior vena cava and may be associated with several types of paraneoplastic syndromes, such as polycythemia, hypoglycemia, and hypercalcemia. There is a microscopic fibrolamellar variant of hepatocellular carcinoma that is seen more often in females, is not associated with AFP, is grossly encapsulated, and has a better prognosis. It is important to compare the characteristics of hepatocellular carcinomas with those of another type of primary tumor of the liver, namely cholangiocarcinoma, which is a malignancy of bile ducts. This tumor is associated with Thorotrast and infection with the liver fluke (*C. sinensis*), but it is not associated with cirrhosis. Histologically, the tumor cells contain cytoplasmic mucin, which is not found in hepatomas. Instead, these malignant cells may contain cytoplasmic bile. Malignant metastatic tumors are the most common tumors found in the liver. Grossly there may be multiple or single nodules, which microscopically usually resemble the primary tumor. For example, metastatic colon cancer to the liver histologically reveals adenocarcinoma. Metastatic disease to the liver usually does not cause functional abnormalities of the liver itself, and the liver enzymes and bilirubin levels in the blood are usually normal. Angiosarcomas are highly aggressive malignant tumors that arise from the endothelial cells of the sinusoids of the liver. Their development is associated with certain chemicals, such as vinyl chloride, arsenic, and Thorotrast. A malignant tumor of the liver that is found in children is the hepatoblastoma. Microscopically, these tumors consist of ribbons and rosettes of fetal embryonal cells.

315. The answer is a. (*Kumar, pp 928–931. Rubin, pp 831–835.*) Gallstones, which affect 10 to 20% of the adult population in developed countries, are divided into two main types: cholesterol stones and bilirubin stones. Cholesterol stones are more common overall, but bilirubin stones are more frequent in individuals with chronic hemolytic disorders, such as sickle cell anemia and thalassemia. These pigment stones are brown or black in color and are composed of bilirubin calcium salts. They are also found more commonly in Asian populations and are related to diseases of the small intestines and bacterial infections of the biliary tree. In contrast to pigment stones, cholesterol stones are pale yellow, hard, round, radiographically translucent stones that are most often multiple. Their formation is related to multiple factors including female sex hormones (such as with oral contraceptives), obesity, rapid weight reduction, and hyperlipidemic states. Their prevalence approaches 75% in some native American populations. 7-alpha-hydroxylase is an enzyme involved in converting cholesterol to bile acids. Decreased functioning of this enzyme, such as with a congenital deficiency or inhibition by clofibrate, causes excess secretion of cholesterol and an increased incidence of cholesterol gallstones. Finally note that struvite stones and urate stones are types of kidney stones (urolithiasis).

316. The answer is c. (*Kumar, pp 934–935. Chandrasoma, pp 663, 665–667.*) Patients with obstruction of the common bile duct present clinically with Charcot's triad, which consists of biliary colic, high fever (secondary to cholangitis), and jaundice. Jaundice secondary to extrahepatic obstruction is associated with normal hemoglobin levels, normal serum indirect bilirubin levels, and increased levels of direct bilirubin and alkaline phosphatase. Common causes of obstruction of the common bile duct include cancer in the head of the pancreas and obstruction by a gallstone. Clinically, these two can be differentiated using Courvoisier's law, which states that in a patient with obstructive jaundice, the presence of a palpable gallbladder is indicative of obstruction due to a cancer of the head of the pancreas. This is because the obstruction causes the gallbladder to dilate. In contrast, most patients with gallstones have cholecystitis, which is associated with a thickened gallbladder wall that prevents the gallbladder from dilating. Therefore, if the obstruction is due to a gallstone, the gallbladder will not dilate and will not be palpable. Cholecystitis (inflammation of the gallbladder) may be either an acute or a chronic response. In acute cholecystitis, which may be associated with a stone (calculous type) or lack a stone (acalculous type), there is an acute inflammatory response that consists mainly of neutrophils. Acute cholecystitis usually presents with right upper quadrant pain and may constitute a surgical emergency. Chronic cholecystitis, which is associated with stones in more than 90% of cases, has a variable histologic appearance, but findings include a thickened muscular wall, scattered chronic inflammatory cells (lymphocytes), and outpouchings of the mucosa (Rokitansky-Aschoff sinuses).

317. The answer is c. (*Kumar, pp 489–495. Rubin, pp 246–249.*) Cystic fibrosis (CF) is one of the most common lethal genetic diseases that affect white populations (1/2000). The primary abnormality in patients with cystic fibrosis involves the epithelial transport of chloride. Normally, binding of a ligand to a membrane surface receptor activates adenyl cyclase, which leads to increased intracellular cAMP. This in turn activates protein kinase A, which phosphorylates the cystic fibrosis transmembrane conductance regulator (CFTR), causing it to open and release chloride ions. Sodium ions and water then follow the chloride ions to maintain the normal viscosity of mucus. The most common abnormality in patients with CF involves decreased glycosylation of the CFTR, which then does not become incorporated into the cell membrane. A lack of chloride channels then causes decreased chloride, sodium, and water secretion, all of which together results in a very thick mucus (the other name of CF is mucoviscidosis). These thick mucus plugs can block the pancreatic ducts, causing fibrosis and cystic dilation of the ducts (hence the name cystic fibrosis). Decreased excretion of pancreatic lipase leads to malabsorption of fat and steatorrhea, which may lead to deficiency of fat-soluble vitamins. Thick mucus may also cause intestinal obstruction in neonates, a condition called meconium ileus. Abnormal mucus in the pulmonary tree leads to atelectasis, fibrosis, bronchiectasis, and recurrent pulmonary infections, especially with *Staphylococcus aureus* and *Pseudomonas* species. Obstruction of the vas deferens and seminal vesicles in males leads to sterility, while obstruction of the bile duct produces jaundice. This child's skin tasted salty because of increased sweat electrolytes, the result of decreased reabsorption of electrolytes from the lumina of sweat ducts.

318. The answer is c. (*Kumar, pp 942–946. Goldman, pp 752–757.*) Inflammation of the pancreas (pancreatitis) may be either acute or chronic. Patients with acute pancreatitis typically present with abdominal pain that is associated with increased serum levels of pancreatic enzymes (amylase and lipase). Most cases of acute pancreatitis are associated with either alcohol ingestion or biliary tract disease (gallstones). Alcohol ingestion is the most common cause, and pancreatitis usually follows an episode of heavy drinking. Other, less frequent causes include hypercalcemia, hyperlipidemias, shock, infections (CMV and mumps), trauma, and drugs. Still, about 10 to 20% of individuals with pancreatitis have no obvious predisposing cause, and in a minority of patients there is a genetic (familial) abnormality that is associated with the development of pancreatitis. These familial disorders involve mutations of one of two genes involved in regulating the activation of trypsin: the cationic trypsinogen (PRSS1) gene or the serine protease inhibitor, Kazal type 1 (SPINK1). The PRSS1 gene codes for a site on trypsin that enables it to normally inactivate itself. Mutations of this gene result in the abnormal prolonged activation of trypsin which leads to recurrent bouts of severe pancreatitis. Germ line mutations in this gene produce an autosomal dominant disorder that usually begins in childhood. Similarly mutations of the SPINK1 gene, which normally codes for a trypsin inhibitor, can produce pancreatitis.

Acute pancreatitis usually presents as a medical emergency. Symptoms of acute pancreatitis include abdominal pain that is localized to the epigastrium and radiates to the back, vomiting, and shock, the latter being the result of hemorrhage and kinins released into the blood. In severe pancreatitis, there may be hemorrhage in the subcutaneous tissue around the umbilicus (Cullen's sign) and in the flanks (Turner's sign). Activation of the plasma coagulation cascade may lead to disseminated intravascular coagulopathy (DIC). Laboratory confirmation of pancreatic disease involves the finding of elevated serum amylase levels in the first 24 h and rising lipase levels over the next several days. Other pancreatic enzymes, such as trypsin, chymotrypsin, and carboxypeptidases, have not been as useful for diagnosis as have amylase and lipase. Complications seen in patients who survive the acute attack include pancreatic abscess formation, pseudocyst formation, or duodenal obstruction. Diabetes mellitus almost never occurs after a single attack of pancreatitis.

319. The answer is b. (*Kumar, pp 945–946. Goldman, pp 757–759.*) Chronic pancreatitis is characterized histologically by chronic inflammation and irregular fibrosis of the pancreas. The major cause of chronic pancreatitis in adults is chronic alcoholism, while in children the major cause is cystic fibrosis. Recurrent attacks of acute pancreatitis also result in the changes of chronic pancreatitis. Hypercalcemia and hyperlipidemia also predispose to chronic pancreatitis (since they are causes of acute pancreatitis), while in as many as 10% of patients, recurrent pancreatitis is associated with pancreas divisum. This condition refers to the finding of the accessory duct being the major excretory duct of the pancreas. Chronic ductal obstruction may be a cause of chronic pancreatitis and may be associated with gallstones, but it is more appropriate to relate gallstones with acute ductal obstruction and resultant acute pancreatitis. Complications of chronic pancreatitis include pancreatic calcifications, pancreatic cysts and pseudocysts, stones within the pancreatic ducts, diabetes, and fat malabsorption, which results in steatorrhea and decreased vitamin K levels.

320. The answer is c. (*Kumar, pp 946–948. Townsend, pp 1129–1130.*) Pseudocysts of the pancreas are so named because the cystic structure is essentially unlined by any type of epithelium. True cysts, wherever they are found in the body, are always lined by some type of epithelium, whether columnar cell, glandular, squamous, or flattened cuboidal cell. The pancreatic pseudocyst is most commonly found against a background of repeated episodes of pancreatitis. Eventual mechanical large duct obstruction by an inflammatory process per se, periductal fibrosis, or an abscess along with inspissated duct fluid from secretions and enzymes leads to the expanding mass. The mass lesion may be located between the stomach and liver, between the stomach and the colon or transverse mesocolon, or in the lesser sac. Drainage or excision is necessary for adequate treatment. Acute bacterial infection may complicate the clinical course.

In contrast, a hydrocystoma is a benign cyst filled with clear fluid. They are found on the skin, especially the eyelids. Cylindromas and syringomas are two types of benign skin tumors, while pseudomyxoma is a condition where mucinous tumors are found in the abdomen (pseudo-myxoma peritonnei). This condition is most commonly associated with a mucocele of the appendix, but is also found with mucus-secreting tumors of the ovaries.

321. The answer is b. (*Kumar, pp 948–952. Rubin, pp 850–852.*) Most carcinomas of the pancreas arise from the ductal epithelium of the pancreas and are adenocarcinomas. Pancreatic cancers are highly malignant tumors that account for about 5% of cancer deaths in the United States. Their occurrence has increased threefold in the past 40 years, mainly as a result of smoking and exposure to chemical carcinogens. They are more frequent in diabetics than nondiabetics. Most cases are found in the head of the pancreas (70%) and produce symptoms such as obstructive jaundice and migratory thrombophlebitis, usually in the superficial veins of the leg (Trousseau's sign). Courvoisier's law states that obstructive jaundice in the presence of a dilated gallbladder is most suggestive of cancer of the head of the pancreas. About 20% of pancreatic adenocarcinomas are found in the body and 10% are found in the tail. Tumors located in the tail of the pancreas present late, when therapy is no longer possible. The major symptoms of pancreatic carcinomas in general include weight loss, abdominal pain (usually the first symptom), back pain, and malaise. Surgery for a tumor of the head of the pancreas may involve pancreatoduodenectomy, which is called a Whipple procedure.

322. The answer is a. (*Kumar, pp 811, 1205–1207. Rubin, pp 855–856.*) Functional islet cell tumors of the pancreas secrete specific substances that result in several syndromes. Glucagonomas (islet cell tumors of the α cells of the pancreas) secrete glucagon and are characterized by mild non-ketotic diabetes mellitus, anemia, venous thrombosis, severe infections, and a migratory, necrotizing, erythematous skin rash. Insulinomas (tumors of β cells of the pancreas) are the most common islet cell neoplasm and are usually benign. Symptoms include low blood sugar, hunger, sweating, and nervousness. δ cell tumors, which secrete somatostatin, produce a syndrome associated with mild diabetes, gallstones, steatorrhea, and hypochlorhydria. The majority of δ cell tumors are malignant. Finally gastrinomas are a cause of the Zollinger-Ellison syndrome. This syndrome consists of intractable gastric hypersecretion, severe peptic ulceration of the duodenum and jejunum, and high serum levels of gastrin. The majority of gastrinomas are malignant and arise from the so-called gastrinoma triangle, which encompasses the duodenum and peripancreatic soft tissue. The G cells of the stomach also secrete gastrin. In contrast, the C cells of the thyroid, which normally secrete calcitonin, are the cell of origin for medullary thyroid carcinomas.

323. The answer is e. (*Kumar, pp 1205–1206. Goldman, p 1287.*) Insulinomas are tumors that originate from the beta cells of the islets of Langerhan in the pancreas. Symptoms that result from the excess and uncontrolled secretion of insulin include low blood sugar (hypoglycemia) with subsequent hunger, sweating, and nervousness. These symptoms are usually produced by fasting, alcohol, or exercise. The classic triad of symptoms associated with insulinomas is called Whipple's triad and consists of hypoglycemia, symptoms of hypoglycemia, and relief of these symptoms with glucose intake. C peptide, a product of insulin synthesis, has no known physiologic function; however, its levels can be useful in the evaluation of patients who present with decreased serum glucose levels and increased insulin levels. In these patients, increased levels of C peptide indicate endogenous insulin secretion, such as from an insulinoma. In contrast, decreased levels of C peptide indicate that the insulin that is present is exogenous insulin, because in the process of manufacturing insulin the C peptide is removed. Exogenous insulin injection may be fictitious injection, such as with Munchausen syndrome.

In contrast, Beck's triad, which is seen with acute tamponade, consists of high venous pressure, low arterial pressure, and muffled heart sounds. Charcot's triad, seen with acute inflammation of the gallbladder, consists of fever, jaundice, and right upper abdominal pain. Another Charcot's triad, consisting of nystagmus, intention tremor, and scanning speech, is seen with multiple sclerosis. Marchiafava's triad, seen with overwhelming sepsis, consists of meningitis, endocardial ulcer, and bacterial pneumonia, while Virchow's triad, seen with increased risks for thrombosis, consists of endothelial damage, turbulent blood flow, and hypercoagulable states.

324. The answer is b. (*Kumar, p 1196. Goldman, pp 1263–1264.*) Diabetes mellitus (DM) results from the clinical effects of decreased action of insulin, such as increased serum glucose levels (hyperglycemia). Previously the two major types of DM, which were given names based on their clinical presentation, were insulin-dependent diabetes mellitus (IDDM) and non–insulin-dependent diabetes mellitus (NIDDM). Any patient with DM, however, may need insulin treatment at some time, so this classification has recently been changed. Currently DM is classified into four clinical types: type 1 DM, type 2 DM, "other specific types," and gestation diabetes. Type 1 DM was formerly called IDDM or "juvenile-onset diabetes," because it is primarily found in children, the peak incidence being at the time of puberty. This type is associated with the presence of anti-islet cell autoantibodies. Type 2 DM was formerly called NIDDM or "adult-onset diabetes."

With this brief overview, note that genetic defects of beta-cell function or insulin action are two important causes of DM that are classified in the "other specific types" category. An example of a disorder that results from genetic defects of beta-cell function is maturity-onset diabetes of the young (MODY), formerly classified as a form of type 2 DM. Several genetic defects can lead to MODY, but the most common form, MODY type 3, is associated with a mutation for a transcription factor called hepatocyte nuclear factor 1alpha. MODY type 2 is associated with mutations of the gene that codes for glucokinase. The most common clinical presentation of MODY is a mild increase in blood glucose in an asymptomatic young person with a prominent familial history of diabetes, often in an autosomal dominant pattern of inheritance.

Finally note that the category "other specific types" also includes the following: diseases of the exocrine pancreas (such as pancreatitis, hemochromatosis, cystic fibrosis, or tumors), endocrinopathies (substances that have antagonistic effects to insulin include corticosteroids, growth hormone, or glucagon), drug or chemical induced DM, infections, or genetic syndromes (such as Down syndrome or Klinefelter's syndrome).

325. The answer is d. (*Kumar, pp 1192–1194, 1199–1202. Rubin, pp 1209–1211.*) There are many clinical and pathophysiologic differences between type 1 and type 2 diabetes mellitus (DM). Type 1 DM occurs most often in children, while type 2 DM is found in adults. Type 2 DM is often associated with obesity (and also decreased numbers of insulin receptors on adipocytes), but children with IDDM are of normal weight, even though they have an increased appetite (polyphagia). The basic defect in type 1 DM is decreased blood insulin levels due to a decrease in the number of insulin-producing beta cells. The mechanisms involved in this beta cell destruction include genetic susceptibility, autoimmunity, and environmental factors. Type 1 DM is more common in genetically susceptible individuals, that is, type 1 DM is more common in individuals of Northern European descent, and it is also linked to HLA types DR3, DR4, and DR3/4. In contrast, type 2 DM is not linked to any HLA type. The destruction of the beta cells is thought to be autoimmune-mediated, as the majority of patients with type 1 DM have circulating islet cell antibodies [including anti–glutamic acid decarboxylase (anti-GAD)]. Additionally, histologic examination of the islets of patients with type 1 DM reveals a lymphocytic infiltrate (insulitis). In contrast, the islets of patients with type 2 DM lack the inflammation, but may show focal atrophy with amyloid deposition. This amyloid is composed of amylin, a normal product of the beta cells. Finally, it is thought that environmental factors may trigger the autoimmunity that produces type 1 DM in genetically susceptible individuals. Possible causes for this are being investigated and include viruses (especially group B coxsackievirus), chemical toxins, and even cow's milk ingested early in life.

326. The answer is a. (*Kumar, pp 1194–1197. Henry, pp 215–218.*) Major factors involved in the pathogenesis of type 2 diabetes mellitus include peripheral insulin resistance and beta cell dysfunction. Indeed, insulin resistance may be one of the best predictors for the development of type 2 diabetes. Possible chemical factors or receptors involved in producing insulin resistance include free fatty acids (FFAs), adipokines, peroxisome proliferator-activator receptor-gamma (PPAR-γ), and thiazolidinediones (TZDs). Plasma FFA concentrations are increased in obese patients. High levels of FFAs can inhibit insulin secretion and lead to insulin resistance. Adipokines are a group of cytokines secreted by adipose tissue and include leptin, adiponectin, resistin, plasminogen activator inhibitor-1, tumor necrosis factor-alpha (TNF-α), and visfatin. Leptin and adiponectin are two insulin-sensitizing adipokines. Leptin reduces food intake and low levels may be associated with the development of insulin resistance. Similarly, low levels of adiponectin, which is downregulated with obesity, are associated with an increased risk of type 2 diabetes. Leptin acts via receptors in the hypothalamus while adiponectin works peripherally. Resistin, a signaling molecule secreted by adipocytes, decreases insulin-mediated glucose uptake by fat cells. That is, increased levels of resistin are associated with insulin resistance, as is increased release of TNF-α from adipocytes, a substance that impairs the actions of insulin. Amylin (islet amyloid protein) is stored within the beta cells of the pancreas and deposits can be seen microscopically in the islets of patients with type 2 diabetes. Pramlintide is a synthetic analog of human amylin.

Peripheral insulin resistance is closely associated with obesity, and the risk of developing type 2 diabetes increases as the body fat increases, especially abdominal fat (central obesity). One theory about the possible role of fat distribution in insulin resistance is the "thrifty" gene hypothesis, which involves abnormal functioning of PPAR-γ, a receptor that is found in adipose tissue and is important for adipocyte differentiation. This "thrifty" gene hypothesis is somewhat based on humans' ability to gain weight quickly ("thrifty") when food is abundant between times of famine. With too much food available, however, fat gets deposited in wrong places, such as the liver, muscle, and islet cells of the pancreas, which in turn can modulate PPAR-γ, and lead to insulin resistance.

327. The answer is d. (*Kumar, pp 1197–1199, 1202. Henry, pp 215–218.*) The major complications of hyperglycemia, as seen in individuals with diabetes mellitus, are related to two mechanisms, nonenzymatic glycosylation of proteins and abnormalities in polyol pathways. Nonenzymatic glycosylation involves the attachment of glucose to proteins forming unstable Schiff bases, which may rearrange to form more stable Amadori-type products that eventually may form irreversible advanced glycosylation end products (AGEs). These end products may then cause cross-linking between collagen molecules. This cross-linking in the BM of endothelial cells can trap LDL in vessel walls, accelerating atherosclerosis. In addition, albumin and IgG may bind to glycosylated basement membranes, causing the increased thickness of basement membranes that is characteristic of diabetic microangiopathy. Binding of AGEs to different receptors may have many different effects, such as stimulation of monocyte emigration, release of cytokines, increased endothelial permeability, and increased proliferation of fibroblasts and smooth-muscle cells. Glycosylation of hemoglobin produces glycosylated hemoglobin (Hb A_{1c}), which can be used to measure long-term control of an individual with diabetes mellitus.

Hyperglycemia can also affect the polyol pathways of many cells (such as nerves, lens, and kidneys) that do not require insulin for glucose transport. Excess intracellular glucose is metabolized by aldose reductase to sorbitol (a polyol) and then to fructose. Increases in both of these substances increase intracellular osmolarity, which leads to water influx and osmotic cell injury. These abnormalities will lead to many complications, including cataracts (formed by excess water influx into the lens), diabetic retinopathy (due to damage to pericytes of retinal capillaries), and peripheral neuropathy (due to damage to Schwann cells). Drugs that inhibit aldolase reductase will prevent excess sorbitol formation and may reduce these complications.

In contrast to the pathomechanisms of diabetes mellitus, deposition of immune complexes in the subendothelial space of the kidneys can be seen with type 1 membranoproliferative glomerulonephritis of lupus nephritis, while loss of glomerular polyanions is seen with minimal change disease, and antibodies to type IV collagen is seen with Goodpasture's syndrome.

Urinary System

Questions

DIRECTIONS: Each item below contains a question or incomplete statement followed by suggested responses. Select the **one best** response to each question.

328. A 55-year-old man presents with prolonged epigastric pain and severe vomiting. Laboratory evaluation finds that his blood pH is increased to 7.46, while his serum bicarbonate is increased to 30 mM. Blood gases also reveal the arterial carbon dioxide to be increased. Physical examination finds the man to be afebrile with dry mucous membranes and decreased skin turgor. His heart rate is increased, but his respiratory rate is decreased in frequency. Which of the following is the most likely diagnosis?

a. Metabolic alkalosis with respiratory compensation
b. Mixed metabolic acidosis and metabolic alkalosis
c. Respiratory acidosis with renal compensation
d. Respiratory alkalosis with no compensation
e. Respiratory alkalosis with renal compensation

329. An anxious 19-year-old woman presents with perioral numbness and carpopedal spasm. Laboratory examination reveals decreased P_{CO_2} and decreased bicarbonate. Which of the following is the most likely diagnosis?

a. Metabolic acidosis due to ketoacidosis
b. Metabolic acidosis due to renal tubular acidosis
c. Metabolic alkalosis due to thiazide diuretic
d. Respiratory acidosis due to hypoventilation
e. Respiratory alkalosis due to hyperventilation

330. A 35-year-old woman during her first pregnancy develops oligohydramnios. At 34 weeks of gestation she delivers a stillborn infant with abnormal facial features consisting of wide-set eyes, low-set floppy ears, and a broad-flat nose. Which of the following abnormalities is most likely to be present in this still-born infant?

a. Absence of the thymus
b. Bilateral renal agenesis
c. Congenital biliary atresia
d. Cystic renal dysplasia
e. Urinary bladder exstrophy

331. An 8-month-old male infant presents with progressive renal and hepatic failure. Despite intensive medical therapy, the infant dies. At the time of autopsy, the external surfaces of his kidneys are found to be smooth, but cut section reveals numerous cysts that are lined up in a row. Which of the following is the mode of inheritance of this renal abnormality?

a. Autosomal dominant
b. Autosomal recessive
c. X-linked dominant
d. X-linked recessive
e. Mitochondrial

332. Which of the following is the most likely cause of the clinical combination of generalized edema, hypoalbuminemia, and hypercholesterolemia in an adult whose urinalysis demonstrated marked proteinuria, with fatty casts and oval fat bodies?

a. Nephritic syndrome
b. Nephrotic syndrome
c. Acute renal failure
d. Renal tubular defect
e. Urinary tract infection

333. A 35-year-old woman recovering from hepatitis B develops hematuria, proteinuria, and red cell casts in the urine. Which one of the following statements best describes the expected renal changes in this patient?

a. Plasma cell interstitial nephritis
b. IgG linear fluorescence along the glomerular basement membrane
c. Granular deposits of antibodies in the glomerular basement membrane
d. Diffuse thickening of the glomerular basement membrane by subepithelial immune deposits
e. Nodular hyaline glomerulosclerosis

334. A 2-year-old boy is being evaluated for the development of progressive peripheral edema. Physical examination finds that he is afebrile, and his blood pressure is within normal limits. Laboratory examination finds decreased serum albumin, increased serum cholesterol, and normal BUN and creatinine levels. Examination of his urine finds massive proteinuria and lipiduria, but no red blood cells are seen. The loss of albumin in the urine is much greater than the loss of globulins. A histologic section from a renal biopsy examined with a routine H&E stain is unremarkable, but electron microscopic examination finds flattening and fusion of the foot processes of the podocytes. The basement membrane is not fragmented and electron dense deposits are not found. What is the best diagnosis?

a. Diffuse proliferative glomerulonephritis (DPGN)
b. Heymann glomerulonephritis (HGN)
c. Membranoproliferative glomerulonephritis (MPGN)
d. Membranous glomerulopathy (MGN)
e. Minimal change disease (MCD)

335. A 28-year-old man presents with moderate proteinuria and hypertension. Histologic sections of a kidney biopsy reveal the combination of normal-appearing glomeruli and occasional glomeruli that have deposits of hyaline material. No increased cellularity or necrosis is noted in the abnormal glomeruli. Additionally, there is cystic dilation of the renal tubules, some of which are filled with proteinaceous material. Electron microscopy reveals focal fusion of podocytes, and immunofluorescence examination finds granular IgM/C3 deposits. Further workup finds a mutation involving the NPHS2 gene, the product of which is found within the slit diaphragm of the glomerulus. What is the normal protein product of this gene?

a. Cubilin
b. Megalin
c. Nephrin
d. Podocin
e. Polycystin

336. A 6-year-old boy presents with bilateral swelling around his eyes. His parents state that the child's eyes have become "puffy" over the past several weeks, and his urine has become smoky-colored. Physical examination reveals mild bilateral periorbital edema, but peripheral edema is not found. The boy is afebrile and his blood pressure is slightly elevated. A urinary dipstick reveals mild proteinuria, while microscopic examination of the boy's urine reveals hematuria with red blood cell casts. Laboratory tests reveal increased ASO titers and decreased serum C3 levels, but C2 and C4 levels are normal. A microscopic section from the kidney reveals increased numbers of cells within the glomeruli. An electron microscopic section of the kidney reveals large electron-dense deposits in the glomeruli that are located between the basement membrane and the podocytes. The foot processes of the podocytes are otherwise unremarkable. Which one of the listed infections did this child most like recently have that precipitated this renal disease?

a. An *E. coli* infection of the small or large intestines
b. A fungal infection of the urethra or urinary bladder
c. A staphylococcal infection of the skin or mouth
d. A streptococcal infection of the pharynx or skin
e. A viral infection of the upper or lower respiratory tract

337. A 47-year-old man presents with increasing peripheral edema and dark, tea-colored urine. Laboratory examination finds decreased serum albumin, while examination of a 24-h urine specimen reveals marked proteinuria. Microscopic examination of this patient's urine reveals numerous red cells along with rare red cell casts. Electron microscopic examination of a renal biopsy from this patient reveals dense, ribbon-like deposits in the lamina densa of the glomerular basement membrane. Which of the following is the most likely diagnosis?

a. Acute glomerulonephritis
b. IgA nephropathy
c. Lipoid nephrosis
d. Membranoproliferative glomerulonephritis
e. Membranous glomerulopathy

338. A 21-year-old woman presents because her urine has turned a brown color. She states that about 2 months ago her urine turned brown 2 days after a cold and stayed brown for about 3 days. At the current time a urinalysis reveals 2+ blood with red cells and red cell casts. Further laboratory tests include a complete blood count (CBC), serum electrolytes, BUN, creatinine, glucose, antinuclear antibodies (ANAs), and serum complement levels (C3 and C4). All of these tests are within normal limits. Immunofluorescence examination of a renal biopsy from this patient reveals the presence of large, irregular deposits of IgA/C3 in the mesangium. A linear staining pattern is not found. Which of the following is the most likely diagnosis?

a. Berger's disease
b. Focal segmental glomerulosclerosis
c. Goodpasture's syndrome
d. Lipoid nephrosis
e. Membranoproliferative glomerulonephritis

339. A 43-year-old man with a history of microscopic polyarteritis acutely develops renal failure with oliguria and hematuria. Laboratory examination reveals the presence of serum p-ANCA (antineutrophil cytoplasmic antibodies). A renal biopsy is diagnostic of type III rapidly progressive glomerulonephritis. Which of the following histologic changes is most likely to have been present in this biopsy specimen?

a. Eosinophilic masses were seen attached to the capsule of Bowman's space
b. Fibrinoid necrosis was present in many of the afferent arterioles
c. Large numbers of neutrophils were seen in the interstitium and tubules
d. Numerous crescents were present in the glomeruli
e. The basement membrane was seen to be split by mesangial cells

340. A 28-year-old man with a history of malaise and hemoptysis presents with the acute onset of renal failure. Laboratory examination reveals increased serum creatinine and BUN, but no antineutrophil cytoplasmic antibodies (ANCA) nor antinuclear (ANA) antibodies are present. Urinalysis reveals the microscopic presence of red blood cells and red blood cell casts, while a renal biopsy reveals crescents within Bowman's space of many glomeruli. Immunofluorescence reveals linear deposits of IgG and C3 along the glomerular basement membrane. Which of the following is the most likely diagnosis?

a. Alport's syndrome
b. Diabetic glomerulopathy
c. Goodpasture's syndrome
d. Henoch-Schönlein purpura
e. Wegener's granulomatosis

341. A 26-year-old woman presents with increasing fatigue and malaise. She states that recently she develops a red facial rash whenever she goes outside on a sunny day. Physical examination finds that she is afebrile, but her blood pressure is slightly increased and slight peripheral edema is found. Laboratory evaluation finds slightly elevated BUN and creatinine, while dipstick examination of her urine reveals slight proteinuria with microscopic hematuria. Very rare granular and red cell casts are seen. Laboratory examination is also positive for serum antinuclear antibodies, one of which is anti–double-stranded DNA. A renal biopsy reveals changes of diffuse proliferative glomerulonephritis, and the diagnosis of class IV lupus nephritis is made. Which of the following histologic changes is most characteristic of class IV lupus nephritis?

a. Mesangial deposits form a "holly leaf" pattern
b. Positive immunofluorescence staining forms a "string of popcorn" pattern
c. Splitting of the basement membrane forms a "tram-track" pattern
d. Thickening of the basement membrane forms a "spike and dome" appearance
e. Thickening of the glomerular capillaries forms a "wire-loop" appearance

342. An asymptomatic 24-year-old woman is found to have microscopic hematuria with a routine urinalysis. Her blood pressure and kidney function are within normal limits, but it is discovered that several members of her family also have asymptomatic microscopic hematuria. Which of the following abnormalities is most likely to be present in this woman?

a. A hereditary defect in the renal transport of neutral amino acids
b. A lack of the globular domain of type IV collagen
c. A mutation involving the cytoplasmic btk gene
d. Diffuse thinning of the glomerular basement membrane
e. The presence of C3 nephritic factor in the serum

343. Histologic sections of a kidney reveal patchy necrosis of epithelial cells of both the proximal and distal tubules with flattening of the epithelial cells, rupture of the basement membrane (tubulorrhexis), and marked interstitial edema. Acute inflammatory cells are not seen. Which of the following is the most likely diagnosis?

a. Acute pyelonephritis
b. Acute tubular necrosis
c. Chronic glomerulonephritis
d. Chronic pyelonephritis
e. Diffuse cortical necrosis

344. A 67-year-old woman presents with signs of slowly progressive renal failure. Physical examination reveals mild hypertension, while laboratory tests find increased serum creatinine and BUN with mild proteinuria. A few scattered neutrophils and rare bacteria are seen microscopically in her urine. Grossly both of her kidneys are small and irregular with dilation of the renal pelvis and clubbing of the calyces, these changes being similar in appearance to those seen in the picture below. Histologic sections from her kidneys revealed chronic inflammation of the interstitium. Which one of the following additional microscopic findings should be present in these histologic sections?

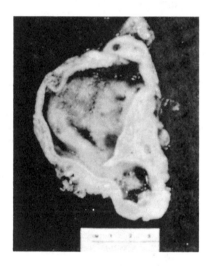

a. The renal papillae should have numerous activated macrophages
b. The tubules should be dilated and filled with colloid casts
c. The afferent and efferent arterioles should demonstrate fibroelastic hyperplasia
d. The glomeruli should have multiple fibrin microthrombi
e. The interstitium should have needle-shaped crystals

345. During a routine physical examination, a 42-year-old woman is found to have an elevated blood pressure of 150/100 mmHg. Workup reveals a small left kidney and a normal-sized right kidney. Laboratory examination reveals elevated serum renin levels. Further workup reveals that renal vein renin levels are increased on the left but decreased on the right. Which of the following is the most likely cause of this patient's hypertension?

a. Atherosclerotic narrowing of the left renal artery
b. Atherosclerotic narrowing of the right renal artery
c. Fibromuscular hyperplasia of the left renal artery
d. Fibromuscular hyperplasia of the right renal artery
e. Hyaline arteriolosclerosis

346. A 53-year-old man presents with severe headaches, nausea, and vomiting. He also relates seeing spots before his eyes and is found to have a diastolic blood pressure of 160 mmHg. Microscopic examination of a renal biopsy demonstrates hyperplastic arteriolitis. Gross examination of his kidneys is most likely to reveal which one of the following changes?

a. A finely granular appearance to the surface
b. Multiple small petechial hemorrhages on the surface
c. Diffuse, irregular cortical scars overlying dilated calyces
d. Cortical scars overlying dilated calyces in renal poles
e. Depressed cortical areas overlying necrotic papillae of varying stages

347. A 35-year-old woman presents with the sudden onset of severe, colicky pain on the right side of her abdomen. She does not relate the pain to food, but says that she cannot find a pain-free position. Physical examination finds marked tenderness over the right costovertebral angle, but rebound tenderness is not present. A pelvic examination is unremarkable. Microscopic examination of her urine reveals the presence of numerous red blood cells. The urine is negative for esterase and nitrite, and no bacteria are seen. Which of the following is the most likely cause of her signs and symptoms?

a. Bilirubin gallstones
b. Calcium oxalate kidney stones
c. Cholesterol gallstones
d. Magnesium ammonium phosphate kidney stones
e. Acute uric acid nephropathy

348. A 54-year-old man presents with left-sided costovertebral pain and gross hematuria. A large mass is found in the upper pole of one of his kidneys, as seen in the picture. Which of the following histologic changes is most likely to be seen when examining microscopic sections from this mass?

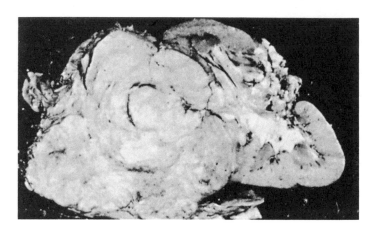

a. Groups and sheets of transitional epithelial cells
b. Immature tubules and abortive glomerular formation
c. Large cells with prominent eosinophilic cytoplasm containing numerous mitochondria
d. Malignant undifferentiated mesenchymal cells
e. Uniform cells with clear cytoplasm containing glycogen and lipid

349. An 8-month-old infant boy presents with an enlarging abdominal mass. Laboratory evaluation finds normal urinary levels of vanillylmandelic acid (VMA). The mass is removed surgically and microscopic sections reveal undifferentiated mesenchymal cells, immature tubules, and abortive glomerular formation. This tumor is most closely associated with abnormalities involving which one of the listed genes?

a. MET gene
b. PRCC gene
c. p16INK4a gene
d. VHL gene
e. WT-1 gene

350. Physical examination of a 3-day-old male infant reveals urine leaking from the area of the umbilicus. Which of the following is the most likely diagnosis?

a. Balanoposthitis
b. Meckel's cyst
c. Meckel's diverticulum
d. Omphalocele
e. Urachal fistula

351. A 19-year-old man presents with dysuria and a mucoid or watery urethral discharge. No prostatic pain is present. Microscopic examination of the discharge reveals numerous neutrophils, but no organisms are seen. Which of the following organisms is the most likely cause of this patient's signs and symptoms?

a. *Chlamydia trachomatis*
b. *Escherchia coli*
c. *Mycoplasma genitalium*
d. *Mycoplasma hominis*
e. *Trichomonas vaginalis*

352. Which of the following histologic changes is most likely to be seen when examining a mucosal biopsy of the urinary bladder from an individual with acute cystitis due to infection with *Escherichia coli*?

a. An infiltrate of lymphocytes and plasma cells
b. An infiltrate of neutrophils
c. Inflammation with eosinophils
d. Noncaseating granulomas
e. Sheets of macrophages with granular cytoplasm

353. A 49-year-old man who is a long-term smoker presents with frequency and hematuria. Histologic examination of sections taken from an exophytic lesion of the urinary bladder reveals groups of atypical cells with frequent mitoses forming finger-like projections that have thin, fibrovascular cores. These groups of atypical cells do not extend into the lamina propria and muscularis. No glands or keratin production are found. Which of the following is the most likely diagnosis?

a. Adenocarcinoma, noninvasive
b. Inverted papilloma, noninvasive
c. Transitional cell carcinoma in situ
d. Papillary transitional cell carcinoma, noninvasive
e. Squamous cell carcinoma in situ

Urinary System

Answers

328. The answer is a. (*Goldman, pp 554–556, 558–559, 563–565. Ayala, pp 121–124.*) The uncomplicated acid-base disorders, which may be of metabolic or respiratory origin, are classified as being metabolic acidosis, metabolic alkalosis, respiratory acidosis, or respiratory alkalosis. The pH (normal 7.38 to 7.44) determines whether the primary process is an acidemia (pH < 7.38) or an alkalemia (pH > 7.44). (Note that compensation for an alkalosis is always acidosis, while compensation for acidosis is always alkalosis, but in either case, compensation does not bring the pH into the normal range.) With metabolic disorders, examine the bicarbonate (normal 21 to 28 mM). Bicarbonate levels in metabolic acidosis are <21 mM, while those in metabolic alkalosis are >28 mM. Similarly, with respiratory disorders, examine the $Paco_2$ (normal Pco_2 is 35 to 40 mmHg arterial, 40 to 45 mmHg venous). In a patient with respiratory alkalosis the $Paco_2$ is <35, while with respiratory acidosis the $Paco_2$ is >40.

Patients with metabolic alkalosis lose acid, and this causes an increase in the blood pH and $[HCO_3^-]$. The body compensates for this increased pH by decreasing the respiratory rate, which increases blood CO_2 levels (hypercapnia) and increases the renal excretion of bicarbonate. Causes of metabolic alkalosis include vomiting (losing gastric acid), increased aldosterone secretion (which causes increased $[H^-]$ excretion by the kidneys), and certain diuretics.

In contrast, metabolic acidosis increases serum acid (increased hydrogen ion concentration), which decreases serum pH and decreases serum bicarbonate concentration. The causes of metabolic acidosis are broken down clinically into two groups: those with a normal anion gap and those with an increased anion gap. (The serum anion gap is found by taking the serum sodium concentration and subtracting the concentration of two anions, namely, chloride and bicarbonate. Normally, the anion gap is between 10 and 16 meq/L.) Increased anion gaps result from increased unmeasured anions, such as may occur in the following clinical situations: ketoacidosis (increased beta-hydroxybutyric acid and acetoacetic acid, seen with diabetic ketoacidosis); lactic acidosis (hypoxic conditions); chronic renal failure (uremia); and ingestion of certain substances such as salicylates, ethylene glycol, methanol, and formaldehyde. A normal anion gap metabolic acidosis may result from either loss of bicarbonate (diarrhea) or loss of renal regeneration of bicarbonate, seen with renal tubular acidosis type 1 (decreased excretion of titratable acid, i.e., NH_4^+) and renal tubular acidosis type 4. In a patient with metabolic acidosis, the body tries to combat the decreased pH by increasing the respiratory rate (tachypnea), which helps to raise the pH by blowing off CO_2 and decreasing the serum CO_2 (hypocapnia). The body also compensates through renal mechanisms that increase H^-excretion and increase bicarbonate reabsorption.

329. The answer is e. (*Goldman, pp 560, 566. Ayala, pp 121, 125.*) Respiratory alkalosis results from an increase in the respiratory rate that decreases blood CO_2 (hypocapnia) and results in decreased arterial $[H^+]$ and $[HCO_3^-]$. The body tries to compensate for the increased pH through renal mechanisms, namely, decreased H^+excretion and decreased reabsorption of HCO_3^-. Note that there is also no respiratory compensation for respiratory alkalosis. Causes of respiratory alkalosis include diseases or states that cause hypoxemia (such as living at high altitude), psychogenic causes, and ingestion of salicylates (which can cause a mixed respiratory alkalosis and metabolic acidosis).

Respiratory acidosis is caused by a decrease in the respiratory rate, which increases blood CO_2 (hypercapnia) and results in increased arterial $[H^+]$ and $[HCO_3^-]$. The body tries to compensate for the decreased pH through renal mechanisms, namely, increased H^+ excretion (through titratable H^+) and increased reabsorption of HCO_3^-. Note that there is no respiratory compensation for respiratory acidosis. Causes of respiratory acidosis include substances that inhibit the medullary respiratory center (such as opiates, sedatives, and anesthetics), impairment of the respiratory muscles (due to neurologic diseases such as multiple sclerosis), airway obstruction, and other pulmonary diseases, such as ARDS and COPD.

330. The answer is b. (*Kumar, pp 471–472, 961. Rubin, pp 217, 865.*) Failure of the metanephric diverticulum to develop normally leads to bilateral renal agenesis, which in turn leads to a constellation of symptoms called Potter's syndrome (sequence). The kidneys are important for the circulation of amniotic fluid. The fetus swallows amniotic fluid (about 400 mL/day), and then absorbs it in the respiratory and digestive tracts. Waste products cross the placental membrane and enter maternal blood in the intervillous space. Excess water is excreted by the fetal kidneys into the amniotic fluid.

Developmental abnormalities that impair fetal swallowing of amniotic fluid, such as esophageal atresia or severe anomalies of the CNS, lead to polyhydramnios (too much amniotic fluid), while agenesis of the kidneys or urinary obstruction leads to oligohydramnios (too little amniotic fluid). The oligohydramnios leads to characteristic facial features that include wide-set eyes; low-set, floppy ears; and a broad, flat nose.

In contrast to absence of the kidneys, absence of the thymus is seen with DiGeorge's syndrome, and congenital biliary atresia is a cause of neonatal jaundice. Urinary bladder exstrophy results from persistence of the cloacal membrane, while multicystic dysplasia of the kidney (MCDK) is the most common cause of an abdominal mass in a newborn. Most cases of unilateral MCDK involute spontaneously.

331. The answer is b. (*Kumar, pp 962–966. Rubin, pp 866–868.*) Cystic diseases of the kidney, which may be congenital, acquired, or inherited, have characteristic gross appearances. In two types of cystic renal disease, the numerous cysts are found in both the cortex and medulla. These two types of polycystic disease of the kidney are the infantile type and the adult type. Adult polycystic kidney disease typically presents in adulthood and has an autosomal dominant inheritance pattern. Histologically, the cysts are lined by tubular epithelium, while the stroma between the cysts is normal. Adult polycystic renal disease is associated with liver cysts and berry aneurysms, which may rupture and cause a subarachnoid hemorrhage. About one-half of patients with adult polycystic renal disease eventually develop uremia. Infantile polycystic kidney disease typically presents in newborns, has an autosomal recessive pattern of inheritance, and is associated with hepatic cysts (microhamartomas) and congenital hepatic fibrosis. Grossly, these renal cysts have a radial spoke arrangement.

In two types of cystic renal disease, the cysts are limited to the medulla. Medullary sponge kidney is usually asymptomatic, is not familial, and is characterized by normal-sized kidneys with small cysts in the renal papillae. In medullary cystic disease complex (nephronophthisis), kidneys are small and sclerotic with multiple cysts at the corticomedullary junction. Individuals with this abnormality present in the first two decades of life with salt-wasting polyuria and progressive renal failure. Most cases are familial and display both recessive and dominant inheritance patterns. Two other types of cysts that are not limited to the medulla are simple cysts and acquired cysts. Simple cortical cysts are single, unilateral cysts, found in adults, that are benign. Patients are usually asymptomatic, but they may present with microscopic hematuria. Acquired polycystic renal disease is associated with chronic renal dialysis. These kidneys are shrunken and have multiple cysts and an irregular surface.

332. The answer is b. (*Kumar, pp 966–968. Rubin, pp 868–870.*) Glomerular diseases may clinically produce either nephrotic syndrome or nephritic syndrome. Nephrotic syndrome is characterized by marked proteinuria, that is, proteinuria greater than 3.5 g/24 h. Because of this marked proteinuria, patients lose albumin (hypoalbuminemia), which leads to peripheral edema. Patients also characteristically have increased serum lipid levels (hyperlipidemia) due to increased hepatic synthesis of cholesterol. The cholesterol is carried within LDL and spills into the urine (lipiduria), where it produces microscopic fatty casts and oval fat bodies. The latter are renal tubular epithelial cells or macrophages that have excess cholesterol in the cytoplasm. Polarization of this excess cholesterol produces Maltese crosses. In contrast to nephrotic syndrome, nephritic syndrome is mainly caused by inflammatory glomerular diseases and produces hematuria (blood in the urine). Red blood cell casts may be present. These patients also may have proteinuria, but it is generally less severe than that in patients with nephrotic syndrome and is generally less than 3.5 g/24 h. Patients also retain salt and water, which leads to hypertension and peripheral edema. In contrast to these two glomerular syndromes, renal tubular defects produce symptoms of polyuria, nocturia, and electrolyte abnormalities (such as metabolic acidosis), while infections of the urinary tract cause bacteriuria and pyuria (bacteria and leukocytes in the urine).

333. The answer is c. (*Kumar, pp 967–973. Rubin, pp 870–872.*) Glomerular injury caused by circulating antigen-antibody complexes is a secondary effect from a nonrenal primary source. Numerous clinical examples exist of a serum sickness-like nephritis as a consequence of systemic infection, with classic clinical models such as syphilis, hepatitis B, malaria, and bacterial endocarditis leading to renal disease. Immune complexes to antigens from any of these sources are circulating within the vascular system and become entrapped within the filtration system of the glomerular basement membranes. This can be seen as granular, bumpy deposits by immunofluorescence within the basement membranes of the glomeruli. Linear fluorescence, on the other hand, is seen in primary antiglomerular basement membrane disease, in which antibodies are directed against the glomerular basement membrane itself. Plasma cell interstitial nephritis is seen in immunologic rejection of transplanted kidneys. Nodular glomerulosclerosis is an effect of diabetes mellitus. The presence of red blood cell casts in the urine nearly always indicates that there has been glomerular injury but is not specific for any given cause. Thickening of the glomerular basement membrane caused by subepithelial immune deposits is seen in membranous glomerulonephritis. While the morphology of membranous glomerulonephritis is different from that of nephritis caused by circulating antigen-antibody complexes (immune complexes), there are similarities in the pathogenesis in that both disorders may be a consequence of or exist in association with infections such as hepatitis B, syphilis, or malaria. Other causes of membranous glomerulonephritis include reactions to penicillamine and gold, and certain malignancies such as malignant melanoma.

334. The answer is e. (*Damjanov, pp 2089–2090. Kumar, pp 981–982.*) There are numerous causes of nephrotic syndrome (NS), including immune complex diseases, diabetes, amyloidosis, toxemia of pregnancy, and such circulating disturbances as bilateral renal vein thrombosis, but the most common cause of the nephrotic syndrome children is minimal change disease (MCD), which is synonymous with foot process disease or nil disease. MCD presents clinically as the nephrotic syndrome, characteristically occurring in younger children but also seen in adults (rarely), with hypoalbuminemia, edema, hyperlipidemia, massive selective proteinuria, and lipiduria (lipoid nephrosis). MCD is a selective proteinuria because it results from decreased amounts of polyanions (mainly heparan sulfate) in the glomerular basement membrane. These polyanions normally block the filtration of the small but negatively charged albumin molecules. The glomeruli in patients with MCD are known for their rather normal appearance on light microscopy. Electron microscopy is necessary for demonstrating the characteristic flattening and fusion of the foot processes of the podocytes attached to the Bowman's space side of the glomerular basement membrane. The podocytes may revert to normal (with steroid immunosuppressive therapy), or the foot process attenuation may persist to some extent, in which case the proteinuria also persists.

The glomeruli in patients with MCD lack electron-dense deposits, and immunofluorescence (IF) tests are negative. In contrast, subepithelial deposits are seen in diffuse proliferative glomerulonephritis (GN), such as poststreptococcal glomerulonephritis (GN). Epimembranous deposits (similar to subepithelial deposits) are found in patients with membranous GN or in the experimental disease Heymann GN. Note that the deposits in MGN are relatively small and are deposited in a very uniform fashion, while the deposits in poststreptococcal GN are comparably large (subepithelial humps) and are not uniformly distributed. Subendothelial deposits are seen with systemic lupus erythematosus, while ribbon-like electron-dense deposits in the basement membrane are seen with type 2 membranoproliferative GN (dense deposit disease). Finally, diffuse thinning with fragmentation of the glomerular basement membrane can be seen with Alport's syndrome (hereditary nephritis).

335. The answer is d. (*Kumar, pp 962–965, 982–984. Rubin, pp 874–875.*) The protein podocin is a component of the slit diaphragm of the glomerulus that is abnormal in a minority of cases of focal segmental glomerulosclerosis (FSGS), a type of glomerular disease that accounts for about 10% of the cases of nephrotic syndrome. FSGS, which affects children and adults, begins as a focal process, affecting only some glomeruli. In the earliest stage, only some of the juxtamedullary glomeruli show changes. Eventually, some glomeruli in other parts of the cortex are affected. In the late stages of the disease, the process may become diffuse, affecting most or all glomeruli. Initially, the process is also segmental, involving some but not all of the lobules within an individual glomerular tuft. The involved area shows sclerosis and may show hyalinosis lesions. Eventually some glomeruli show sclerosis of the entire tuft (global sclerosis). Electron microscopy shows increased mesangial matrix and dense granular mesangial deposits. Immunofluorescence typically shows granular mesangial fluorescence for IgM and C3. Because of the focal nature of FSGS, early cases can be difficult to distinguish from minimal change disease (MCD). Clinically, the nephrotic syndrome of FSGS is more severe than that of MCD and is nonselective. The process is much less responsive to steroids and is much more prone to progress to chronic renal failure. It tends to recur in transplanted kidneys.

Although FSGS can be associated with several disorders such as HIV infection, heroin use, and sickle cell disease, it can also be primary (idiopathic) disorder. Some of these primary cases in fact have a genetic basis and are related to mutations of genes coding for protein products of the slit diaphragm of the glomerulus. One of these is the protein podocin, which is coded for by the NPHS2 gene. Mutations involving this gene have been found in an autosomal recessive form of FSGS and a steroid-resistant nephrotic syndrome of childhood. Nephrin, which is coded for by the NPHS1 gene, is also an important component of the slit diaphragm. Mutations of this gene have been found in the congenital nephrotic syndrome of the Finnish type. In contrast, megalin and cubilin are two receptors on the luminal side of proximal tubular epithelial cells that are important for the reabsorption of albumin and low molecular weight proteins that have been filtered in the glomerulus. Finally, defects in polycystin-1 and polycystin-2 are seen with the autosomal dominant (adult) form of polycystic kidney disease (PKD), while defects in fibrocystin are seen with the autosomal recessive (childhood) form of PKD.

336. The answer is d. (*Kumar, pp 974–976. Rubin, pp 882–884.*) The most common cause of the nephritic syndrome in children is acute proliferative glomerulonephritis (APGN). In children, this illness typically begins 1 to 4 weeks after a group A β-hemolytic streptococcal infection of the pharynx or skin (impetigo or scarlet fever). As such, it is also called acute poststreptococcal glomerulonephritis (PSGN). Patients develop hematuria, red cell casts, mild periorbital edema, and increased blood pressure. Laboratory tests reveal increased ASO titers and decreased C3. Throat cultures taken at the time of presentation with renal symptoms are negative. Light microscopy reveals diffuse endothelial and mesangial cell proliferation with neutrophil infiltration, so that narrowing of capillary lumina and enlargement of the glomerular tuft to fill the Bowman's space occur. Electron microscopy reveals the mesangial deposits and large, hump-shaped subepithelial deposits in peripheral capillary loops that are characteristic. Immunofluorescence shows granular deposits containing IgG, C3, and often fibrin in glomerular capillary walls and mesangium. Children with poststreptococcal glomerulonephritis usually recover, and therapy is supportive only.

337. The answer is d. (*Kumar, pp 984–986. Rubin, pp 884–887.*) Electron-dense deposits composed of immunoglobulin and complement within the basement membrane are seen in type II membranoproliferative glomerulonephritis (MPGN or "dense deposit disease"), while subendothelial deposits are seen in type I MPGN. Note that MPGN occurs in two types. Type I, which is associated with nephrotic syndrome, is driven by immune complexes; type II is associated with hematuria and chronic renal failure and, in addition to immune complexes, involves alternate complement activation. In both types there is mesangial proliferation accompanied by thickening of the glomerular basement membranes, and a special finding that often supports the diagnosis of MPGN is the presence of actual splitting of the glomerular basement membranes. In type I there are subendothelial deposits of IgG, C3, C1, and C4. In type II there are dense deposits of C3 with or without IgG and no C1.

In contrast, IgA (Berger's) nephropathy has IgA deposits in the mesangium and is a common cause of focal segmental glomerulonephritis (FSGN), while membranous glomerulopathy has uniform electron-dense deposits in the subendothelial space. Lipoid nephrosis, also known as minimal change disease, does not have electron-dense deposits.

338. The answer is a. (*Kumar, pp 986–988. Rubin, pp 889–890.*) Many diseases involve hematuria, and a few of these diseases occur in the setting of an upper respiratory infection or of upper respiratory signs and symptoms. When hematuria follows within 2 days of the onset of an upper respiratory infection without skin lesions in a young patient, IgA nephropathy (Berger's disease) should be considered. This disease involves the deposition of IgA in the mesangium of the glomeruli. Light microscopic examination may suggest the disease, but renal biopsy immunofluorescence (IF) must be performed to confirm it. This disorder may be the most common cause of nephritic syndrome worldwide. The hematuria may become recurrent, with proteinuria that may approach nephrotic syndrome proportions. Serum levels of IgA may be elevated. A small percentage of patients may progress to renal failure over a period of years. In contrast to Berger's disease, a linear IF pattern suggests a type II hypersensitivity reaction, such as Goodpasture's syndrome, while a granular pattern is seen with poststreptococcal glomerulonephritis (GN), membranous GN, focal segmental glomerulosclerosis, and membranoproliferative GN. Most positive immunofluorescence patterns involve IgG and C3, except that a granular IgM pattern is present in focal segmental glomerulosclerosis, while mesangial IgA is seen in IgA nephropathy (Berger's disease). Lipoid nephrosis would have a negative IF pattern; that is, there would be no staining present.

339. The answer is d. (*Kumar, pp 976–978. Rubin, pp 892–893.*) Rapidly progressive glomerulonephritis (RPGN) is characterized by the microscopic presence of numerous crescents within the Bowman's space. These crescents are composed of visceral and parietal epithelial cells, inflammatory cells, and fibrin. These are indicative of severe damage to the glomerular basement membrane. RPGN may be subdivided into three types based on the immuno-fluorescence (IF) staining pattern. Type I RPGN reveals linear staining of IgG and C3, while type II RPGN reveals immune complex deposition (granular staining). These patients may have other glomerular or systemic diseases, including poststreptococcal GN, membranoproliferative GN, IgA nephropathy (Berger's disease), and SLE. Type III RPGN reveals minimal immune changes and is referred to as pauci-immune crescentic GN. Antineutrophil cytoplasmic antibodies (ANCAs), which are found in some patients with vasculitis, are found in many of these patients with pauci-immune GN. ANCAs are either perinuclear (P-ANCAs, against myeloperoxidase) or cytoplasmic (C-ANCAs, against proteinase 3). P-ANCAs are found in patients with microscopic polyarteritis and idiopathic crescentic GN, while C-ANCAs are found in patients with Wegener's granulomatosis, a disorder that is characterized by acute necrotizing granulomas of the respiratory tract, focal necrotizing vasculitis, and diffuse necrotizing GN.

In contrast to the histologic findings of RPGN, eosinophilic masses attached to the capsule of Bowman's space ("capsular drops") are seen in patients with diabetic renal disease, while fibrinoid necrosis of arterioles is seen with several different types of angiitis. Large numbers of neutrophils in the interstitium and tubules of the kidneys is diagnostic for acute pyelonephritis, while splitting of the glomerular basement membrane by mesangial cells is characteristic of membranoproliferative glomerulonephritis.

340. The answer is c. (*Kumar, pp 968, 976–978, 993. Rubin, pp 890–892.*) Type I rapidly progressive glomerulonephritis reveals linear staining of IgG and C3 along the glomerular basement membrane, this being a classic type II hypersensitivity reaction. The majority of these patients are found to have Goodpasture's syndrome, which is characterized by the presence of autoantibodies against the noncollagenous portion of type IV collagen. Patients with Goodpasture's syndrome are usually males aged 20 to 40. The lungs and kidneys are most often involved with this disease. Pulmonary hemorrhage produces hemoptysis and renal involvement produces hematuria; the chronic hemorrhage leads to anemia. Treatment is plasmapheresis or plasma exchange to remove autoantibodies from serum.

None of the other possible answers for this question have linear immuno-fluorescence patterns. Alport's syndrome is characterized clinically by recurrent hematuria, progressive hearing impairment, and ocular abnormalities, such as cataracts and dislocated lens. Henoch-Schönlein glomerulonephritis is a cause of focal segmental glomerulonephritis, and deposits may be found within the mesangial matrix. Finally, Wegener's granulomatosis, a disorder that is characterized by acute necrotizing granulomas of the respiratory tract along with focal necrotizing vasculitis, is a cause of type III rapidly progressive glomerulonephritis (pauci-immune crescentic GN).

341. The answer is e. (*Kumar, pp 227–235, 990. Rubin, pp 887–889.*) The glomerular diseases of patients with systemic lupus erythematosus (SLE) are many and include mesangial lupus glomerulonephritis (GN), focal or diffuse proliferative GN, and membranous GN. The World Health Organization (WHO) classifies SLE renal disease into five classes as follows: class I = no changes; class II = mesangial GN; class III = focal proliferative GN; class IV = diffuse proliferative GN (the most common class); class V = diffuse membranous GN. All of these glomerular diseases are the result of the deposition of immune complexes (DNA-anti-DNA complexes) that may be in a mesangial, intramembranous, subepithelial, or subendothelial location. In membranous lupus GN, the deposits are in a subepithelial location, while in diffuse proliferative lupus GN (WHO class IV) the deposits are mainly in a subendothelial location and produce a characteristic "wire-loop" appearance due to thickening of the capillary wall. None of these changes are specific for lupus.

In contrast to the "wire-loop" appearance of the glomerular capillaries with lupus nephritis, "holly leaf" mesangial deposits are seen with focal segmental GN (IgA deposits suggests Berger disease), a "string of popcorn" immunofluorescence pattern is also seen with membranous glomerulonephropathy, "tram-track" splitting of the basement membrane is seen with both types of membranoproliferative GN, and a "spike and dome" appearance of the basement membrane is seen with membranous glomerulonephropathy.

342. The answer is d. (*Kumar, pp 988–989. Rubin, pp 881–882.*) Two of the most common renal causes of asymptomatic hematuria are IgA nephropathy and thin basement membrane disease (benign familial hematuria). Most patients with thin basement disease do not have symptoms and microscopic hematuria is incidentally found with urinalysis. Blood pressure and kidney function are usually within normal limits, and the prognosis is excellent. Gross hematuria with or without pain is not seen with benign familial hematuria and if present, other causes to be considered include renal stones.

Alport's syndrome is also in the differential of an individual with microscopic hematuria. This disease is characterized by glomerular injury (resulting in recurrent hematuria), progressive hearing impairment (especially to high frequencies), and ocular abnormalities (such as cataracts and dislocated lens). Alport's syndrome is particularly common in the Mormon population (i.e., Salt Lake City) and is also called hereditary nephritis, as most cases have an X-linked dominant inheritance pattern. Microscopic sections from the kidney reveal thinning, splitting, and fragmentation of basement membrane and foam cells in glomeruli and tubules. This disease results from defective GBM synthesis, which may cause an absence of the globular region of the alpha 3 chain of type IV collagen. Since this is the region to which the antibodies in Goodpasture's syndrome react, sera from a patient with Goodpasture's syndrome would fail to react with the glomeruli from a patient with Alport's syndrome.

In contrast to the etiology of benign familial hematuria and Alport's syndrome, a hereditary defect in the renal transport of neutral amino acids can be seen with Fanconi syndrome, which is associated with cystinosis, glucosuria, phosphaturia, and bicarbonate wasting. A mutation involving the cytoplasmic btk gene is seen with X-linked agammaglobulinemia, while the presence of C3 nephritic factor in the serum is seen with dense deposit disease (type 2 membranoproliferative glomerulonephritis).

343. The answer is b. (*Kumar, pp 993–996. Rubin, pp 900–902.*) Acute tubular necrosis (ATN) may produce oliguria, decreased glomerular filtration rate (GFR), increased fractional excretion of sodium, and an abnormal urinary sediment. ATN may be caused by renal ischemia (ischemic ATN) or chemical toxins (toxic ATN). Renal ischemia is the most common cause of ATN, while toxic ATN may be caused by antibiotics (such as aminoglycosides and amphotericin B), heavy metals (such as cisplatin), radiographic agents, and endogenous toxins (such as myoglobin and hemoglobin). Both ischemic ATN and toxic ATN are characterized by the finding of eosinophilic hyalin or pigmented granular casts in the urine. Histologically, both ischemic and toxic ATN reveal interstitial edema, flattening of the tubular epithelial cells, and tubular epithelial cell necrosis. One difference between these two etiologies is that the tubular epithelial cell necrosis is extensive with toxic ATN, while the necrosis with ischemic ATN is patchy with interposed unaffected segments. This can be quite variable, however, and certain causes may be associated with damage to specific portions of the kidney. Both ischemia and heavy metals primarily damage the epithelial cells of the proximal straight tubules, while aminoglycosides primarily affect the proximal convoluted tubule.

344. The answer is b. (*Kumar, pp 1000–1002. Rubin, pp 904–906.*)
Chronic pyelonephritis is an asymmetric, irregularly scarring process of the
kidneys that may be unilateral or bilateral. Chronic pyelonephritis results
from chronic infection of the kidney, due to ascending infection secondary
to chronic obstruction or chronic vesicoureteral reflux (causing chronic,
recurrent infections). Clinically patients develop hypertension, chronic
renal failure, pyuria (neutrophils in the urine), mild proteinuria, and bacteriuria. Grossly the kidneys develop deep, coarse scars overlying
deformed calyxes and are asymmetrically contracted. These U-shaped cortical scars contrast with the V-shaped scars produced by vascular disease
(such as vascular occlusion). Microscopically there is interstitial fibrosis
with chronic inflammatory cells (lymphocytes and plasma cells). Many of
the glomeruli are totally fibrotic (global sclerosis), while many of the
tubules are dilated and contain amorphic, eosinophilic material (called
"thyroidization"). Chronic pyelonephritis may be similar to chronic
glomerulonephritis, but the renal involvement is asymmetric in chronic
pyelonephritis, and the cortical scars are larger in chronic pyelonephritis.

In contrast to the histologic findings with chronic pyelonephritis,
groups of activated macrophages are diagnostic for granulomatous inflammation, while fibroelastic hyperplasia of arterioles (intimal fibrosis) can be
seen with hypertension or it can be an aging change. Multiple fibrin
microthrombi within the glomeruli is suggestive of a microangiopathic
hemolytic anemia, such as disseminated intravascular coagulation, while
urate crystals appear microscopically as needle-shaped crystals, and may
be found in the interstitium of the kidneys in urate nephropathy.

345. The answer is c. (*Kumar, pp 1008–1009.*) A rare cause of hypertension is renal artery stenosis, which may occur secondary to either an athero-
matous plaque at the orifice of the renal artery or fibromuscular dysplasia of
the renal artery. The former is more common in elderly men, while the latter
is more common in young women. The decrease in blood flow to the kidney
with the renal artery obstruction (Goldblatt's kidney) causes hyperplasia of
the juxtaglomerular apparatus and increased renin production. This produces increased secretion of angiotensin and aldosterone, which leads to
retention of sodium and water and produces hypertension. Increased levels
of aldosterone also produce a hyperkalemic alkalosis. The kidney with stenosis of the renal artery becomes small and shrunken due to the effects of
chronic ischemia, but the stenosis protects this kidney from the effects of the

increased blood pressure. The other kidney, however, is not protected and may develop microscopic changes of benign nephrosclerosis (hyaline arteriolosclerosis).

346. The answer is b. (*Kumar, pp 1006–1008. Rubin, pp 894–895.*) Malignant hypertension is characterized clinically by finding a diastolic blood pressure greater than 130 mmHg. Additional clinical signs and symptoms of malignant hypertension include severe headache, ear noises, flame-shaped retinal hemorrhages with AV-nicking, and papilledema. The renal changes associated with malignant hypertension are called malignant nephrosclerosis. These characteristic changes include fibrinoid necrosis of arterioles (necrotizing arteriolitis), hyperplastic arteriolosclerosis (onion-skinning), necrotizing glomerulitis, and often a thrombotic microangiopathy. Grossly the kidney has a "flea-bitten" appearance with multiple red petechiae. The clinical course is often downhill, with only 50% of patients surviving 5 years; marked proteinuria, hematuria, cardiovascular problems, and finally renal failure contribute to death. The disease is often associated with accelerated preexisting benign essential hypertension, chronic renal disease (glomerulonephritis), or scleroderma.

In contrast to malignant nephrosclerosis, benign nephrosclerosis (renal disease occurring in benign hypertension) is characterized by hyaline arteriolosclerosis with thickened, hyalinized arteriolar walls and narrowed lumina. Fibroelastic hyperplasia occurs in the larger muscular arteries. Small kidneys with a finely granular surface often result because of ischemic atrophy of nephrons. Broad U-shaped cortical scars overlying dilated calyces in the renal poles are seen with chronic pyelonephritis (reflux causes scars involving poles only, while obstruction produces scars all over the kidney), depressed cortical areas overlying necrotic papillae of varying stages are seen with analgesic nephropathy and diabetes mellitus, multiple small white areas on the surface are seen with acute pyelonephritis, and wedge-shaped (i.e., V-shaped) pale cortical scars are seen with renal infarcts.

347. The answer is b. (*Kumar, pp 1004–1005. Rubin, pp 908–910.*) The combination of severe flank pain (renal colic) and hematuria is highly suggestive of urolithiasis. The formation of urinary stones relates to decreased urine volume and increased urine concentrations of certain substances. Most stones contain calcium (either calcium oxalate or calcium phosphate) and are seen in patients with hypercalcinuria (with or without hypercalcemia), such as with hyperparathyroidism or diffuse bone disease. Magnesium ammonium phosphate stones are formed in alkaline urine as the result of urease-producing (urea-splitting) bacteria such as *Proteus*. The ammonia released from the breakdown of urea combines with magnesium and phosphate. These stones are large and may fill the renal pelvis (staghorn or struvite calculi). Examination of the urine with a dipstick reveals an alkaline urine that is positive for esterase (from the leukocytes in the urine) and nitrite (since *Proteus* reduces nitrate). Uric acid stones may form in patients with hyperuricemia, such as patients with gout or patients being treated for leukemias or lymphomas. Precipitation of uric acid within the tubules of the kidney could produce urinary obstruction and acute renal failure. This condition is referred to as acute uric acid nephropathy.

In contrast to the signs and symptoms produced by kidney stones, gallstones may be asymptomatic, or they may produce fever, jaundice, and right upper abdominal pain (Charcot's triad), due to acute inflammation of the gallbladder. Gallstones are either composed of cholesterol, bilirubin, or a combination of both.

348. The answer is e. (*Kumar, pp 1016–1018. Rubin, pp 915–916.*) Renal cell carcinoma accounts for 85% of primary renal tumors and usually occurs in the sixth decade, although sometimes at a much younger age. The combination of costovertebral pain, a palpable mass, and hematuria is the classic triad of symptoms seen in about 10% of patients with renal cell carcinoma. Hematuria is often the first symptom, but it often occurs late, after invasion of the renal vein or widespread metastases, frequently to lung, bone, or brain. Histologically, renal cell carcinoma is predominantly of the clear cell type (clear cell carcinoma) with intracytoplasmic glycogen and lipid, but less often granular cells with numerous mitochondria or spindle cells occur. Grossly, the lesions are greater than 3 cm in diameter and are yellow in color (similar to tumors of the adrenal cortex; thus another name for renal cell carcinoma is hypernephroma). These tumors arise from the renal epithelial cells and thus may be classified as adenocarcinomas, but tubular formation, not glandular formation, may be present. Renal cell carcinomas may produce hormones or hormone-like substances: for example, renin (hypertension), glucocorticoids (Cushing's syndrome), and gonadotropins (feminization and masculinization). More frequently, though in only 5 to 10% of patients, polycythemia or erythrocytosis occurs owing to production of erythropoietin. Renal cell carcinoma is associated with von Hippel-Lindau syndrome, in which many patients develop bilateral renal cell carcinomas. Translocations between chromosomes 3 and 8 and between 3 and 11 have been found in some cases of familial renal cancer and in a few sporadic cases of renal cancer.

In contrast, carcinomas originating from the renal pelvis (not the cortex) arise from transitional epithelial cells and microscopically are similar to tumors arising in the urinary bladder, i.e., transitional cell carcinomas. Finally, immature tubules and abortive glomerular formation are characteristic features of nephroblastoma (Wilms' tumor).

349. The answer is e. (*Kumar, pp 504–505, 1016–1018, 1032. Rubin, pp 913–915.*) Malignant tumors of the kidney in children are called nephroblastomas (Wilms' tumor) and histologically reveal a combination of metanephric blastema, undifferentiated mesenchymal cells, and immature tubule or glomerular formation. Children present with an enlarging abdominal mass that, in contrast to adrenal neuroblastoma, is associated with normal urinary vanillylmandelic acid (VMA) levels. Deletions involving WT1, located on chromosome 11, are associated with the development of Wilms' tumor (nephroblastoma). Several syndromes are associated with genetic deletions of WT1, that lead to an increased incidence of Wilms' tumor. These include WAGR syndrome (characterized by aniridia, genital abnormalities, and mental retardation) and Denys-Drash syndrome (characterized by gonadal dysgenesis and renal failure). Deletions involving a second Wilms' tumor gene (WT2) are associated with Beckwith-Wiedemann syndrome (characterized by hemihypertrophy, renal medullary cysts, and adrenal cytomegaly).

In contrast, the development of renal cell carcinoma (adenocarcinoma of the kidney) is associated with defects involving several different genes, including the VHL gene, the MET protooncogene, and the PRCC (papillary renal cell carcinoma) gene. Defects of the p16INK4a tumor-suppressor gene are associated with the development of urothelial (transitional cell) tumors.

350. The answer is e. (*Kumar, p 1026. Damjanov, pp 1710–1711, 2190–2191. Sadler, pp 333, 335–336.*) The cloaca is an embryonic structure that connects ventrally to the allantoic stalk and laterally to the mesonephric ducts. At about the eighth week of development a cloacal membrane forms within the cloaca and separates the cloaca into a dorsal rectum and a ventral urogenital sinus. The latter is the origin of the urachus, urinary bladder, and proximal urethra. Initially the urinary bladder is continuous with the allantois, which constricts and forms the thick, fibrous urachus. The urachus in turn becomes attenuated, but still remains attached to the bladder dome and forms the median umbilical ligament in the adult. Incomplete attenuation of the urachus (persistent urachus) can lead to formation of a urachal cyst, urachal sinus, or urachal fistula. The end attached to the bladder can remain and form a bladder diverticulum, while the central portion can remain and form a urachal cyst. Urachal sinuses and fistulas still connect the umbilicus to the urinary bladder, and therefore urine can leak at the site of the umbilicus.

Normally, mesodermal tissue grows onto the cloacal membrane to form the muscles of the lower abdominal wall. During this process the cloacal membrane is obliterated and disappears. In some embryos mesoderm does not grow onto the cloacal membrane. This leads to persistence of the cloacal membrane, which can become quite thin and rupture. This in turn causes the posterior bladder mucosa to evert through this defect in the anterior abdominal wall. This condition is called exstrophy and is associated with recurrent urinary infections and epispadias in males. There is also an increased incidence of neoplastic transformation, most commonly adenocarcinoma.

Meckel's diverticulum is a diverticulum found in the terminal ileum that is the result of persistence of the omphalomesenteric duct. It is usually about 2 in long and is located less than 2 ft from the ileocecal valve. An omphalocele refers to protrusion of the intestines through an unclosed umbilical ring. This abnormality results from incomplete internalization of the intestines during fetal growth. A similar defect, gastroschisis, does not involve the umbilicus. Instead, viscera herniate through a defect in the anterior abdominal wall just lateral to the umbilicus.

351. The answer is a. (*Kumar, pp 394–395, 1034. Rubin, p 925.*) Urethritis can be classified based on its etiology into either gonococcal and nongonococcal urethritis (NGU). The latter may be the most common cause of dysuria in sexually active males. Causes of NGU include some bacteria, such as *E. coli* and streptococci, but at least half of the cases of NGU are caused by *Chlamydia trachomatis*, a small Gram-negative obligate intracellular bacterium. This organism is probably the most common cause of bacterial sexually transmitted disease in both men and women. Unlike gonococcal urethritis, *C. trachomatis* urethritis may be asymptomatic. Diagnosis of chlamydial urethritis is made by using PCR tests using nucleic acid amplification. Other organisms that cause NGU include *Ureaplasma urealyticum*,

Mycoplasma hominis, Mycoplasma genitalium, and *Trichomonas vaginalis,* but infection with these organisms is less frequent than with *C. trachomatis.*

352. The answer is b. (*Kumar, pp 1027–1028. Rubin, p 925.*) Inflammation of the urinary bladder (cystitis) may be caused by many different etiologies, all of which produce symptoms of frequency, dysuria, and lower abdominal pain. Acute cystitis histologically reveals stromal edema and an infiltrate of neutrophils. Grossly, the bladder mucosa is hyperemic. In most cases cystitis is secondary to infections of the bladder, usually by coliform bacteria, e.g., *E. coli.* Cystitis occurs more commonly in females and is associated with sexual intercourse, pregnancy, and instrumentation. Hemorrhage may also be present (hemorrhagic cystitis) and is usually the result of radiation injury, chemotherapy, or an adenovirus infection.

353. The answer is d. (*Kumar, pp 1028–1033.*) Neoplastic lesions of the urinary bladder may either be benign or malignant. There is some controversy involving some types of benign lesions of the bladder. In particular, there is disagreement as to whether papillary lesions may be benign (papillomas). Many pathologists would classify papillary transitional lesions that lack cellular atypia or numerous mitoses as grade I (low-grade) papillary transitional cell carcinomas (TCCs) and not papillomas. Pathologists do agree, however, on the existence of a rare type of benign lesion called an inverted papilloma, which is characterized by nodular mucosal lesions that histologically have an endophytic growth pattern. Malignant neoplasms of the bladder may be transitional cell carcinomas, which are by far the most common type of tumor of the urinary bladder; squamous cell carcinomas, which produce keratin; or adenocarcinomas, which form glandular structures. TCCs may be either papillary or flat lesions. Papillary TCCs, which are the most common type of bladder cancer, may be either invasive or noninvasive. Noninvasive papillary TCCs are not referred to as being in situ, as that term implies a noninvasive, nonpapillary lesion. Nonpapillary (flat) TCCs may also be invasive (into the lamina propria or muscularis) or noninvasive (in situ). In contrast, squamous cell carcinomas of the urinary bladder are quite rare except in Egypt and other areas of the Middle East, where they are associated with schistosomiasis. Similarly, adenocarcinomas of the urinary bladder are quite rare, except that they may be associated with urachal epithelial remnants located in the dome of the bladder, glandular metaplasia, or cystitis glandularis.

Reproductive Systems

Questions

DIRECTIONS: Each item below contains a question or incomplete statement followed by suggested responses. Select the **one best** response to each question.

354. A 24-year-old man is being evaluated for infertility, and during physical examination the urethral orifice is noted to be on the ventral surface of the penis. Which of the following is the basic defect that caused this abnormality?

a. Abnormal development of the prepuce
b. Abnormal fusion of the paramesonephric ducts
c. Exstrophy of the bladder
d. Failure of the urethral folds to close
e. Repeated inflammation of the glans and prepuce

355. An uncircumcised 49-year-old man presents with the sudden onset of severe pain in the distal portion of his penis. The emergency room physician examines the patient and finds that the foreskin is retracted but cannot be rolled back over the glans penis. The ER physician calls the urologist, who performs an emergency resection of this patient's foreskin. Which of the following is the most likely diagnosis?

a. Balanoposthitis
b. Epispadias
c. Omphalocele
d. Paraphimosis
e. Phimosis

356. Histologic examination of an excision specimen from a lesion on the dorsal surface of the penis reveals a papillary lesion with clear vacuolization of epithelial cells on the surface and extension of the hyperplastic epithelium into the underlying tissue along a broad front. Which of the following is the most likely diagnosis?

a. Condyloma acuminatum
b. Bowen's disease
c. Erythroplasia of Queyrat
d. Verrucous carcinoma
e. Squamous cell carcinoma

357. The photomicrograph is of a section from a testis removed from the inguinal region of a man aged 25. Which of the following statements about this condition is true?

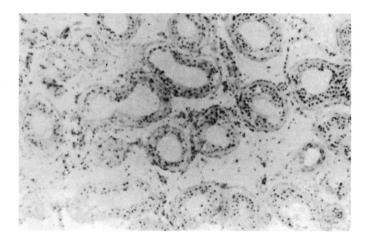

a. It is bilateral in the majority of cases
b. Teratoma is the most common malignancy to arise
c. Risk of associated malignancy is reduced by orchiopexy
d. There is increased risk of malignancy in the contralateral testis
e. Both Leydig and Sertoli cells are reduced in number

358. A 27-year-old man presents with painless scrotal enlargement. He reports a sensation of "heaviness" in his scrotum. He denies any history of fever, chills, nausea, or vomiting. Physical examination finds an approximate 1-cm mass in the superior portion of the scrotum, anteriorly located to the testis. Because the mass transilluminates, the diagnosis of hydrocele is considered. Which of the following is the best method to confirm that this mass is in fact a benign cyst and not a solid tumor?

a. Doppler flow study
b. Fine needle aspiration
c. Imaging ultrasound
d. Surgical biopsy
e. Testicular scintigraphy

359. A 44-year-old man presents with painless enlargement of one testicle. Physical examination reveals a single testicular mass that does not transilluminate. The mass is resected, examined histologically, and radiation therapy is subsequently given based on the pathologist's diagnosis. Which of the following best describes the expected microscopic appearance of this tumor?

a. A mixture of malignant cytotrophoblasts and syncytiotrophoblasts
b. Abnormal tissue derived from all three germ levels with scattered immature neural elements
c. Large tumor cells with abundant eosinophilic, granular cytoplasm, and rare intracytoplasmic rhomboid crystals
d. Numerous lymphocytes in the fibrous stroma between groups of tumor cells having distinct cell membranes and clear cytoplasm
e. Sheets of undifferentiated tumor cells having focal glandular differentiation

360. A 27-year-old man presents with a testicular mass, which is resected and diagnosed as being a yolk sac tumor. Which of the following substances is most likely to be increased in this patient's serum as a result of being secreted from the cells of this tumor?

a. Acid phosphatase
b. α-fetoprotein (AFP)
c. Alkaline phosphatase
d. β-human chorionic gonadotropin (β-hCG)
e. Prostate-specific antigen (PSA)

361. A 47-year-old man presents with the sudden onset of fever, chills, and dysuria. Rectal examination finds the prostate gland to be edematous and very sensitive; examination is quite painful. Microscopic examination of prostatic secretions reveals the presence of numerous neutrophils. Which of the following organisms is the most likely cause of this illness?

a. Bacillus Calmette-Guerin
b. *Escherichia coli.*
c. *Proteus mirabillis*
d. *Staphylococcus aureus*
e. *Ureaplasma urealyticum*

362. A 69-year-old man presents with urinary frequency, nocturia, dribbling, and difficulty in starting and stopping urination. Rectal examination reveals the prostate to be enlarged, firm, and rubbery. A needle biopsy reveals increased numbers of glandular elements and stromal tissue. The glands are found to have a double layer of epithelial cells. Prominent nuclei or back-to-back glands are not seen. Which of the following is the most likely diagnosis?

a. Atrophic prostatitis
b. Atypical small acinar proliferation
c. High-grade prostatic intraepithelial neoplasia
d. Benign prostatic hyperplasia
e. Prostatic adenocarcinoma

363. A 67-year-old man is found on rectal examination to have a single, hard, irregular nodule within his prostate. A biopsy of this lesion reveals the presence of small glands lined by a single layer of cells with enlarged, prominent nucleoli. From what portion of the prostate did this lesion most likely originate?

a. Anterior zone
b. Central zone
c. Peripheral zone
d. Periurethral glands
e. Transition zone

364. A female newborn is being worked up clinically for several congenital abnormalities. During this workup, it is discovered that normal development of the vagina and uterus in this female infant has not occurred. Failure of the uterus to develop (agenesis) is directly related to the failure of which one of the following embryonic structures to develop?

a. Urogenital ridge
b. Mesonephric duct
c. Paramesonephric duct
d. Metanephric duct
e. Epoophoron

365. Which of the following describes multiple small mucinous cysts of the endocervix that result from blockage of the endocervical glands by overlying squamous metaplastic epithelium?

a. Bartholin's cysts
b. Chocolate cysts
c. Follicular cysts
d. Gartner's duct cysts
e. Nabothian cysts

366. A 75-year-old woman presents with a pruritic vulvar lesion. Physical examination reveals an irregular white, rough area involving her vulva. Which one of the following histologic changes is most consistent with the diagnosis of lichen sclerosis?

a. Atrophy of the epidermis with dermal fibrosis
b. Atypia of the epidermis with dysplasia
c. Hyperplasia of the epidermis with hyperkeratosis
d. Invasion of the epidermis by individual malignant cells
e. Loss of pigment in the basal layers of the epidermis

367. A 65-year-old woman presents with a pruritic red, crusted, sharply demarcated map-like lesion involving a large portion of her labia majora. Histologic sections from this lesion reveal individual anaplastic tumor cells infiltrating the epidermis. Distinctive clear spaces are noted between these anaplastic cells and the surrounding normal epithelial cells. These malignant cells stain positively for mucin and negatively with S100. Which of the following is the most likely diagnosis?

a. Clear cell adenocarcinoma
b. Malignant melanoma
c. Extramammary Paget's disease
d. Sarcoma botryoides
e. Squamous cell carcinoma

368. A 25-year-old woman being evaluated for infertility is found to have an abnormal ridge of red, moist granules located in the upper third of her vagina. Pertinent medical history is that her mother was treated with diethylstilbestrol (DES) during her pregnancy. A biopsy from the abnormal vaginal ridge reveals the presence of benign glands underneath stratified squamous epithelium. Which of the following is the most serious long-term complication of this abnormality?

a. Clear cell carcinoma
b. Condyloma acuminatum
c. Extramammary Paget's disease
d. Multiple papillary hidradenomas
e. Verrucous carcinoma

369. A 23-year-old woman presents to her gynecologist for a routine phys-ical examination that includes a Pap smear. Her sexual history includes many sexual partners beginning at an early age, but she has never been pregnant. Physical examination is unremarkable. The Pap smear returns as abnormal with the presence of atypical squamous epithelial cells of unde-termined significance (ASCUS). She returns for a 6-month follow-up and a repeat pelvic exam is performed. Her cervix is painted with iodine and an area near the cervical os is present that does not stain with iodine. This area is flat and not papillary. Several biopsies are obtained from this pale area, and a representative histologic section is seen in the picture below. This histologic section shows koilocytosis, which is most characteristic of infec-tion with which one of the following organisms?

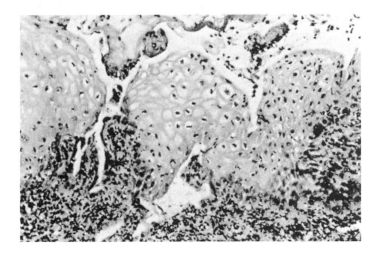

   a. Cytomegalovirus
   b. Epstein-Barr virus
   c. Herpes simplex virus
   d. Human papillomavirus
   e. Parvovirus B19

370. A 29-year-old woman presents with severe pain during menstruation (dysmenorrhea). During workup, an endometrial biopsy is obtained. The pathology report from this specimen makes the diagnosis of chronic endometritis. Based on this pathology report, which of the following was present in the biopsy sample of the endometrium?

a. Neutrophils
b. Lymphocytes
c. Lymphoid follicles
d. Plasma cells
e. Decidualized stromal cells

371. A 39-year-old woman presents with severe menorrhagia and colicky dysmenorrhea. A hysterectomy including resection of the fallopian tubes and ovaries is performed and the pathologist who examines the specimen makes the diagnosis of "adenomyosis." Which one of the listed abnormalities was present in this resected specimen?

a. Ectocervical tissue was present within the wall of the fallopian tube
b. Endocervical tissue was present on the surface of the ovary
c. Endometrial tissue was present within the hilum of the ovary
d. Endometrial tissue was present within the wall of uterus
e. Ovarian tissue was present on the surface of the uterus

372. A 23-year-old woman presents with urinary frequency and abnormal uterine bleeding. A careful medical history finds that her abnormal menstrual bleeding is characterized by excessive bleeding at irregular intervals. A pelvic examination finds a single mass in the anterior wall of the uterus, this being confirmed by ultrasonography. Which one of the following clinical terms best describes the abnormal uterine bleeding in this woman?

a. Amenorrhea
b. Dysmenorrhea
c. Menometrorrhagia
d. Oligomenorrhea
e. Polymenorrhea

373. A 24-year-old woman presents with a 2-year history of infertility. An endometrial biopsy is obtained approximately 5 to 6 days after the predicted time of ovulation. This biopsy specimen reveals secretory endometrium, but there is a significant difference (asynchrony) between the estimated chronologic menstrual date and the estimated histologic menstrual date. No proliferative endometrium is seen. Which of the following is the most likely diagnosis?

a. Anovulatory cycle (no corpus luteum formed)
b. Inadequate luteal phase (decreased functioning of the corpus luteum)
c. Irregular shedding (prolonged functioning of the corpus luteum)
d. Normal endometrium during the follicular phase of the cycle (no corpus luteum formed)
e. Normal endometrium during the luteal phase of the cycle (normal corpus luteum)

374. A 60-year-old postmenopausal woman presents with the new onset of uterine bleeding. An endometrial biopsy is diagnosed as atypical hyperplasia. Which of the following histologic changes is most characteristic of this abnormality?

a. Crowding of endometrial glands with budding and epithelial atypia
b. Lymphatic invasion by interlacing bundles of atypical spindle-shaped cells
c. Menstrual-type endometrial glands with focal atypical cystic dilatation
d. Secretory-type endometrial glands with hyperplasia of atypical polygonal cells having clear cytoplasm
e. Stromal invasion by malignant glands with focal areas of atypical squamous differentiation

375. Prolonged unopposed estrogen stimulation in an adult woman increases the risk of development of endometrial hyperplasia and subsequent carcinoma. Which of the following is the most common histologic appearance for this type of cancer?

a. Adenocarcinoma
b. Clear cell carcinoma
c. Small cell carcinoma
d. Squamous cell carcinoma
e. Transitional cell carcinoma

376. A 46-year-old woman undergoes an abdominal hysterectomy for a "fibroid" uterus. The surgeon requests a frozen section on the tumor, which is deferred because of the lesion's degree of cellularity. Which of the following criteria will be used by the pathologist in determining benignancy versus malignancy in permanent sections?

a. Mitotic rate
b. Cell pleomorphism
c. Cell necrosis
d. Nucleus-to-cytoplasm ratio
e. Tumor size

377. A 25-year-old woman presents with lower abdominal pain, fever, and a vaginal discharge. Pelvic examination reveals bilateral adnexal (ovarian) tenderness and pain when the cervix is manipulated. Cultures taken from the vaginal discharge grow *Neisseria gonorrhoeae*. Which of the following is the most likely cause of this patient's adnexal pain?

a. Adenomatoid tumor
b. Ectopic pregnancy
c. Endometriosis
d. Luteoma of pregnancy
e. Pelvic inflammatory disease

378. A 19-year-old woman presents with oligomenorrhea. Physical examination reveals an obese young woman with acne and increased facial hair. A pelvic examination is essentially within normal limits, excluding the adnexal regions, which could not be palpated secondary to obesity. Ultrasound examination reveals bilateral enlargement of the ovaries with multiple subcortical cysts. Which of the following sets of serum laboratory values is most likely to be present in this individual?

	Serum Luteinizing Hormone (LH)	Serum Follicle-Stimulating Hormone (FSH)	LH/FSH Ratio
a.	Decreased	Decreased	High
b.	Decreased	Decreased	Low
c.	Decreased	Increased	Low
d.	Increased	Decreased	High
e.	Increased	Increased	Low

379. A 23-year-old woman presents with pelvic pain and is found to have an ovarian mass of the left ovary that measures 3 cm in diameter. Grossly, the mass consists of multiple cystic spaces. Histologically, these cysts are lined by tall columnar epithelium, with some of the cells being ciliated. Which of the following is the correct diagnosis for this ovarian tumor, which histologically recapitulates the histology of the fallopian tubes?

a. Serous tumor
b. Mucinous tumor
c. Endometrioid tumor
d. Clear cell tumor
e. Brenner tumor

380. A 32-year-old woman presents with the recent onset of oligomenorrhea followed by amenorrhea. She has also developed acne, deepening of her voice, and temporal balding. Physical examination finds the loss of female secondary characteristics and slight abdominal distention. She is found to have a 4.0-cm mass within her left ovary. This mass is resected surgically and a histologic section reveals the tumor cells to stain positively with an immunoperoxidase stain against inhibin. Rare Call-Exner bodies are present. What is the correct diagnosis?

a. Androblastoma
b. Borderline mucinous tumor
c. Granulosa cell tumor
d. Pseudomyxoma peritonei
e. Sertoli cell tumor

381. A 29-year-old woman presents with intermittent lower abdominal pain. A pelvic examination finds an ovarian mass involving her right ovary. This ovarian mass is resected and gross examination reveals a cystic tumor that measures about 4 cm in diameter. A histologic section from this tumor reveals a mixture of elements as seen in the picture. Immature or neural tissue is not found. Which of the following is the most likely diagnosis?

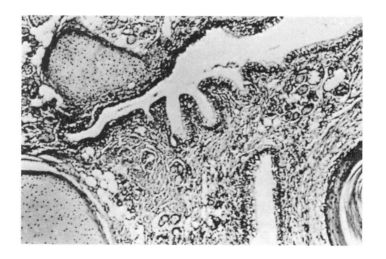

a. Brenner tumor
b. Chronic salpingitis
c. Dermoid cyst
d. Ectopic pregnancy
e. Mucinous cystadenoma

382. A 39-year-old woman presents with increasing abdominal distention and pelvic pain. A CT scan finds a slight amount of fluid in the pleural cavity and also a 3.5-cm tumor of the right ovary. The tumor is resected and histologic sections reveal the tumor to be composed of spindle-shaped cells. These cells did not stain with an oil red O special stain. Which of the following types of ovarian tumor is most likely to produce this constellation of findings?

a. Epithelial tumor
b. Stromal tumor
c. Germ cell tumor
d. Surface tumor
e. Metastatic tumor

383. An 18-year-old woman presents with amenorrhea and is found to have normal secondary sex characteristics and normal-appearing external genitalia. Her first menstrual period was at age 13, and her cycle has been unremarkable until now. She states that her last menstrual period was 8 weeks prior to this visit. A urine test for hCG is positive. Which of the following is the most likely diagnosis?

a. Ectopic pregnancy
b. Intrauterine pregnancy
c. Stein-Leventhal syndrome
d. Turner's syndrome
e. Weight loss syndrome

384. A 24-year-old woman delivers a normal 8-lb baby boy at 40 weeks of gestation. She has no history of drug abuse, and her pregnancy was unremarkable. Examination had revealed the placenta to be located normally, but following delivery the woman fails to deliver the placenta and subsequently develops massive postpartum hemorrhage and shock. Emergency surgery is performed to stop the bleeding. Which of the following is the most likely cause of her postpartum bleeding?

a. An abruptio placenta
b. A placenta previa
c. A placenta accreta
d. A hydatidiform mole
e. An invasive mole

385. A 26-year-old woman acutely develops lower abdominal pain and vaginal bleeding. While in the bathroom she passes a cast of tissue composed of clot material and then collapses. She is brought to the hospital, where a physical examination reveals a soft, tender mass in right adnexa and pouch of Douglas. Histologic examination of the tissue passed in the bathroom reveals blood clots and decidualized tissue. No chorionic villi or trophoblastic tissue are present. Which of the following conditions is most likely present in this individual?

a. Aborted intrauterine pregnancy
b. Complete hydatidiform mole
c. Ectopic pregnancy
d. Endometrial hyperplasia
e. Partial hydatidiform mole

386. A 26-year-old woman in the third trimester of her first pregnancy develops persistent headaches and swelling of her legs and face. Early during her pregnancy a physical examination was unremarkable; however, now her blood pressure is 170/105 mmHg and urinalysis reveals slight proteinuria. Which of the following is the most likely diagnosis?

a. Eclampsia
b. Gestational trophoblastic disease
c. Nephritic syndrome
d. Nephrotic syndrome
e. Preeclampsia

387. A 25-year-old woman in her fifteenth week of pregnancy presents with uterine bleeding and passage of a small amount of watery fluid and tissue. She is found to have a uterus that is much larger than estimated by her gestational dates. Her uterus is found to be filled with cystic, avascular, grapelike structures that do not penetrate the uterine wall. No fetal parts are found. Immunostaining for p57 was negative in the cytotrophoblasts and villi mesenchyme. Which of the following is the best diagnosis?

a. Partial hydatidiform mole
b. Complete hydatidiform mole
c. Invasive mole
d. Placental site trophoblastic tumor
e. Choriocarcinoma

388. A 50-year-old woman presents with fatigue, insomnia, hot flashes, night sweats, and absence of menses for the last 5 months (secondary amenorrhea). Her urine hCG test is negative. Laboratory tests reveal decreased serum estrogen and increased serum FSH and LH levels. Which of the following is the most likely cause of this individual's clinical signs and symptoms?

a. 17-hydroxylase deficiency of the adrenal cortex
b. Prolactin-secreting tumor of the anterior pituitary
c. Gonadotropin-releasing hormone–secreting tumor of the hypothalamus
d. Menopause
e. Menarche

389. A 27-year-old woman who is actively training for a marathon presents with the new onset of a painful lump in the upper outer quadrant of her right breast. A mammogram shows an irregular mass with focal areas of calcification. An excisional biopsy reveals a localized area of granulation tissue and numerous lipid-laden macrophages surrounding necrotic adipocytes. Which of the following is the most likely diagnosis?

a. Acute mastitis
b. Ectasia
c. Enzymatic fat necrosis
d. Foreign-body reaction
e. Traumatic fat necrosis

390. During a routine breast self-examination, a 35-year-old woman is concerned because her breasts feel "lumpy." She consults you as her primary care physician. After performing an examination, you reassure her that no masses are present and that the "lumpiness" is due to fibrocystic changes. Which of the following pathologic findings is a type of nonproliferative fibrocystic change?

a. A blue-domed cyst
b. A radial scar
c. Atypical ductal hyperplasia
d. Papillomatosis
e. Sclerosing adenosis

391. A 23-year-old woman presents with a rubbery, freely movable 2-cm mass in the upper outer quadrant of the left breast. Which of the following histologic features is most likely to be seen when examining a biopsy specimen from this mass?

a. Large numbers of neutrophils
b. Large numbers of plasma cells
c. Duct ectasia with inspissation of breast secretions
d. Necrotic fat surrounded by lipid-laden macrophages
e. A mixture of fibrous tissue and ducts

392. A 39-year-old woman presents with the new onset of a bloody discharge from her right nipple. Physical examination reveals a 1-cm freely movable mass that is located directly beneath the nipple. Sections from this mass reveal multiple fibrovascular cores lined by several layers of epithelial cells. Atypia is minimal. The lesion is completely contained within the duct and no invasion into underlying tissue is seen. Which of the following is the most likely diagnosis?

a. Benign phyllodes tumor
b. Ductal papilloma
c. Intraductal carcinoma
d. Paget's disease
e. Papillary carcinoma

393. A 35-year-old woman presents with a 2.2-cm mass in her left breast. The mass is excised, and histologic sections reveal a tumor composed of a mixture of ducts and cells, as seen in the photomicrograph. The epithelial cells within the ducts are not atypical in appearance. There is a marked increase in the stromal cellularity, but the stromal cells are not atypical in appearance and mitoses are not found. Which of the following is the most likely diagnosis?

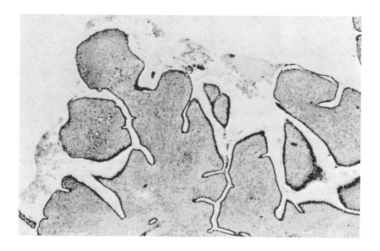

a. Atypical epithelial hyperplasia
b. Benign phyllodes tumor
c. Fibroadenoma
d. Malignant phyllodes tumor
e. Medullary carcinoma

394. A 48-year-old woman presents with a painless mass located in her left breast. Physical examination finds a firm, nontender, 3-cm mass in the upper outer quadrant of her left breast. There was retraction of the skin overlying this mass, and several enlarged lymph nodes were found in her left axilla. The mass was resected and histologic sections revealed an invasive ductal carcinoma. Biopsies from her axillary lymph nodes revealed the presence of metastatic disease to 4 of 18 examined axillary lymph nodes. The expression of which one of the following by the tumor cells would best predict a response to therapy with Trastuzumab?

a.   BRCA1
b.   Estrogen receptors
c.   HER2/neu
d.   Progesterone receptors
e.   Urokinase plasminogen activator

395. A 48-year-old woman presents with a 1.5-cm firm mass in the upper outer quadrant of her left breast. A biopsy from this mass reveals many of the ducts to be filled with atypical cells. In the center of these ducts there is extensive necrosis. No invasion into the surrounding fibrous tissue is seen. Which of the following is the most likely diagnosis?

a.   Colloid carcinoma
b.   Comedocarcinoma
c.   Infiltrating ductal carcinoma
d.   Infiltrating lobular carcinoma
e.   Lobular carcinoma in situ

396. A 60-year-old woman presents with a slowly enlarging 2.5-cm firm, irregular mass in the upper outer quadrant of her left breast. A biopsy from this mass is interpreted by the pathologist as being an infiltrating lobular carcinoma of the breast. Which of the following histologic features is most characteristic of this tumor?

a.   Expansion of lobules by monotonous proliferation of epithelial cells
b.   Large cells with clear cytoplasm within the epidermis
c.   Large syncytium-like sheets of pleomorphic cells surrounded by aggregates of lymphocytes
d.   Small individual malignant cells dispersed within extracellular pools of mucin
e.   Small tumor cells with little cytoplasm infiltrating in a single-file pattern

397. A 46-year-old woman presents with a 4-month history of a discharge from the nipple. An excisional biopsy of the nipple area reveals infiltration of the nipple by large cells with clear cytoplasm. These cells are found both singly and in small clusters in the epidermis and are PAS-positive and diastase-resistant. Which of the following is the most likely diagnosis?

a. Ductal papilloma
b. Eczematous inflammation
c. Mammary duct ectasia
d. Paget's disease
e. Phyllodes tumor, malignant

398. A 35-year-old woman who underwent a modified radical mastectomy of her right breast for infiltrating ductal carcinoma 2 years ago presents with enlargement of her right breast. The breast has a swollen, red-discolored appearance. It is diffusely indurated and tender on palpation. Multiple axillary lymph nodes are palpable in the lower axilla. The working clinical diagnosis is inflammatory carcinoma. Which of the following histologic features is most characteristic of this clinical diagnosis?

a. Duct ectasia with numerous plasma cells
b. Extensive invasion of dermal lymphatics
c. Infiltrating malignant ducts surrounded by numerous neutrophils
d. Malignant vascular tumor forming slit-like spaces
e. Marked dermal desmoplasia

399. A 51-year-old man presents with bilateral enlargement of his breasts. Physical examination is otherwise unremarkable, and the diagnosis of gynecomastia is made. Which of the following histologic features is most likely to be seen when examining a biopsy specimen from this man's breast tissue?

a. Atrophic ductal structures with increased numbers of lipocytes
b. Dilated ducts filled with granular, necrotic, acidophilic debris
c. Expansion of lobules by monotonous proliferation of epithelial cells
d. Granulomatous inflammation surrounding ducts with numerous plasma cells
e. Proliferation of ducts in hyalinized fibrous tissue with periductal edema

Reproductive Systems

Answers

354. The answer is d. (*Kumar, p 1035. Rubin, pp 935, 938–939.*) Genital malformations affecting the penis include abnormal locations of the urethral opening and phimosis. Because of a malformation the urethral opening may be located either on the ventral (inferior) surface of the penis (hypospadias) or the dorsal (superior) surface (epispadias). These abnormal locations may produce obstruction, urinary tract infection, or problems with infertility. Hypospadias, which is more common, results from failure of the urethral folds to close, while epispadias results from faulty positioning of the genital tubercle. Epispadias is also associated with exstrophy of the urinary bladder. In contrast, abnormal development of the prepuce (foreskin) may result in the inability for it to retract over the glans penis, this condition being called phimosis. Repeated inflammation of the glans and prepuce can lead to scarring. Abnormal fusion of the paramesonephric ducts can produce uterine abnormalities, such as a double uterus or a bicornuate uterus.

355. The answer is d. (*Kumar, p 1035. Rubin, p 936. Damjanov, pp 1710–1711, 2190–2191. Sadler, pp 351–352.*) Phimosis occurs when the orifice of the prepuce (foreskin) is too small to permit normal retraction. This may be due to inflammatory scarring or abnormal development of the prepuce. If a phimotic prepuce is forcibly retracted over the glans penis, a condition called paraphimosis may develop. This condition is extremely painful and may cause obstruction of the urinary tract or blood flow, which may lead to necrosis of the penis. Nonspecific infection of the glans and prepuce is called balanoposthitis. Genital malformations may cause an abnormal location of the urethral opening, either on the ventral surface of the penis (hypospadias) or the dorsal surface (epispadias). These abnormal developments may cause problems with infertility. Hypospadias is the result of failure of the urethral folds to close, while epispadias is the result of faulty positioning of the genital tubercle. The latter is also associated with exstrophy of the urinary bladder.

356. The answer is d. (*Kumar, pp 1035–1037. Rubin, pp 936–938.*) Clear vacuolization of the superficial layers of the epithelial cells (koilocytosis) is characteristic of infection by human papillomavirus (HPV). These changes are found in both condyloma acuminatum and verrucous carcinoma, but condyloma is a benign papillary lesion that does not grow into the underlying tissue, while verrucous carcinoma, also known as giant condyloma or Buschke-Löwenstein tumor, invades the underlying tissue along a broad front. This type of invasion is in contrast to squamous cell carcinomas, which invade tissue as finger-like projections of atypical squamous epithelial cells. Three dysplastic, precancerous intraepithelial lesions of the penis that do not invade into the underlying tissue are Bowen's disease, erythroplasia of Queyrat, and Bowenoid papulosis.

357. The answer is d. (*Kumar, pp 1037–1039. Rubin, pp 939–941.*) The condition illustrated is cryptorchidism (failure of the testis to descend into the scrotum). It is present in up to 1% of males after puberty and is unilateral in the majority of cases. The testis is small, brown, and atrophic grossly. Microscopically, the tubules are atrophic with thickened basement membranes. The interstitial cells are usually prominent and occasional focal proliferations of Sertoli cells may be seen. The incidence of malignancy is increased 7- to 11-fold, and this risk is greater for abdominal than for inguinal locations. Seminoma is the most common malignancy. The risk of malignancy is not reduced by orchiopexy. There is a smaller but definite risk of malignancy in the contralateral, correctly placed testis.

358. The answer is c. (*Kumar, p 1047. Townsend, pp 1686–1692.*) Scrotal enlargement may be caused by cysts, tumors, inflammatory processes, or abnormalities of the blood vessels. Transillumination is helpful in differentiating between cysts (which transilluminate) and tumors (which do not), but an inguinal-scrotal imaging ultrasound is used to confirm the diagnosis. Benign scrotal cysts may form from abnormalities of the tunica vaginalis. Recall that the processus vaginalis is an outpouching of the peritoneum that enters into the scrotum. When the testis reaches the scrotum, the proximal portion of the processus vaginalis obliterates, but the distal portion persists and does not fuse. This forms the tunica vaginalis of the testis. Examples of cysts that involve this tunica vaginalis include hydroceles, hematoceles, chyloceles, and spermatoceles. Hydroceles contain clear fluid and result from developmental abnormalities or inflammatory processes. Hematoceles result from hemorrhage into a hydrocele, while chyloceles result from the accumulation of lymph fluid within the tunica as a result of elephantiasis.

Spermatoceles refer to cystic enlargements of the efferent ducts or the rete testis with numerous spermatocytes present.

In contrast to transillumination and imaging ultrasound, Doppler flow studies are used to assess perfusion to the testis, while testicular scintigraphy is a type of nuclear scan. Both of these tests are quite useful if testicular torsion is suspected clinically. A surgical biopsy or fine needle aspiration (FNA) of the testis may be performed for a testicular tumor or for the workup of infertility.

359. The answer is d. (*Kumar, pp 1040–1046. Rubin, pp 943–948.*) Germ cell tumors of the testis are clinically divided into two categories—seminomas and nonseminomatous germ cell tumors (NSGCTs)—because of their differences in presentation, metastasis, prognosis, and therapy. The NSGCTs include embryonal carcinomas, yolk sac tumors (infantile embryonal carcinomas or endodermal sinus tumors), choriocarcinomas, and immature teratomas. When compared with NSGCTs, seminomas are extremely radiosensitive, and they are more commonly present with stage I disease. NSGCTs are relatively radioresistant, are more aggressive, and have a worse prognosis. Seminomas typically spread via lymphatics after having remained localized for a long time. Embryonal carcinoma, choriocarcinoma, and mixed tumors with an element of choriocarcinoma tend to metastasize early via the blood. Choriocarcinomas are the most aggressive variant.

Seminomas are characterized histologically by large cells with distinct cell membranes and clear cytoplasm. An important, distinct variant of seminoma is the spermatocytic seminoma. It is characterized by being found in older individuals and by the fact that it does not metastasize. Histologically, a spermatocytic seminoma is characterized by maturation of the tumor cells, some of which histologically resemble secondary spermatocytes. In contrast to the histologic appearance of seminomas and spermatocytic seminomas, choriocarcinomas have a mixture of malignant cytotrophoblasts and syncytiotrophoblasts, malignant teratomas have tissue derived from all three germ levels with scattered immature neural elements, Leydig cells tumors have large tumor cells with abundant eosinophilic, granular cytoplasm, and rare intracytoplasmic rhomboid crystals, and finally, embryonal carcinomas have sheets of undifferentiated tumor cells. Focal glandular differentiation may be present.

360. The answer is b. (*Kumar, pp 1040–1046.*) Germ cell tumors of the testis often secrete enzymes or polypeptide hormones, examples of which include α-fetoprotein (AFP) and human chorionic gonadotropin (hCG). AFP is synthesized by the fetal gut, liver, and yolk sac. It may be secreted by either yolk sac tumors (endodermal sinus tumors) or embryonal carcinomas. AFP may also be secreted by liver cell carcinomas. β-hCG is a glycoprotein that is normally synthesized by placental syncytiotrophoblasts. Markedly elevated serum levels are most often associated with choriocarcinomas, which are characterized histologically by a mixture of malignant cytotrophoblasts and syncytiotrophoblasts. Mildly elevated serum levels of β-hCG may be found in patients with other types of germ cell tumors if they contain syncytiotrophoblast-like giant cells. This is found in about 10% of classic seminomas.

To summarize: markedly elevated levels of hCG are associated with choriocarcinomas, while elevated levels of AFP are most characteristic of yolk sac tumors and embryonal carcinomas. But there are many areas of overlap between tumors, and many tumors are composed of multiple types of germ cell cancers. The only definitive statement that can be made is that elevated serum levels of AFP cannot be seen in a tumor that is a pure seminoma.

361. The answer is b. (*Kumar, pp 1047–1048. Rubin, pp 952–953.*) Inflammation of the prostate (prostatitis) is characterized by finding at least 15 leukocytes per high-power field in prostatic secretions. Prostatitis is classified as being either acute or chronic. Patients with acute prostatitis present with the sudden onset of fever, chills, and dysuria. Acute prostatitis is usually caused by bacteria that cause urinary tract infections and urethritis, most commonly gram-negative infections, especially with *Escherichia coli.*

Chronic prostatitis presents clinically as low back pain, dysuria, and suprapubic discomfort. It is divided into chronic bacterial prostatitis, which is associated with recurrent urinary tract infections (UTIs) with the same organism, and chronic abacterial prostatitis, which is not associated with recurrent UTIs. Instead, chronic abacterial prostatitis is associated with infections with either *Chlamydia trachomatis* or *Ureaplasma urealyticum. Chlamydia trachomatis* should be suspected in patients with chronic prostatitis with negative cultures of urine and prostatic secretions. Granulomatous prostatitis causes vague symptoms and is diagnosed histologically. The most common cause of granulomatous prostatitis in the United States is Bacillus Calmette-Guerin, which is used for the treatment of superficial cancer of the urinary bladder.

362. The answer is d. (*Kumar, pp 1052–1053. Rubin, pp 953–956.*) Benign enlargement of the prostate is caused by benign prostatic hyperplasia

(BPH) and produces clinical symptoms of urinary frequency, nocturia, difficulty in starting and stopping urination, dribbling, and dysuria. Histologically, the hyperplastic nodules are composed of a variable mixture of hyperplastic glands and hyperplastic stromal cells. Histologic signs of malignancy are not present. The development of BPH is associated with increased age and higher testosterone levels. BPH results from androgen-induced glandular proliferation, but estrogen also sensitizes the tissue to androgens. Urinary obstruction results because the inner, periurethral portions of the prostate (the middle and lateral lobes) are affected most commonly. BPH does not predispose the individual to cancer. In contrast to the benign histology of BPH, the histologic signs characteristic of prostatic adenocarcinoma include small glands that appear "back to back" without intervening stroma or that appear to be infiltrating beyond the normal prostate lobules. Histologically, these malignant glands are composed of a single layer of cuboidal epithelial cells, because the outer basal layer of epithelial cells, seen in normal and hyperplastic glands, is not present. These malignant cells often contain one or more enlarged nucleoli.

363. The answer is c. (*Kumar, pp 1050–1056.*) Knowledge of the anatomic division of the prostate is important in understanding the locations of the major pathologic diseases of the prostate. Most adenocarcinomas of the prostate originate in the peripheral zone, while hyperplastic nodules originate in the transition zone. This anatomic differentiation is the result of the physiologic fact that the transition zone is particularly estrogen-sensitive, while the peripheral zone is particularly androgen-sensitive. Dihydrotestosterone (DHT), which is formed from testosterone by the action of 5-α-reductase, is responsible for the development of the prostate during fetal growth and also at the time of puberty. With aging, DHT levels are increased in the prostate, where DHT binds to nuclear DNA and causes prostatic hyperplasia. This hyperplastic effect by DHT is augmented by estrogen, which appears to function by induction of androgen receptors, and therefore this hyperplasia occurs in the portion of the prostate that is particularly estrogen-sensitive.

364. The answer is c. (*Kumar, pp 1060–1061. Sadler, pp 322–327.*) The paired genital ducts consist of the mesonephric (Wolffian) duct, which extends from the mesonephros to the cloaca, and the paramesonephric (Müllerian) duct, which runs parallel and lateral to the Wolffian duct. The mesonephric ducts in males, if stimulated by testosterone secreted by the

Leydig cells, develop into the vas deferens, epididymis, and seminal vesicles. In contrast, because normal females do not secrete testosterone, the Wolffian ducts regress and form vestigial structures. They may, however, form mesonephric cysts in the cervix or vulva, or they may form Gartner duct cysts in the vagina. The cranial group of mesonephric tubules (the epoophoron) remains as vestigial structures in the broad ligament above the ovary, while the caudal group of mesonephric tubules (the paroophoron) forms vestigial structures in the broad ligament beside the ovary. The paramesonephric (Müllerian) ducts in the female form the fallopian tubes, the uterus, the uppermost vaginal wall, and the hydatid of Morgagni. The lower portion of the vagina and the vestibule develop from the urogenital sinus. Males secrete Müllerian-inhibiting factor (MIF) from the Sertoli cells of the testes, which causes regression of the Müllerian ducts. This results in the formation of the vestigial appendix testis. The metanephric duct in both sexes forms the ureter, renal pelvis, calyces, and renal collecting tubules. Several abnormalities result from abnormal embryonic development of the Müllerian ducts. Uterine agenesis may result from abnormal development or fusion of these paired paramesonephric ducts. Developmental failure of the inferior portions of the Müllerian ducts results in a double uterus, while failure of the superior portions to fuse (incomplete fusion) may form a bicornuate uterus. Retarded growth of one of the paramesonephric ducts along with incomplete fusion to the other paramesonephric ducts results in the formation of a bicornuate uterus with a rudimentary horn.

365. The answer is e. (*Kumar, pp 1060, 1065, 1070, 1072–1073.*) Obstruction of the ducts of any of the glands found within the female genitalia may cause the formation of a genital cyst. The paired Bartholin's glands, which are analogous to the bulbourethral glands of the male, are located in the lateral wall of the vestibule. If these are obstructed, a cyst may form that is usually lined with transitional epithelium. Gartner's duct cysts, derived from Wolffian (mesonephric) duct remnants, are located in the lateral walls of the vagina. Cysts derived from the same Wolffian duct may also be found on the lateral aspect of the vulva and are called mesonephric cysts. Obstruction of the ducts of the mucous glands in the endocervix may result in small mucous (Nabothian) cysts. Cysts may also be found within the skin of the vulva. These cysts, which contain white, cheesy material, are called keratinous (epithelial inclusion) cysts. Clinically they are referred to as sebaceous cysts, which is a misnomer. Follicular cysts are benign cysts of the ovary, while "chocolate cysts" refers to cystic areas of endometriosis that include hemorrhages and blood clots.

366. The answer is a. (*Kumar, pp 1065–1066. Rubin, pp 970–972.*) Several pathologic conditions are associated with the formation of white plaques on the vulva, which are clinically referred to as leukoplakia. Lichen sclerosis is seen histologically as atrophy of the epidermis with underlying dermal fibrosis. This abnormality is seen in postmenopausal women, who develop pruritic white plaques of the vulva. It is not thought to be premalignant. Loss of pigment in the epidermis (vitiligo) can also produce leukoplakia. Inflammatory skin diseases, such as chronic dermal inflammation, squamous hyperplasia (characterized by epithelial hyperplasia and hyperkeratosis), and vulvar intraepithelial neoplasia (characterized by epithelial atypia or dysplasia), can also present with leukoplakia. A term related to leukoplakia is vulvar dystrophy, but this refers specifically to either lichen sclerosis or squamous hyperplasia. Because the latter is sometimes associated with epithelial dysplasia, it is also referred to as hyperplastic dystrophy. It is most commonly seen in postmenopausal women. The male counterpart of lichen sclerosis, called balanitis xerotica obliterans, is found on the penis. Paget's disease is a malignant tumor that can be found in the breast or the vulva. The latter is seen clinically as pruritic, red, crusted, sharply demarcated map-like areas. Histologically, these malignant lesions reveal single anaplastic tumor cells surrounded by clear spaces ("halos") infiltrating the epidermis. These malignant cells stain positively with PAS and mucicarmine stains.

367. The answer is c. (*Kumar, pp 1066–1070. Rubin, p 973.*) Two rare vulvar malignancies, characterized by malignant cells that individually infiltrate the epidermis, are Paget's disease and malignant melanoma. Paget's disease, which manifests grossly as pruritic, red, crusted, sharply demarcated map-like areas, histologically reveals single anaplastic tumor cells infiltrating the epidermis. These cells are characterized by having clear spaces ("halos") between them and the adjacent epithelial cells. These malignant cells stain positively with PAS or mucicarmine stains. Paget's disease of the vulva (extramammary Paget's disease) is similar to Paget's disease of the nipple except that 100% of cases of Paget's disease of the nipple are associated with an underlying ductal carcinoma of the breast, while vulvar lesions are most commonly confined to the skin. Malignant melanoma of the vulva may resemble Paget's disease both grossly and microscopically; however, these malignant cells stain positively with a melanin stain or an S100 immunoperoxidase stain. In contrast to these rare vulvar malignancies, squamous cell carcinoma is the most common histologic type of vulvar cancer. Clear cell adenocarcinoma and sarcoma botryoides are two rare vaginal malignancies. Clear cell carcinoma is associated with previous maternal DES exposure, while sarcoma botryoides is a type of rhabdomyosarcoma found in girls.

368. The answer is a. (*Kumar, pp 1071–1072. Rubin, p 975.*) Adenocarcinomas of the vagina and cervix have always existed, but rates are increased in young women whose mothers received diethylstilbestrol (DES) while pregnant. DES, which has estrogenic activity, was used in the past to terminate an attack of threatened abortion and thereby stabilize the pregnancy. However, a side effect of this therapy proved to be a particular form of adenocarcinoma, clear cell carcinoma. The tumor, which carries a poor prognosis, has at least three histologic patterns. One is a tubulopapillary configuration, followed by sheets of clear cells and glands lined by clear cells, and solid areas of relatively undifferentiated cells. Many of the cells have cytoplasm that protrudes into the lumen and produces a "hobnail" (nodular) appearance. Prior to the development of adenocarcinoma, a form of adenosis consisting of glands with clear cytoplasm that resembles that of the endocervix can be seen. This has been termed vaginal adenosis and may be a precursor of clear cell carcinoma. Clinically, adenosis of the vagina is manifested by red, moist granules superimposed on the pink-white vaginal mucosa.

369. The answer is d. (*Kumar, pp 1073–1079. Rubin, pp 980–983.*) Cervical condylomata and cervical intraepithelial neoplasia (CIN), which comprises both dysplasia and carcinoma in situ (CIS), are associated with human papillomavirus (HPV) infection. More than 50 genotypes of HPV are known at present, and condylomata acuminata are associated with types 6 to 11, while types 16 to 18 are usually present in CIN. Histologically, HPV infection is characterized by prominent perinuclear cytoplasmic vacuolization with shrunken, dark, irregular nuclei (koilocytosis). Following an abnormal Pap smear report suggesting condyloma, CIN, or possible invasive carcinoma, workup of the patient should include colposcopy, multiple cervical punch biopsies, and endocervical curettage to distinguish among patients who have invasive cancer, CIN, or flat condylomata. In contrast, Epstein-Barr virus is a cause of infectious mononucleosis ("mono"), herpes simplex virus is a cause of "herpes," and parvovirus B19 is a cause of "fifth disease."

370. The answer is d. (*Kumar, p 1083.*) The endometrium and myometrium are relatively resistant to infections. Therefore, inflammation of the endometrium (endometritis) is rare. The diagnosis of endometritis depends on finding inflammatory cells within the endometrium that are not present during the normal menstrual cycle. Polymorphonuclear leukocytes (neutrophils) are normally present during menstruation, while a stromal lymphocytic infiltrate can be seen at other times during the menstrual cycle. Lymphoid aggregates and lymphoid follicles may also be seen in normal endometrium. Therefore the presence of any of these types of leukocytes is not diagnostic of endometritis. Acute endometritis is usually caused by bacterial infection following delivery or miscarriage and is characterized by the presence of neutrophils in endometrial tissue that is not menstrual endometrium. The histologic diagnosis of chronic endometritis depends on finding plasma cells within the endometrium. All it takes is one plasma cell to make the diagnosis. Chronic endometritis may be seen in patients with intrauterine devices (IUDs), pelvic inflammatory disease (PID), retained products of conception (postpartum), or tuberculosis. The latter is characterized histologically by the presence of caseating granulomas with Langhans giant cells. These are secondary causes of chronic endometritis. In a significant number of cases, no underlying cause is found. Decidualized stromal cells are the result of the effects of progesterone and are seen normally in the late secretory phase or in patients who are pregnant. Histologically, these stromal cells contain abundant eosinophilic cytoplasm.

371. The answer is d. (*Kumar, pp 1083–1084. Rubin, pp 988–991.*) Endometrial tissue located in abnormal locations is still under the cyclic influence of hormones and may produce menorrhagia, dysmenorrhea, and cyclic pelvic pain. The ectopic endometrial tissue may be located within the myometrium or it may be found outside of the uterus. The former type, consisting of nests of endometrial stroma within the myometrium, is called adenomyosis. It is thought to result from the abnormal down growth of the endometrium into the myometrium. Symptoms produced by adenomyosis include menorrhagia, colicky dysmenorrhea, dyspareunia, and pelvic pain.

Ectopic endometrial tissue outside of the uterus is called endometriosis and histologically reveals endometrial glands, stroma, and hemosiderin pigment (from the cyclic bleeding). Repeated cyclic bleeding in patients with endometriosis can lead to the formation of cysts that contain areas of new and old hemorrhages. Because they grossly contain blood clots, these cysts have been called "chocolate cysts." Endometriosis is thought to possibly arise from metaplasia of celomic epithelium into endometrial tissue, or implantation of normal fragments of menstrual endometrium either via the fallopian tubes or via the blood vessels. Other sites of endometriosis include the uterine ligaments (associated with dyspareunia), the rectovaginal pouch (associated with pain on defecation and low back pain), the fallopian tubes (associated with peritubular adhesions, infertility, and ectopic pregnancies), the urinary bladder (associated with hematuria), the GI tract (associated with pain, adhesions, bleeding, and obstruction), and the vagina (associated with bleeding).

372. The answer is c. (*Kumar, pp 1080–1083. Rubin, pp 991–992.*) With normal menstruation about 30 to 40 mL of blood is lost. Amounts greater than 80 mL lost on a continued basis are considered to be abnormal. Menorrhagia refers to excessive bleeding at the time of menstruation, either in the number of days or the amount of blood. A submucosal leiomyoma could produce menorrhagia. Metrorrhagia refers to bleeding that occurs at irregular intervals, while menometrorrhagia refers to excessive bleeding that occurs at irregular intervals. Causes of either of these include cervical polyps, cervical carcinoma, endometrial carcinoma, or exogenous estrogens. Postmenopausal bleeding occurs more than 1 year after the normal cessation of menses at menopause. Oligomenorrhea refers to infrequent bleeding that occurs at intervals greater than 35 days. Causes include polycystic ovarian syndrome and too low a total body weight. Polymenorrhea refers to frequent, regular menses that are less than 22 days apart. It is commonly associated with anovulatory cycles, which can occur at menarche. Dysmenorrhea refers to painful menses. It is associated with increased levels of prostaglandin F in the menstrual fluid.

373. The answer is b. (*Kumar, pp 1080–1083. Rubin, pp 991–992.*) Dysfunctional uterine bleeding (DUB) is defined as abnormal uterine bleeding that is due to a functional abnormality rather than an organic lesion of the uterus. In contrast, secondary dysmenorrhea refers to painful menses associated with an organic cause, such as endometriosis, which is the most common cause. Most cases of DUB are related to an endocrine abnormality affecting the hypothalamic-pituitary-ovarian axis. The three main categories of DUB are anovulatory cycles (the most common form), inadequate luteal phase, and irregular shedding. Anovulatory cycles consist of persistence of the Graafian follicle without ovulation. This results in continued and excess estrogen production without the normal postovulatory rise in progesterone levels. With no progesterone production, no secretory endometrium is formed. Instead, biopsies reveal nonsecretory (proliferative) endometrium with mild hyperplasia. The mucosa becomes too thick and is sloughed off, resulting in the abnormal bleeding. Anovulatory cycles characteristically occur at menarche and menopause. They are also associated with polycystic ovary (Stein-Leventhal) syndrome. It is important to note that other causes of unopposed estrogen effect can lead to this appearance of a proliferative endometrium with mild hyperplasia. These causes include exogenous estrogen administration or estrogen-secreting neoplasms, such as a granulosa cell tumor of the ovary or an adrenal cortical neoplasm. If there is ovulation but the functioning of the corpus luteum is inadequate, then the levels of progesterone are decreased, resulting in asynchrony between the chronologic dates and the histologic appearance of the secretory endometrium. This is referred to as an inadequate luteal phase (luteal phase defect) and is an important cause of infertility. Biopsies are usually performed several days after the predicted time of ovulation. If the histologic dating of the endometrium lags 4 or more days behind the chronologic date predicted by the menstrual history, the diagnosis of luteal phase defect can be made. Clinically, these patients exhibit low serum progesterone, FSH, and LH levels. In contrast, prolonged functioning of the corpus luteum (persistent luteal phase with continued progesterone production) results in prolonged heavy bleeding at the time of menses. Histologically, there is a combination of secretory glands mixed with proliferative glands (irregular shedding). Clinically, these patients have regular periods, but the menstrual bleeding is excessive and prolonged (lasting 10 to 14 days). Current oral contraceptives, being a combination of estrogen and progesterone, cause the endometrium to include inactive glands with predecidualized stroma. The endometrium in postmenopausal women reveals an atrophic pattern with atrophic or inactive glands.

374. The answer is a. (*Kumar, pp 1085–1088. Rubin, p 993.*) Endometrial hyperplasia, related to excess estrogens, is important clinically because of its relation to the development of endometrial adenocarcinoma. The types of endometrial hyperplasia include simple hyperplasia, complex hyperplasia, and atypical hyperplasia. Simple hyperplasia, which histologically resembles proliferative-type endometrium, was previously classified as mild hyperplasia or cystic hyperplasia. In cystic hyperplasia, some glands become dilated or form cysts. Complex hyperplasia consists of crowded endometrial glands having budding, but no cytologic atypia, while atypical hyperplasia is characterized by complex glandular crowding with cellular atypia. The most important prognostic feature is the presence of cytologic atypia. Therefore, both simple hyperplasia and complex hyperplasia are lower-grade hyperplasias, while atypical hyperplasia, which used to be called adenomatous hyperplasia with atypia, is a higher-grade hyperplasia. In contrast to the types of hyperplasia, endometrial adenocarcinoma is characterized by stromal invasion by malignant glands.

375. The answer is a. (*Kumar, pp 1086–1089. Damjanov, pp 2269–2271.*) Cancers that originate from the endometrium grossly may present as a polypoid mass within the uterine cavity or a diffuse tumor involving the endometrium with possible spread into the myometrium. Histologically they are adenocarcinomas that are composed of malignant, infiltrating glandular structures. If there are areas of squamous differentiation within these tumors, they are called adenoacanthomas. If there are areas of malignant squamous differentiation, they are called adenosquamous carcinomas. Endometrial carcinoma affects menopausal and postmenopausal women, with the peak incidence at 55 to 65 years of age. Although it was much less common than squamous cervical cancer several decades ago, it has not been controlled as effectively as cervical cancer by the Papanicolaou smear technique and therapy, so that it is now more common than invasive cervical cancer. However, the major symptom of endometrial carcinoma—postmenopausal bleeding—results in diagnosis while the tumor is still confined to the uterus (stage I or II), which permits cure by surgery or radiotherapy. The annual death rate in the United States from endometrial cancer is 3000, while more than 6000 deaths result from squamous cervical cancer. Risk factors for endometrial cancer include obesity and glucose intolerance or diabetes.

376. The answer is a. (*Damjanov, pp 2273–2275. Rubin, pp 998–1000.*) "Fibroids" of the uterus are among the most common abnormalities seen in uteri surgically removed in the United States in women of reproductive age. They arise in the myometrium, submucosally, subserosally, and mid-wall, both singly and several at a time. Sharply circumscribed, they are benign smooth-muscle tumors that are firm, gray-white, and whorled on cut section. Their malignant counterpart, leiomyosarcoma of the uterus, is quite rare in the de novo state and arises even more rarely from an antecedent leiomyoma. Whereas cell pleomorphism, tissue necrosis, and cytologic atypia per se are established criteria in assessing malignancy in tumors generally, they are important to the pathologist in uterine fibroids only if mitoses are also present. Regardless of cellularity or atypia, if 10 or more mitoses are present in 10 separate high-power microscopic fields, the lesion is a leiomyosarcoma. If five or fewer mitoses are present in 10 fields with bland morphology, the leiomyoma will behave in a benign fashion. Problems arise when the mitotic counts range between three and seven per 10 fields with varying degrees of cell and tissue atypia. These equivocal lesions should be regarded by both pathologist and clinician as "gray-area" smooth-muscle tumors of unpredictable biologic behavior. Fortunately, the gray-area leiomyoma of the uterus is rarely seen. Thus mitoses are the most important criteria in assessing malignancy in smooth-muscle tumors of the uterus.

377. The answer is e. (*Kumar, pp 1065–1066. Rubin, pp 964–966, 1000–1001.*) Pelvic inflammatory disease (PID) is a common disorder caused by infection with either gonococci (the most common cause), chlamydiae, or enteric bacteria. Gonococcal infection, seen microscopically as gram-negative intracellular diplococci, begins in the Bartholin's glands and then spreads upward to involve the fallopian tubes and tuboovarian regions. This produces PID, which is characterized by pelvic pain, fever, adnexal tenderness, and pain when the cervix is manipulated. Complications of PID include peritonitis from rupture of a tuboovarian abscess, infertility, and intestinal obstruction.

378. The answer is d. (*Kumar, pp 1092–1093. Chandrasoma, pp 764–767.*) Infertility affects close to 20% of married couples in the United States, and in many of these cases the infertility is related to polycystic ovary (Stein-Leventhal) syndrome in the female. The symptoms of patients with this syndrome are related to increased androgen production, which causes hirsutism, and decreased ovarian follicle maturation, which can lead to amenorrhea. These patients typically have excess androgens (andro-stenedione), increased estrogen levels, increased LH levels, increased GnRH levels, and decreased FSH levels (with a high LH/FSH ratio). The cause of this syndrome is thought to be the abnormal secretion of gonadotropins by the pituitary. Increased secretion of LH stimulates the thecal cells to secrete excess amounts of androgens, which are converted to estrone by the peripheral aromatization of androgens by the adrenal gland. Excess estrogens in turn increase the levels of gonadotropin-releasing hormone (GnRH) but decrease the levels of FSH. The GnRH increases the levels of LH, which then stimulate the thecal cells of the ovary to secrete more androgens, and the hormonal cycle begins again. The ovaries in these patients are enlarged and show thick capsules, hyperplastic ovarian stroma, and numerous follicular cysts, which are lined by a hyperplastic theca interna. Because these patients do not ovulate, there is a markedly decreased number of corpora lutea, which in turn results in decreased progesterone levels. These patients also have an increased risk of developing endometrial hyperplasia and endometrial carcinoma because of the excess estrogen production. Treatment for these patients in the past involved surgical wedge resection of the ovary, but now clomiphene, which stimulates ovulation, is used.

379. The answer is a. (*Kumar, pp 1093–1099. Rubin, pp 1004–1010.*) The surface epithelial tumors of the ovary are derived from the surface celomic epithelium, which embryonically gives rise to the Müllerian epithelium. Therefore these ovarian epithelial tumors may recapitulate the histology of organs derived from the Müllerian epithelium. For example, serous ovarian tumors are composed of ciliated columnar serous epithelial cells, which are similar to the lining cells of the fallopian tubes. Endometrioid ovarian tumors are composed of nonciliated columnar cells, which are similar to the lining cells of the endometrium. Mucinous ovarian tumors are composed of mucinous nonciliated columnar cells, which are similar to the epithelial cells of the endocervical glands. Other epithelial ovarian tumors are similar histologically to other organs of the urogenital tract, such as the clear cell ovarian carcinoma and the Brenner tumor. Clear cell carcinoma of the ovary is similar histologically to clear cell carcinoma of the kidney, or more accurately, the clear cell variant of endometrial adenocarcinoma or the glycogen-rich cells associated with pregnancy. The Brenner tumor is similar to the transitional lining of the renal pelvis or bladder. This ovarian tumor is associated with benign mucinous cystadenomas of the ovary.

380. The answer is c. (*Kumar, pp 1102–1104. Rubin, p 1006.*) The most common type of ovarian tumor that is composed of cells that stain positively with inhibin is a granulosa cell tumor. Histologically the cells may form Call-Exner bodies, which are gland-like structures formed by the tumor cells aligning themselves around a central space that is filled with acidophilic material. The tumor cells may secrete estrogens and cause precocious sexual development in girls or increase the risk for endometrial hyperplasia and carcinoma in women. Less commonly granulosa cell tumors can secrete androgens and produce masculinization. Sertoli-Leydig tumors (androblastomas) also may secrete androgens and produce virilization in women. The tumor cells may stain positively with inhibin, but Call-Exner bodies are not present. Granulosa cell tumors vary in their clinical behavior, but they are considered to be potentially malignant.

Pseudomyxoma peritonei refers to the formation of multiple mucinous masses within the peritoneum. This condition results from the spread of mucinous tumors, either from metastasis or rupture of an ovarian mucinous cyst. Most cases, however, probably result from spread of a mucinous tumor located in the appendix (mucocele). This condition is difficult to treat surgically and if widespread can lead to intestinal obstruction and possibly death.

381. The answer is c. (*Damjanov, pp 2293–2294. Kumar, pp 1099–1100.*) Benign cystic teratomas constitute about 10% of cystic ovarian tumors. The cysts contain greasy sebaceous material mixed with a variable amount of hair. The cysts' walls contain skin and skin appendages, including sebaceous glands and hair follicles. A variety of other tissues—such as cartilage, bone, tooth, thyroid, respiratory tract epithelium, and intestinal tissue—may be found. The presence of skin and skin appendages gives the tumor its other name, dermoid cyst. Dermoid cysts are benign, but in less than 2%, one element may become malignant, most frequently the squamous epithelium.

In contrast to the characteristic histologic findings with a dermoid cyst, an ovarian Brenner tumor histologically is similar to the transitional lining of the renal pelvis or bladder. Chronic salpingitis would reveal the presence of chronic inflammatory cells, such as lymphocytes and macrophages, within the fallopian tubes, while histologic sections from an ectopic pregnancy would reveal chorionic villi, and possibly, fetal tissue.

382. The answer is b. (*Kumar, pp 1093–1094, 1102–1104. Chandrasoma, pp 775–776.*) Ovarian neoplasms are divided into four main categories: epithelial tumors, sex cord-stromal tumors, germ cell tumors, and metastases. Examples of ovarian stromal tumors include thecomas, fibromas, granulosa cell tumors, and Sertoli-Leydig cell tumors. Histologically, the-comas are composed of spindle-shaped cells with vacuolated cytoplasm. They are vacuolate because of steroid hormone (estrogen) production, which can be stained with an oil red O stain. Fibromas are also composed of spindle-shaped cells, but they do not produce steroid hormones and are oil red O–negative. Fibromas are associated with Meigs' syndrome, which consists of an ovarian fibroma, ascites, and hydrothorax.

The stromal cells of the ovary are the precursors of endocrine-active cells, so it is easy to understand that neoplasms derived from these stromal cells are often associated with hormone production. For example, granu-losa cells normally secrete estrogens, thecal cells normally secrete andro-gens, and hilar cells (Leydig cells) may secrete androgens. Excess androgen production in females may lead to masculinization and produce symptoms such as amenorrhea, loss of secondary female sex characteristics, and the development of secondary male characteristics, such as hirsutism, tempo-ral balding, and deepening of the voice. Ovarian tumors associated with excess androgen production include androblastomas (Sertoli-Leydig cell tumors). Other ovarian diseases associated with excess androgen produc-tion include polycystic ovarian disease and hyperthecosis. Excess estrogen production is associated with precocious puberty in the young and with endometrial hyperplasia and cancer in older women. Ovarian tumors that may secrete estrogens include granulosa cell tumors and thecomas.

383. The answer is b. (*McPhee, pp 630–634. Kumar, pp 1104–1105.*) Sec-ondary amenorrhea refers to absent menses for 3 months in a woman who had previously had menses. Causes of secondary amenorrhea include preg-nancy (the most common cause), hypothalamic/pituitary abnormalities, ovarian disorders, and end organ (uterine) disease. Pregnancy can be diag-nosed by obtaining a clinical history along with a pregnancy test that deter-mines serum or urine β-human chorionic gonadotropin (β-hCG) levels. Placental human chorionic gonadotropin (hCG), secreted by syncytiotro-phoblasts, functions early in pregnancy to stimulate the corpus luteum to continue secreting progesterone until the mature placenta, working together with the mother and the fetus, can produce progesterone. Levels of hCG reach a peak at approximately 8 to 10 weeks of development and then rapidly decline.

The remainder of the disorders causing secondary amenorrhea can be differentiated by examining gonadotropin (FSH and LH) levels along with the results of a progesterone challenge test. Withdrawal bleeding following progesterone administration indicates that the endometrial mucosa had been primed with estrogen, which in turn indicates that the hypothalamus/pituitary axis and ovaries are normal. Hypothalamic/pituitary disorders, which are characterized by decreased FSH and LH levels, include functional gonadotropin deficiencies, such as can be seen in patients with a weight loss syndrome. In these patients, markedly decreased body weight (>15% below ideal weight) causes decreased secretion of GnRH from the hypothalamus. Decreased gonadotropin levels decrease estrogen levels, which results in amenorrhea and an increased risk for osteoporosis. Because of the decreased estrogen levels, a progesterone challenge does not result in withdrawal bleeding. Ovarian conditions, such as surgical removal of the ovaries, would most likely produce elevated gonadotropin levels due to the lack of negative feedback from estrogen and progesterone. Because of the decreased estrogen levels, a progesterone challenge would not result in withdrawal bleeding. Uterine (end organ) disorders are characterized by normal FSH and LH levels. An example is Asherman's syndrome, in which numerous and overly aggressive dilatation and curettage of the endometrium for menorrhagia removes the stratum basalis and no glandular epithelium remains. A patient with Asherman's syndrome would have no response to progesterone.

384. The answer is c. (*Kumar, pp 1105–1106. Chandrasoma, pp 809–811.*) Abruptio placenta refers to premature separation of a normally located placenta. This abnormality produces marked hemorrhage, premature labor, and fetal demise. Factors that predispose an individual to abruptio placenta include use of certain drugs (cocaine, alcohol, tobacco), maternal hypertension, preeclampsia, multiparity, and increasing maternal age. Placenta previa occurs when the placenta implants in the lower uterine segment. This may also result in severe bleeding problems at the time of delivery. Vaginal examination of a patient with this condition could also be dangerous. Placenta accreta refers to the absence of the decidua and the direct attachment of the placenta to the myometrium. There is no plane of separation between the placental villi and the myometrium. It is an important cause of postpartum hemorrhage because the placenta fails to separate from the myometrium at the time of labor. The hemorrhage can be life-threatening, and a total hysterectomy is the treatment of choice. In both placenta accreta and placenta previa the villi are histologically normal and there is no trophoblastic proliferation.

In contrast, gestational trophoblastic disease refers to abnormal proliferation of trophoblastic tissue and includes hydatidiform mole, invasive mole, and malignant choriocarcinoma. These neoplasms all secrete β-human chorionic gonadotropin (β-hCG) and should be suspected clinically whenever the uterus is too large for the estimated gestational age and no fetal movement or heart sounds are present.

385. The answer is c. (*Kumar, p 1105. Rubin, p 1001.*) Ectopic pregnancy is a potentially life-threatening condition if it is not treated by removal before rupture and hemorrhage with fatal exsanguination. The most common location for extrauterine implantation is the fallopian tube (85% of cases), with rare implantation in the ovary or abdomen. If the tubal implantation has existed for 1 to 4 weeks, the β-hCG test result is likely to be negative; thus a negative result does not exclude pregnancy. It is always worthwhile to repeat a laboratory test when the result is unexpected. Tubal pregnancy is not uncommon and should always be considered if endometrial samples suggest gestational change without chorionic villi.

386. The answer is e. (*Kumar, pp 1106–1110. Chandrasoma, pp 811–814.*) Toxemia of pregnancy refers to the combination of hypertension, proteinuria, and pitting edema. This combination of signs is also called preeclampsia. When convulsions develop in an individual with preeclampsia, the condition is then referred to as eclampsia. These signs and symptoms result from abnormal placental implantation with incomplete conversion of the blood vessels of the decidua. Both of these result in placental ischemia. Normally the blood vessels of the uterine wall at the site of implantation increase in diameter and lose their muscular components. These changes increase the blood flow to the placenta and are the result of increased production of prostacyclin (a strong vasodilator) and decreased production of thromboxane (a potent vasoconstrictor). These changes do not take place at the implantation site in patients who develop preeclampsia. This causes placental ischemia and damages the endothelial cells of the blood vessels of the placenta. This endothelial damage disrupts the normal balance between vasodilation and vasoconstriction. As a result, there are increased levels of vasoconstrictors, such as thromboxane, angiotensin, and endothelin, and decreased levels of vasodilators, such as PGI_2, PGE_2, and nitric oxide. This results in arterial vasoconstriction, which produces systemic hypertension and can lead to activation of intravascular coagulation (DIC). Risk factors for the development of preeclampsia include nulliparity, twin gestation, and hydatidiform mole. Other complications associated with preeclampsia include renal disease and liver disease, such as the HELLP syndrome, which refers to hemolytic anemia, elevated liver enzymes, and low platelets.

387. The answer is b. (*Kumar, pp 1110–1114. Rubin, pp 1020–1024.*) Gestational trophoblastic diseases include benign hydatidiform mole (partial and complete), invasive mole (chorioadenoma destruens), placental site trophoblastic tumor, and choriocarcinoma. Hydatidiform moles, both partial and complete, are composed of avascular, grape-like structures that do not invade the myometrium. It is important to differentiate between these two disorders because about 2% of complete moles may develop into choriocarcinoma, but partial moles are rarely followed by malignancy. In complete (classic) moles, all the chorionic villi are abnormal and fetal parts are not found. In partial moles, only some of the villi are abnormal and fetal parts may be seen. Complete moles have a 46,XX diploid pattern and arise from the paternal chromosomes of a single sperm by a process called androgenesis. In contrast, partial moles have a triploid or a tetraploid karyotype and arise from the fertilization of a single egg by two sperm. Another way to differentiate these two disorders is to use immunostaining for p57, which is a gene that is paternally imprinted (inactivated). Because the complete mole arises only from paternal chromosomes, immunostaining for p57 will be negative.

Invasive moles penetrate the myometrium and may even embolize to distant sites. A similar lesion is the placental site trophoblastic tumor, which is characterized by invasion of the myometrium by intermediate trophoblasts. Gestational choriocarcinomas, composed of malignant proliferations of both cytotrophoblasts and syncytiotrophoblasts without the formation of villi, can arise from either normal or abnormal pregnancies: 50% arise in hydatidiform moles, 25% in cases of previous abortion, 22% in normal pregnancies, and the rest in ectopic pregnancies or teratomas. Both hydatidiform moles and choriocarcinomas have high levels of human chorionic gonadotropin (hCG); the levels are extremely high in choriocarcinoma unless considerable tumor necrosis is present.

388. The answer is d. (*McPhee, pp 625–626. Kumar, pp 1082–1083.*) Menopause refers to cessation of menstrual cycles in females, while menarche refers to the first menstrual cycle. Characteristics of menopause include elevated gonadotropins (FSH is the best indicator), secondary amenorrhea, hot flashes, decreased vaginal secretions, and night sweats. In addition, atrophy begins in estrogen-dependent tissues, such as the vagina. Gradual loss of bone density can lead to osteoporosis.

389. The answer is e. (*Kumar, pp 1124–1126. Rubin, pp 1033–1034.*) Fat necrosis of the breast is characterized by necrotic fat surrounded by lipid-laden macrophages and a neutrophilic infiltration. It is associated with trauma to the breasts, usually in women with pendulous breasts. Traumatic fat necrosis differs from enzymatic fat necrosis because it does not involve the pancreatic enzyme lipase. Fat necrosis may be confused clinically with cancer; however, in contrast to cancer, fat necrosis is painful. Numerous neutrophils are seen in acute bacterial infection of the breast (acute mastitis), which is usually seen in the postpartum lactating or involuting breast. Dilation of the breast ducts (ectasia) with inspissation of breast secretions is characteristic of mammary duct ectasia, which is common in elderly women. If large numbers of plasma cells are also present, the lesion is called plasma cell mastitis. Reaction to silicone, as occurs with a ruptured or leaking silicone implant, is characterized histologically by a foreign-body-type granulomatous reaction with multinucleated giant cells and numerous foamy histiocytes.

390. The answer is a. (*Kumar, pp 1126–1129. Rubin, pp 1034–1035.*) Fibrocystic change of the breast is one of the most common features seen in the female breast. It is most likely associated with an endocrine imbalance that causes an abnormality of the normal monthly cyclic events within the breast. These fibrocystic changes are subdivided into nonproliferative and proliferative changes. Nonproliferative changes include fibrosis of the stroma and cystic dilation of the terminal ducts, which when large may form blue-domed cysts. A common feature of the ducts in nonproliferative changes is apocrine metaplasia, which refers to epithelial cells with abundant eosinophilic cytoplasm with apical snouts. Proliferative changes include epithelial hyperplasia of the ducts. This hyperplastic epithelium may form papillary structures (papillomatosis when pronounced) or may be quite abnormal (atypical hyperplasia). Two benign, but clinically important, forms of proliferative fibrocystic change include sclerosing adenosis and radial scar. Both of these may be mistaken histologically for infiltrating ductal carcinoma, but the presence of myoepithelial cells is a helpful sign that points to the benign nature of the proliferation. Sclerosing adenosis is a disease of the terminal lobules that is typically seen in patients 35 to 45 years old. It produces a firm mass, most often located in the upper outer quadrant. Microscopically there is florid proliferation of small ductal structures in a fibrous stroma, which on low power is stellate in appearance and somewhat maintains the normal lobular architecture. A radial scar refers to ductal proliferation around a central fibrotic area.

391. The answer is e. (*Kumar, pp 1149–1151. Rubin, pp 1035–1037.*) The most common benign neoplasm of the breast is fibroadenoma, which typically occurs in the upper outer quadrant of the breast in women between the ages of 20 and 35. These lesions originate from the terminal duct lobular unit and histologically reveal a mixture of fibrous connective tissue and ducts. Clinically, fibroadenomas are rubbery, freely movable, oval nodules that usually measure 2 to 4 cm in diameter. Numerous neutrophils are seen in acute bacterial infection of the breast (acute mastitis), which is usually seen in the postpartum lactating or involuting breast. Dilation of the breast ducts (ectasia) with inspissation of breast secretions is characteristic of mammary duct ectasia, which is common in elderly women. If large numbers of plasma cells are also present, the lesion is called plasma cell mastitis. Fat necrosis of the breast, associated with traumatic injury, is characterized by necrotic fat surrounded by lipid-laden macrophages and a neutrophilic infiltration.

392. The answer is b. (*Damjanov, pp 2365, 2375–2376. Kumar, pp 1128–1129.*) Ductal papillomas are usually found near the nipple and present with a bloody nipple discharge. The histologic distinction between benign cystic intraductal papillomas of the breast and papillary adenocarcinomas is based on multiple criteria. The age of the patient is not of immense importance, since papillomas occur in both younger and older women. Benign papillomas are structured with a complex arrangement of papillary fronds of fibrovascular stalks, covered by one or (usually) two types of cells (epithelial and myoepithelial). Papillary carcinomas are usually of one monotonous cell type and have either no or only a few fibrovascular stalks. Papillary carcinomas show a uniform growth of cells with similar appearance with enclosed tubular spaces; the whole arrangement bridges across the entire lumen at times or simply lines the outer rim of the duct (cribriforming). Peripheral invasion of the stroma, if present at all, makes the diagnosis of carcinoma rather certain. There are lesions in which the differentiation is exceedingly difficult, even in the hands of renowned surgical pathologists. Many competent pathologists understandably prefer to defer the diagnosis on all papillary lesions of the breast on frozen section until well-fixed and optimally prepared permanent sections are available.

393. The answer is b. (*Damjanov, pp 2205–2206, 2363–2364. Kumar, pp 1149–1151.*) Neoplastic proliferations of the stroma of the breast may lead to the formation of either fibroadenomas or phyllodes tumors. Fibroadenomas are characterized histologically by a mixture of fibrous tissue and ducts, with no increase in cellularity or mitoses. Only the stromal cells, not the glandular cells, are clonal proliferations. Another neoplastic tumor that arises from the stromal cells is the phyllodes tumor. It is distinguished from fibroadenomas by a more cellular stroma and the presence of stromal mitoses. The phyllodes tumor, which has been called a cystosarcoma phyllodes, may either be benign or malignant. A benign phyllodes tumor is characterized by increased stromal cells with few mitoses, while a malignant phyllodes tumor has increased numbers of stromal cells that are atypical along with numerous mitoses.

394. The answer is c. (*Kumar, pp 1146–1149. Rubin, pp 1039–1040, 1045–1046.*) Prognostic factors for women with breast cancer have been divided into major prognostic factors and minor prognostic factors. Systemic therapy may be beneficial for most women with nodal metastases or carcinomas larger than 1 cm. Three of the minor prognostic factors are used to help determine the type of chemotherapy to be used. These three factors are the presence of estrogen receptors, the presence of progesterone receptors, and the overexpression of HER2/neu. The evaluation of the hormone receptor status of breast cancer cells is useful to predict the response to hormonal manipulation. Most tumors that are positive for estrogen and progesterone receptors respond to hormone manipulation, such as with tamoxifen, a selective estrogen receptor modulator. Amplification of

HER2/neu, which is a membrane glycoprotein that is involved in control of cell growth, is associated with a poor prognosis. Trastuzumab (Herceptin) is an antibody to HER2/neu. The use of Trastuzumab improved the response to chemotherapy of patients whose tumors overexpressed HER2/neu.

Major prognostic factors include tumor size, the presence of invasion, lymph node metastases, and distant metastases. The presence of metastases to axillary lymph nodes is the single most important prognostic indicator for invasive breast cancers in the absence of distant metastases. The absolute number of involved lymph nodes is directly related to the survival rate. There is a significant decrease in 5-year survival if one to three nodes are positive, but with four or more positive nodes at the time of diagnosis the survival rate is much less. The histologic type and grade of tumor and its size are also important, but minor factors for predicting prognosis. The histologic grade is based on the degree of tubule formation, the number of mitoses present, and the degree of nuclear pleomorphism. Tubule formation is associated with a lower grade and a better prognosis, while nuclear pleomorphism and the number of mitoses are associated with a higher grade and a worse prognosis. Finally, tumors with a high proliferative rate are associated with a worse prognosis, while high levels of urokinase plasminogen activator are associated with a better prognosis.

395. The answer is b. (*Kumar, pp 1139–1142. Rubin, pp 1040–1041.*) Malignant carcinomas of the breast may be either noninvasive or invasive. Noninvasive carcinomas (carcinoma in situ) may be located within the ducts (intraductal carcinoma) or within the lobules (lobular carcinoma in situ). There are several variants of intraductal carcinoma, including comedocarcinoma, cribriform carcinoma, and intraductal papillary carcinoma. Comedocarcinoma grows as a solid intraductal sheet of cells with a central area of necrosis. It is frequently associated with the erb B2/neu oncogene and a poor prognosis. Cribriform carcinoma is characterized by round, ductlike structures within the solid intraductal sheet of epithelial cells, while intraductal papillary carcinoma has a predominant papillary pattern. In contrast, invasive malignancies are characterized by infiltration of the stroma, which may produce a desmoplastic response within the stroma (scirrhous carcinoma). Infiltrating ductal carcinomas also produce yellow-white chalky streaks that result from the deposition of elastic tissue around ducts (elastosis). Other patterns of invasion that produce specific results include infiltration of cells in a single file in infiltrating lobular carcinoma and mucin production in colloid carcinoma.

396. The answer is e. (*Kumar, pp 1142–1146. Rubin, pp 1041, 1044.*) Lobular carcinoma of the breast, both in situ and invasive, is an important lesion clinically because of its tendency to occur multicentrically within the same breast and also because of its association with a high frequency of disease (both ductal and lobular carcinoma) in the opposite breast. Lobular carcinoma in situ is characterized histologically by proliferation of cells of the terminal duct lobular unit, which fills and expands the lobules. Unlike the case with intraductal carcinoma, papillary and cribriform structures are not formed and neither is central necrosis present. Invasive lobular carcinoma is distinguished by its tendency to infiltrate the stroma in a single file. This pattern is not seen with invasive ductal carcinoma, which tends to cause a marked desmoplastic response, causing a scirrhous carcinoma. Infiltrating lobular carcinomas also form concentric "targets" around ducts, and they have an increased frequency of being estrogen receptor-positive.

In contrast to the histologic appearance of infiltrating lobular carcinoma, Paget's disease is characterized by infiltration of the epidermis by malignant cells with clear cytoplasm. Histologic sections of a medullary carcinoma of the breast reveal large syncytium-like sheets of pleomorphic cells surrounded by aggregates of lymphocytes, while colloid breast carcinoma shows small individual malignant cells dispersed within extracellular pools of mucin.

397. The answer is d. (*Kumar, pp 1140–1141. Rubin, pp 1041–1042.*) Infiltration of the nipple by large cells with clear cytoplasm is diagnostic of Paget's disease. These cells are usually found both singly and in small clusters in the epidermis. Paget's disease is always associated with (in fact, it begins with) an underlying intraductal carcinoma that extends to infiltrate the skin of nipple and areola. Paget cells may resemble the cells of superficial spreading melanoma, but they are PAS-positive and diastase-resistant (mucopolysaccharide- or mucin-positive), unlike melanoma cells. Eczematous dermatitis of the nipples is a major differential diagnosis, but is usually bilateral and responds rapidly to topical steroids. Paget's disease should be suspected if the "eczema" persists more than 3 weeks with topical therapy. Paget's disease occurs mainly in middle-aged women but is unusual. In Paget's disease of the vulvar-anal-perineal region, there is very rarely underlying carcinoma. Mammary fibromatosis is a rare, benign spindle cell lesion affecting women in the third decade. Clinically, it may mimic cancer with retraction or dimpling of skin. It should be treated by local excision with wide margins since there is risk of local recurrence.

398. The answer is b. (*Kumar, pp 1146–1149. Rubin, pp 1045–1046.*) Inflammatory breast carcinoma is often misunderstood because of the qualifying adjective inflammatory. The term does not refer to the presence of inflammatory cells, abscess, or any special histologic-type of breast carcinoma; rather, it refers to more of a clinical phenomenon, in that the breast is swollen, erythematous, and indurated and demonstrates a marked increase in warmth. These changes are caused by widespread lymphatic and vascular permeation within the breast itself and in the deep dermis of the overlying skin by breast carcinoma cells. The clinical induration and erythema are presumably related to lymphatic-vascular blockage by tumor cells; if present, these findings mean a worse prognosis.

399. The answer is e. (*Kumar, pp 1151–1152. Rubin, p 1033.*) Gynecomastia (enlargement of the male breast) histologically reveals epithelial hyperplasia within the ducts that is surrounded by hyalinized fibrous tissue. It is caused by an increase in the estrogen-to-androgen ratio. This abnormality may sometimes be found in males at the time of puberty. Other causes of gynecomastia include Klinefelter's syndrome (decreased secretion of testosterone), testicular feminization (androgen insensitivity), testicular tumors, cirrhosis of the liver, alcohol abuse, increased gonadotropin levels (such as choriocarcinoma of the testis), increased prolactin levels, drugs (such as digoxin), or hyperthyroidism. Testicular neoplasms that are associated with gynecomastia are tumors that secrete human chorionic gonadotropin (hCG), which increases the synthesis of estradiol. Testicular tumors associated with the production of hCG include germ cell tumors (choriocarcinoma and seminoma), Leydig cell tumors, and Sertoli cell tumors.

Endocrine System

Questions

DIRECTIONS: Each item below contains a question or incomplete statement followed by suggested responses. Select the **one best** response to each question.

400. A 59-year-old woman presents with headaches and decreasing vision over the past several months. Her children state that she has been bumping into things recently and does not seem to see them when they are not directly in front of her. Physical examination is unremarkable except for the visual field abnormality illustrated in the picture. Her visual problems are most likely to be caused by a tumor originating in which one of the following anatomic areas?

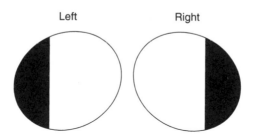

a. Parietal lobe
b. Pineal gland
c. Pituitary gland
d. Posterior orbit
e. Temporal lobe

401. A 25-year-old woman who has never been pregnant presents with amenorrhea for 3 months and a milky discharge from her nipple. She states that her menstrual cycles have been irregular for the past year. Laboratory tests show that her serum LH and estradiol levels are below normal, and a pregnancy test is negative. Which of the following is the most likely cause of these signs and symptoms?

a. Craniopharyngioma of the hypothalamus
b. Germinoma of the pineal gland
c. Islet cell adenoma of the pancreas
d. Medullary carcinoma of the thyroid gland
e. Prolactinoma of the pituitary gland

402. A 42-year-old man presents with increasing fatigue and occasional headaches. He states that recently he has had to change his shoe size from 9 to 10, and he also thinks that his hands and jaw are now slightly larger. Physical examination reveals a prominent forehead and lower jaw, enlarged tongue, and large hands and feet. Initial laboratory examination reveals increased serum glucose. Which of the following is the most likely explanation for this constellation of clinical findings?

a. Acromegaly
b. Apoplexy
c. Cretinism
d. Diabetes
e. Gigantism

403. A 25-year-old woman presents with the acute onset of cessation of lactation. She delivered her first child several months ago and has been breast-feeding since then. She reports that she has not menstruated since the delivery. She also says that lately she has been tired and has been "feeling cold" all of the time. Laboratory workup reveals a deficiency of ACTH and other anterior pituitary hormones. Which of the following is the most likely cause of this patient's signs and symptoms?

a. Craniopharyngioma
b. Cushing's disease
c. Empty sella syndrome
d. Nonsecretory chromophobe adenoma
e. Sheehan's syndrome

404. A 49-year-old man who smokes two packs of cigarettes a day presents with a lung mass on x-ray and recent weight gain. Laboratory examination shows hyponatremia with hyperosmolar urine. Which of the following is the most likely cause of these clinical findings?

a. Renal failure
b. Pituitary failure
c. Conn's syndrome
d. Cardiac failure
e. Excess ADH

405. A 5-year-old girl is brought to the doctor's office by her mother, who states that the girl has been drinking a lot of water lately and has been urinating much more often than normal. Physical examination reveals a young girl whose eyes protrude slightly. An x-ray of her head reveals the presence of multiple lytic bone lesions involving her calvarium and the base of her skull, a biopsy of which reveals aggregates of Langerhans cells with intracytoplasmic Birbeck's granules. Which of the following sets of laboratory values is most consistent with the expected findings for this girl's disorder?

	Serum Sodium	**Urine**
a.	Hypernatremia	Low osmolarity and low specific gravity
b.	Hypernatremia	High osmolarity and high specific gravity
c.	Hyponatremia	Low osmolarity and low specific gravity
d.	Hyponatremia	High osmolarity and high specific gravity
e.	Normal	Normal osmolarity and normal specific gravity

406. A 28-year-old woman at 24 weeks of gestation of her first pregnancy has the following laboratory data: increased serum total thyroxine; normal free thyroxine; decreased resin triiodothyronine uptake; normal free thyroxine index; and normal thyroid-stimulating hormone. Which of the following is the best clinical interpretation of these laboratory findings?

a. Euthyroid individual with increased thyroid-binding globulin
b. Euthyroid individual with decreased thyroid-binding globulin
c. Hyperthyroid individual with decreased thyroid-binding globulin
d. Hypothyroid individual with decreased thyroid-binding globulin
e. Hypothyroid individual with increased thyroid-binding globulin

407. An 8-month-old infant is being evaluated for growth and mental retardation. Physical examination reveals a small infant with dry, rough skin; a protuberant abdomen; periorbital edema; a flattened, broad nose; and a large, protuberant tongue. Which of the following disorders is the most likely cause of this infant's signs and symptoms?

a. Graves' disease
b. Cretinism
c. Toxic multinodular goiter
d. Toxic adenoma
e. Struma ovarii

408. A 35-year-old woman presents with progressive muscle weakness and cold intolerance. Physical examination finds enlargement of her thyroid gland, which is rubbery in consistency. No lymphadenopathy is found. Laboratory evaluation finds decreased serum levels of both triiodothyronine (T3) and thyroxine (T4), but serum levels of thyroid-stimulating hormone (TSH) are increased. No thyroid-stimulating immunoglobulins are identified in the serum, but thyroidal peroxidase autoantibodies are present. Which of the following histologic findings is most consistent with a diagnosis of Hashimoto's thyroiditis?

a. Diffuse fibrous deposition between atrophic follicles
b. Follicular cell hyperplasia with scalloping of colloid
c. Granulomatous inflammation with multinucleated giant cells
d. Lymphoid infiltrate with scattered Hurthle cells
e. Parafollicular hyperplasia with deposition of amyloid

409. A 29-year-old woman presents with nervousness, heat intolerance, and weight loss. Physical examination reveals the presence of exophthalmus, pretibial myxedema, and diffuse enlargement of the thyroid. Laboratory examination reveals elevated serum thyroxine (T4) and triiodothyronine (T3) levels, while the level of serum thyroid-stimulating hormone (TSH) is decreased. Histologic sections from her thyroid gland reveal increased cellularity with scalloping of the colloid at the margins of the follicles. Which of the following types of autoantibodies is most specific for this individual disease?

a. Antimicrosomal antibodies
b. Antithyroglobulin antibodies
c. Antithyroid peroxidase antibodies
d. TSH-receptor-blocking antibodies
e. TSH-receptor-stimulating antibodies

410. A 58-year-old woman presents with increased "fullness" in her neck. Physical examination finds a single, nonfunctioning mass within the thyroid. Clinically she is found to be euthyroid and her serum TSH level is within normal limits. Histologic sections from this mass reveal a single nodule composed of follicles similar to normal thyroid tissue. The nodule is surrounded by a complete fibrous capsule that compresses adjacent normal thyroid tissue. Focal invasion into the capsule is found. Further evaluation of the tumor cells finds the presence of the PAX8-PPAR-gamma fusion gene. Which of the following is the most likely diagnosis?

a. Colloid carcinoma
b. Colloid goiter
c. Diffuse nontoxic goiter
d. Follicular adenoma
e. Follicular carcinoma

411. A 45-year-old woman presents for a routine physical examination and is found to have several small masses within the right lobe of her thyroid gland. No enlarged lymph nodes are found. Her thyroid gland is resected surgically and histologic sections from the tumor masses reveal multiple papillary structures and scattered small, round, laminated calcifications. Which of the following histologic changes is most likely to be present within these tumor masses?

a. Amyloid stromal invasion by malignant C cells
b. Blood vessel and capsular invasion by malignant follicles
c. Optically clear nuclei with longitudinal nuclear grooves
d. Sheets of small round cells with cytoplasmic glycogen
e. Undifferentiated anaplastic cells with giant cell formation

412. A 37-year-old man presents with a single, firm mass within the thyroid gland. This patient's father developed a tumor of the thyroid gland when he was 32 years of age. Histologic examination of the mass in this 37-year-old man reveals organoid nests of tumor cells separated by broad bands of stroma, as seen in the photomicrograph. The stroma stains positively with Congo red stain and demonstrates yellow-green birefringence. Which of the following is the most likely diagnosis?

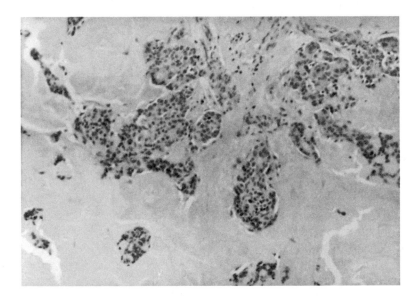

a. Follicular carcinoma
b. Papillary carcinoma
c. Squamous cell carcinoma
d. Medullary carcinoma
e. Anaplastic carcinoma

413. A 21-year-old woman presents with the acute onset of perioral tingling and muscle cramps involving both of her hands. Physical examination finds an anxious woman with an increased respiratory rate, while laboratory examination reveals decreased arterial P_{CO_2}, decreased bicarbonate, and an increased blood pH. The respiratory alkalosis in this individual caused tetany by decreasing the ionized serum levels of what substance?

a. Calcium
b. Chloride
c. Magnesium
d. Potassium
e. Sodium

414. A 52-year-old woman presents with nausea, fatigue, muscle weakness, and intermittent pain in her left flank. Laboratory examination reveals an increased serum calcium and a decreased serum phosphorus. The patient's plasma parathyroid hormone levels are increased, but parathyroid hormone–related peptide levels are within normal limits. Urinary calcium is increased, and microhematuria is present. Which of the following is the most likely cause of this patient's signs and symptoms?

a. Primary hyperparathyroidism
b. Primary hypoparathyroidism
c. Pseudohypoparathyroidism
d. Secondary hyperparathyroidism
e. Secondary hypoparathyroidism

415. A 65-year-old man presents with bone pain and is found to have hypocalcemia and increased parathyroid hormone. Surgical exploration of his neck finds all four of his parathyroid glands to be enlarged. Which of the following disorders is the most likely cause of this patient's enlarged parathyroid glands?

a. Primary hyperplasia
b. Parathyroid adenoma
c. Chronic renal failure
d. Parathyroid carcinoma
e. Lung carcinoma

416. A 65-year-old woman presents with numbness and tingling of her hands, feet, and lips. Physical examination reveals hyperactivity of her muscles, which is illustrated by a positive Chvostek's sign. Which one of the labeled boxes in the graph below best depicts the expected serum levels of calcium and parathyroid hormone in this individual?

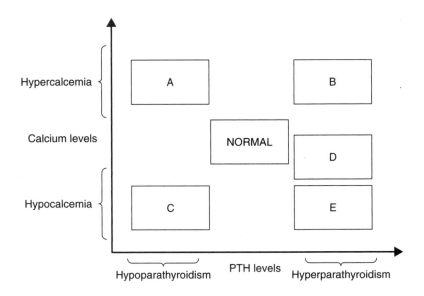

a. Box A
b. Box B
c. Box C
d. Box D
e. Box E

417. A 17-year-old woman with mental retardation presents with cramping in her legs and numbness and tingling around her mouth. Physical examination reveals a short, obese young woman who has several subcutaneous calcified masses. Laboratory examination reveals hypocalcemia despite her PTH being elevated. X-rays of her hands and feet reveal shortened fourth and fifth metacarpal and metatarsal bones. Which of the following is the basic defect causing this disorder?

a. Decreased production of ACTH by the anterior pituitary
b. Defective binding of hormones to guanine nucleotide-binding proteins
c. Malformation of pharyngeal pouches 3 and 4
d. Secretion of parathyroid-related peptide by a benign parathyroid adenoma
e. The presence of autoantibodies to the parathyroid hormone receptor

418. An XX infant is found to have external male genitalia and internal female genitalia. Physical examination reveals decreased blood pressure, while laboratory examination reveals a serum sodium level of 132 meq/L. Additionally, bilateral adrenal cortical hyperplasia is present. A deficiency of which of the following enzymes is most likely to produce the clinical findings in this infant?

a. 3-β-dehydrogenase
b. 11-hydroxylase
c. 17-hydroxylase
d. 21-hydroxylase
e. 1-α-hydroxylase

419. A 55-year-old woman presents with increasing muscle weakness and fatigue. Physical examination finds an obese adult woman with purple abdominal stria and increased facial hair. The excess adipose tissue is mainly distributed in her face, neck, and trunk. Laboratory evaluation finds increased plasma levels of cortisol and glucose. Which of the following is the most likely diagnosis?

a. Addison's disease
b. Bartter's syndrome
c. Conn's syndrome
d. Cushing's syndrome
e. Schmidt's syndrome

420. Which box in the schematic represents the most likely serum findings for an individual on long-term exogenous glucocorticoid administration?

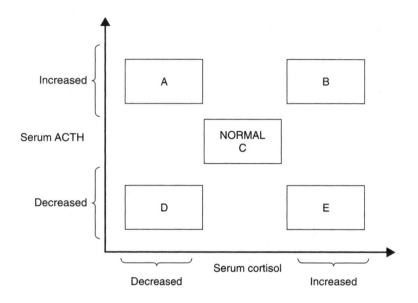

a. Box A
b. Box B
c. Box C
d. Box D
e. Box E

421. A 47-year-old man presents with headaches, muscle weakness, and leg cramps. He is not currently taking any medications. Physical examination finds a thin adult man with mild hypertension. Laboratory examination reveals slightly increased sodium, decreased serum potassium level, and decreased hydrogen ion concentration. Serum glucose levels are within normal limits. A CT scan reveals a large tumor involving the cortex of his left adrenal gland. Which of the following combinations of serum laboratory findings is most likely to be present in this individual?

a. Decreased aldosterone with increased renin
b. Decreased cortisol with decreased ACTH
c. Increased aldosterone with decreased renin
d. Increased cortisol with increased ACTH
e. Increased deoxycorticosterone with increased cortisol

422. A 42-year-old man presents with weakness and dizziness associated with stress. Physical examination reveals a slightly decreased blood pressure along with a diffuse increase in skin pigmentation. Laboratory examination reveals hyponatremia and hyperkalemic acidosis with decreased aldosterone, decreased cortisol, decreased glucose, increased ACTH, decreased sex steroids, and increased LH and FSH. Thyroid function tests are found to be within normal limits. Which of the following is the most likely cause of this patient's signs and symptoms?

a. A benign adenoma of the adrenal cortex
b. A malignant tumor of the adrenal medulla
c. Autoimmune destruction of the adrenal cortex
d. Bilateral hyperplasia of the adrenal cortex
e. Tuberculosis of the adrenal medulla

423. A 41-year-old woman presents with anorexia and weight loss. She has a recent medical history of candida infection of her skin. Physical examination reveals a slightly decreased blood pressure along with increased skin pigmentation. Laboratory examination reveals a low cortisol with increased ACTH. After further workup the diagnosis of adrenal cortical failure is made and a defect in the autoimmune regulator gene is found. Which one of the following abnormalities is most closely associated with this woman's disorder?

a. Hashimoto's thyroiditis
b. Diabetes mellitus
c. Ectodermal dystrophy
d. Parathyroid hyperplasia
e. Pituitary adenoma

424. A 35-year-old man who presents with a neck mass is found to have a serum calcium level of 11.8 mg/dL and periodic elevation of his blood pressure. Extensive workup reveals the presence of a medullary carcinoma of the thyroid, a pheochromocytoma, and hyperplasia of the parathyroid glands. Which of the following is the most likely diagnosis?

a. Multiple endocrine neoplasia syndrome type 1
b. Multiple endocrine neoplasia syndrome type 2A
c. Multiple endocrine neoplasia syndrome type 2B
d. Polyglandular syndrome type I
e. Polyglandular syndrome type II

425. A 34-year-old woman presents with recurrent episodes of severe headaches, palpitations, tachycardia, and sweating. A physical examination reveals her blood pressure to be within normal limits; however, during one of these episodes of headaches, palpitations, and tachycardia, her blood pressure is found to be markedly elevated. Workup finds a small tumor of the right adrenal gland. Which of the following is most likely to be increased in the urine of this individual?

a. Acetone
b. Aminolevulinic acid (ALA)
c. Hydroxy-indoleacetic acid (HIAA)
d. N-formiminoglutamate (FIGlu)
e. Vanillylmandelic acid (VMA)

426. A 2-year-old boy presents with repeated viral and fungal infections and tetany. Workup reveals hypocalcemia and a marked impairment of cell-mediated immunity resulting from an absence of T cells. Because of these signs and symptoms, the diagnosis of DiGeorge's syndrome is made. Considering this diagnosis, the absence of T cells is a direct result of the failure of which embryonic structure to develop?

a. Third pharyngeal pouch
b. Fourth pharyngeal pouch
c. Fifth pharyngeal pouch
d. Ultimobranchial body
e. Foramen cecum

427. A 57-year-old woman presents with difficulty swallowing, drooping eyelids, and double vision. Workup finds a mass in the anterior mediastinum. Biopsies from this mass reveal thymus tissue having scattered reactive lymphoid follicles with germinal centers. Which of the following is the most likely diagnosis?

a. Malignant thymoma
b. Thymic carcinoma
c. Thymic hyperplasia
d. Thymic hypoplasia
e. Thymic lymphoma

428. A 51-year-old woman presents with problems seeing and drooping eyelids. She had been diagnosed 5 years prior as having lupus. A chest x-ray reveals a mass in the anterior mediastinum, which is confirmed by a CT scan. Surgical exploration finds a well-encapsulated tumor. No evidence of invasion is seen. The mass is resected, and histologic sections reveal scattered lymphocytes within a diffuse proliferation of spindle-shaped cells. Which of the following is the cell of origin of this tumor?

a. Epithelial cells of the thymus
b. Fibroblasts of the mediastinal mesenchyme
c. Follicular cells of ectopic thyroid tissue
d. Immature T lymphocytes of the thymus
e. Mesothelial cells of the mediastinal mesothelium

Endocrine System

Answers

400. The answer is c. (*Kumar, p 1158. McPhee, pp 544–546.*) The visual pathway extends from the retina through the optic nerve, then the optic chiasm, through the optic tract, through the lateral geniculate body, and then through the optic radiations of the temporal and parietal lobes to end in the occipital lobes. Lesions in any of these areas produce characteristic visual field defects. For example, bitemporal hemianopsia (loss of vision in the periphery, also called "tunnel vision") is classically produced by lesions that involve the optic chiasm. The pituitary gland, which normally weighs about 0.5 g, lies in a bone depression (the sella turcica) and is covered by dura (diaphragma sellae). Anterior to the diaphragma sellae is the optic chiasm. Pituitary tumors may easily compress the optic chiasm and result in bilateral loss of peripheral vision.

Involvement of the optic nerve produces blindness in one eye (mononuclear anopsia), while involvement of the optic tract on one side results in homonymous hemianopsia (loss of the same side of the visual field in both eyes). A lesion involving the temporal lobe optic radiations produces a homonymous superior field defect, while a lesion involving the parietal lobe optic radiations produces a homonymous inferior field defect.

401. The answer is e. (*Kumar, pp 1158–1161. McPhee, pp 544–548.*) Pituitary adenomas are the most common neoplasms of the pituitary gland. These benign neoplasms are classified according to the hormone or hormones that are produced by the neoplastic cells. The cell types, in order of decreasing frequency, are the following: lactotrope adenomas (which secrete prolactin), null cell adenomas (which do not secrete hormones), somatotrope adenomas (which secrete growth hormone), corticotrophic adenomas (which secrete ACTH), gonadotrope adenomas (which secrete FSH and LH), and thyrotrope cell adenomas (which secrete TSH). Prolactin-secreting tumors (lactotrope adenomas or prolactinomas) produce symptoms of hypogonadism and galactorrhea (milk secretion not associated with pregnancy). In females this hypogonadism produces amenorrhea and infertility, while in males it produces impotence and decreased libido. The same symptoms that are seen with a prolactin-secreting pituitary adenoma can also be produced by certain drugs, such as methyldopa and reserpine.

402. The answer is a. (*Henry, pp 304–306, 1034. Kumar, pp 1161–1162.*) The second most common type of functioning pituitary adenoma is a growth-hormone—secreting somatotropic adenoma. This tumor can produce gigantism if it occurs in children prior to the closure of the epiphyseal plates or acromegaly if it occurs in adults after the closure of the epiphyseal plates. The latter is characterized by cartilaginous-periosteal soft tissue growth of the distal extremities (acromegaly) and growth of the skull and face bones. Additional findings in patients with excess growth hormone production include thickening of the skin, diabetes mellitus, and enlargement of the viscera, including increased size of the heart, kidneys, liver, and spleen. Cardiac failure is usually the mechanism of death. In contrast, cretinism is caused by a deficiency of thyroid hormone in infants, while apoplexy refers to the sudden loss of sensation and consciousness, usually caused by pressure on the brain, or referring to infarction of the pituitary.

403. The answer is e. (*Kumar, pp 1162–1163. Rubin, pp 1156–1158.*) Hypopituitarism results from destructive processes that involve the adenohypophysis (anterior pituitary). These processes may be acute (sudden) or chronic. Sheehan's syndrome, also known as postpartum pituitary necrosis, results from the sudden infarction of the anterior lobe of the pituitary. This can occur with obstetric complications, such as hemorrhage or shock. The pituitary gland normally doubles in size during pregnancy; hypovolemia during delivery decreases blood flow and may result in infarction of the anterior pituitary. Sheehan's syndrome produces symptoms of hypopituitarism. The initial sign is cessation of lactation, which may be followed by secondary amenorrhea due to the loss of gonadotropins. Other signs of hypopituitarism include hypothyroidism and decreased functioning of the adrenal gland. Acute destruction of the pituitary is also associated with DIC and thrombosis of the cavernous sinus. Chronic causes of hypopituitarism include nonsecretory chromophobe pituitary adenomas, empty sella syndrome, and suprasellar (hypothalamic) tumors. Nonsecretory chromophobe adenomas present as space-occupying lesions that cause decreased hormone production. The gonadotropins are lost first, which results in signs of hypogonadism. Types of chromophobe adenomas include null cell adenomas (no cytoplasmic granules), chromophobes (sparse granules), and oncocytic adenomas (increased cytoplasmic mitochondria). The term pituitary apoplexy refers to spontaneous hemorrhage into a pituitary tumor, while the empty sella syndrome is caused by a defective diaphragma sellae, which permits CSF from the third ventricle to enter the sella. It may also be secondary to infarction or necrosis. A CT scan reveals the sella to be enlarged or to appear empty.

404. The answer is e. (*Kumar, pp 1163–1164. Goldman, pp 549–550, 1047–1050.*) The syndrome of inappropriate antidiuretic hormone (SIADH) is an important cause of dilutional hyponatremia that has been identified in tumors of the thymus gland, malignant lymphoma, and pancreatic neoplasms. It occurs predominantly, however, as a result of ectopic secretion of ADH by small cell carcinomas of the lung. Since the tumor cells per se are autonomously producing ADH, there is no feedback inhibition from the hypothalamic osmoreceptors, and the persistent ADH effect on the renal tubules causes water retention even with concentrated urine, hence the term inappropriate ADH. Laboratory findings include low plasma sodium levels (dilutional hyponatremia), low plasma osmolality, and high urine osmolality caused by disproportionate solute excretion without water.

405. The answer is a. (*Kumar, pp 701–702, 1163–1164. Rubin, pp 1161, 1364–1365.*) Diabetes insipidus (DI) results from a deficiency of antidiuretic hormone (ADH) and is characterized by polyuria and polydipsia, but not the polyphagia or hyperglycemia of diabetes mellitus. The hallmark of DI is a dilute urine (low urine osmolarity) with an increased serum sodium (hypernatremia). Many cases of diabetes insipidus are of unknown cause (idiopathic), but DI may be the result of hypothalamic tumors, inflammations, surgery, or radiation therapy. Multifocal Langerhans cell histiocytosis (Hand-Schüller-Christian disease) is one of the Langerhans cell histiocytoses (histiocytosis X). The disorder, which usually begins between the second and sixth years of life, is associated with the characteristic triad of bone lesions (particularly in the calvarium and the base of the skull), diabetes insipidus, and exophthalmos.

406. The answer is a. (*Kumar, pp 1164–1166. Henry, pp 310–313.*) Tests used to determine thyroid function include serum thyroxine (T_4), resin T_3 uptake (RTU), thyroxine uptake (TU), free thyroxine index (FTI), and thyroid-stimulating hormone (TSH) levels. Serum T_4 measures the total T_4, which includes T_4 bound to thyroid-binding globulin (TBG) and free T_4. Therefore, increased total serum T_4 levels can be from increased free T_4 (such as Graves' disease) or from increased TBG. The resin T_3 uptake (RTU) essentially measures the TBG concentration by measuring the binding of radioactive T_3 to TBG; note that this is not the serum T_3 concentration. The same thing is essentially determined using the thyroxine uptake (TU). These values then can be used to artificially determine the free thyroxine index (FTI), which is an estimate of the free thyroxine. The FTI (T_7) can be determined using either T_4 times TU or T_4 times T_3U.

To illustrate, consider the following. If a person is euthyroid, then their free T_4 will be within normal limits. If the TBG in this person is normal, then the serum T_4 will also be normal, but if their TBG is increased, which can be the result of increased estrogen from birth control pills or pregnancy, then the total serum T_4 will be increased. Because the TBG is increased, however, the resin triiodothyronine uptake will be decreased. Because they are euthyroid and their free T_4 is normal, then their TSH will also be normal. Note that the measurement of serum TSH levels is the best test to determine if thyroid function is normal or abnormal. A normal TSH level indicates that free T_3 and free T_4 levels in the serum are normal. Increased serum TSH indicates low free T_3 and T_4 levels (primary hypothyroidism), while decreased serum TSH levels indicate either decreased production by the pituitary (hypopituitarism) or increased thyroid production by the thyroid gland (hyperthyroidism).

407. The answer is b. (*Kumar, pp 1167–1169. McPhee, pp 561, 567–571.*) The consequences of excess or inadequate thyroid hormone are directly attributed to abnormalities involving the normal functioning of thyroid hormones, such as regulation of body processes. For example, excess thyroid hormone (hyperthyroidism) results in weight loss (increased lipolysis) despite increased food intake, heat intolerance, increased heart rate, tremor, nervousness, and weakness (due to loss in muscle mass). Inadequate levels of thyroid hormone (hypothyroidism) produce different signs and symptoms in children than in older children and adults. In young children hypothyroidism produces cretinism, a disease that is characterized by marked retardation of physical and mental growth (severe mental retardation). Patients develop dry, rough skin and a protuberant abdomen. Characteristic facial features include periorbital edema; a flattened, broad nose;

and a large, protuberant tongue. In contrast, hypothyroidism in older children and adults produces myxedema. This disease is characterized by a decrease in the metabolic rate, which can result in multiple signs and symptoms, such as cold intolerance and weight gain. Neurologic features of this abnormality include slowing of intellectual and motor function (fatigue, lethargy, and slow speech), apathy, sleepiness, depression, paranoia, and prolonged relaxation phase in deep tendon reflexes ("hung-up" reflexes). Other signs and symptoms of hypothyroidism include dry skin and brittle hair, which can produce hair loss; decreased erythropoiesis, which produces a normochromic normocytic anemia; increased cholesterol, which increases the risk of atherosclerosis; and myxedema, which is the increased interstitial deposition of mucopolysaccharides. The latter abnormality can result in diffuse nonpitting edema of the skin, hoarseness, and enlargement of the heart. Other systems affected by hypothyroidism include the heart, the GI tract, and the GU tract. Patients may develop a slowed heart rate and decreased stroke volume (resulting in cool, pale skin) and constipation, as well as impotence (in men) or menorrhagia and anovulatory cycles (in women).

408. The answer is d. (*Kumar, pp 1169–1170. Rubin, pp 1171–1173.*) Hashimoto's thyroiditis, one of the autoimmune thyroid diseases, is associated with the HLA-B8 haplotype and high titers of circulating autoantibodies, including antimicrosomal, antithyroglobulin, and anti-TSH receptor antibodies. This abnormality, which is not uncommon in the United States, is characterized histologically by an intense lymphoplasmacytic infiltrate, with the formation of lymphoid follicles and germinal centers. This produces destruction and atrophy of the follicles and transforms the thyroid follicular cells into acidophilic cells. There are many different names for these cells, including oxyphilic cells, oncocytes, and Hürthle cells. Not uncommonly, patients develop hypothyroidism as a result of follicle disruption, and the manifestations consist of fatigue, myxedema, cold intolerance, hair coarsening, and constipation. Rarely, cases of Hashimoto's thyroiditis may develop hyperthyroidism (Hashitoxicosis), while the combination of Hashimoto's disease, pernicious anemia, and type I diabetes mellitus is called Schmidt's syndrome. This is one type of multiglandular syndrome.

Although subacute thyroiditis and Riedel's thyroiditis may have similar symptoms to Hashimoto's thyroiditis, biopsy findings in these disorders are distinctly different. Subacute (de Quervain's, granulomatous, or giant cell) thyroiditis is a self-limited viral infection of the thyroid. It typically follows an upper respiratory tract infection. Patients develop the acute onset of fever and painful thyroid enlargement and may develop a transient hypothyroidism. Histologically there is destruction of the follicles with a granulomatous reaction and multinucleated giant cells that surround fragments of colloid. One-half of patients with Riedel's thyroiditis are hypothyroid, but, in contrast to the other types of thyroiditis, microscopic examination reveals dense fibrosis of the thyroid gland, often extending into extrathyroidal soft tissue. This fibrosis produces a rock-hard enlarged thyroid gland that may produce the feeling of suffocation. This combination of signs and symptoms may be mistaken clinically for a malignant process. Additionally, these patients may develop similar fibrosis in the mediastinum or retroperitoneum. Subacute lymphocytic thyroiditis is also a self-limited, painless enlargement of the thyroid that is associated with hypothyroidism, but that lacks antithyroid antibodies or lymphoid germinal centers within the thyroid. Finally, follicular cell hyperplasia with scalloping of colloid is characteristic of hyperthyroidism due to Graves' disease, while the extracellular deposition of amyloid in the thyroid gland is characteristic of medullary thyroid carcinoma.

409. The answer is e. (*Kumar, pp 1172–1173. Rubin, pp 1167–1171.*) Graves' disease, or diffuse toxic goiter, is one of the three most common disorders associated with thyrotoxicosis or hyperthyroidism (the other two are toxic multinodular goiter and toxic adenoma). This hyperfunctioning and hyperplastic diffuse goiter is accompanied by a characteristic triad of clinical findings: signs of hyperthyroidism, exophthalmus, and pretibial myxedema. Graves' disease is an autoimmune form of goiter caused by thyroid-stimulating immunoglobulins or thyroid-stimulating hormone (TSH) receptor antibodies. Autoantibodies to TSH receptor antigens are produced because of a defect in antigen-specific suppressor T cells. The antibodies bind to TSH receptors on thyroid follicular cells and function as TSH, with resultant thyroid growth and hyperfunction. Such antibodies can be identified in almost all cases of Graves' disease. In contrast to these stimulating autoantibodies, Hashimoto's thyroiditis, an autoimmune cause of hypothyroidism, is associated with high titers of circulating blocking autoantibodies, such as antithyroglobulin, anti-TSH receptor, and antimicrosomal antibodies.

410. The answer is e. (*Kumar, pp 1173–1178, 1180–1181. Rubin, pp 1166–1167.*) Follicular carcinoma is the second most common malignancy of the thyroid gland. These tumors present as slowly enlarging painless nodules that usually are found to be "cold" (nonfunctioning) nodules with thyroid scans. The histology of follicular carcinoma is similar to follicular adenoma and this type of malignancy may have a well-defined capsule. Invasion into blood vessels or the capsule must be present to diagnosis follicular carcinoma. There are two basic pathways that lead to the development of follicular carcinomas of the thyroid. One involves mutations of the RAS family of oncogenes, while the other involves a unique translocation between PAX8 and the peroxisome proliferator–activated receptor gamma (PPAR gamma), which forms a PAX8-PPAR-gamma fusion gene.

The PAX (paired box) genes are a family of related genes that code for transcription factors important for tissue development. Abnormalities of these PAX genes are associated with various diseases: PAX-2 with the "renal-coloboma" syndrome; PAX-3 with the Waardenburg syndrome (white forelocks of hair; eye colors don't match); PAX-5 with lymphoplasmacytoid lymphoma; PAX-6 with aniridia and Wilm's tumor; PAX-8 with follicular thyroid carcinoma; and PAX-9 with congenital absence of teeth.

Note that the clinical term goiter is used to describe any enlargement of the thyroid. Most patients with goiter are euthyroid (nonfunctional goiter), as hyperthyroidism (toxic goiter) is relatively rare. In the early stages of goiter formation, there is diffuse hyperplasia of the small thyroid follicles, which histologically resembles the changes of Graves' disease. This early stage is called a diffuse nontoxic goiter or simple goiter. The thyroid gland then undergoes repeated episodes of involution and hyperplasia. Over time this produces an enlarged multinodular goiter that histologically consists of multiple nodules, some of which consist of colloid-filled enlarged follicles and others of which show hyperplasia of small follicles lined by active epithelium. There are also areas of fibrosis, hemorrhage, calcification, and cystic degeneration. The last stage of goiter formation consists of nodules composed primarily of enlarged colloid-filled follicles. This stage is called a colloid goiter. Finally, note that colloid carcinoma is a type of malignancy of the breast, not the thyroid gland.

411. The answer is c. (*Kumar, pp 1178–1180. Rubin, pp 1174–1179.*) The four major histologic subtypes of thyroid carcinoma are papillary carcinoma, follicular carcinoma, medullary carcinoma, and undifferentiated (anaplastic) carcinoma. Papillary carcinomas of the thyroid are composed of papillary structures with fibrovascular cores, while follicular carcinomas typically show a microfollicular pattern. It is important prognostically to differentiate papillary carcinomas from follicular carcinomas, as papillary carcinomas tend to be indolent (up to 80% survival at 10 years), while follicular carcinomas are much more aggressive (5-year mortality of up to 70%). Follicular areas may be present within a papillary carcinoma and in fact may be quite extensive. If present, these changes can make diagnosis difficult. It is important to recognize this follicular variant of papillary carcinoma because its behavior remains similar to that of indolent papillary carcinoma. Features consistent with papillary carcinoma, even in predominantly follicular areas, include optically clear nuclei ("ground glass," "Orphan Annie eyes"), nuclear grooves, calcospherites (psammoma bodies), and intranuclear cytoplasmic pseudoinclusions.

In contrast to the histologic features of papillary carcinoma, follicular carcinoma of the thyroid has a histology that is similar to a follicular adenoma, but capsular and blood vessel invasion is present. Medullary carcinoma is characterized by its amyloid stroma, its genetic (familial) associations, and its elaboration of calcitonin and other substances. It is a malignancy that originates from the parafollicular C cells. Undifferentiated (anaplastic) carcinoma, seen in individuals over the age of 50, is characterized by anaplastic spindle or giant cells with frequent mitoses. This tumor is characterized by rapid growth and a poor prognosis.

412. The answer is d. (*Kumar, pp 1182–1183. Rubin, p 1177.*) The development of a thyroid mass in a young person who gives a familial history for a similar lesion should raise high clinical suspicion of the possibility that the mass is a medullary carcinoma of the thyroid (MCT). MCT is a tumor of the parafollicular (C) cells of the thyroid and as such is associated with secretion of calcitonin. The procalcitonin is deposited in the stroma of the tumor and appears as amyloid, which stains positively with Congo red stain. The tumor cells have peripheral nuclei that give them a plasmacytoid appearance when viewed cytologically with fine-needle aspiration (FNA). Electron microscopy reveals membrane-bound dense-core neurosecretory granules in the neoplastic cells. MCT may secrete other substances in addition to calcitonin, such as ACTH, CEA, and serotonin. It is also associated with paraneoplastic syndromes, such as carcinoid syndrome (due to serotonin) and Cushing's syndrome (due to ACTH).

413. The answer is a. (*Henry, pp 101, 174, 194–196*.) Hypocalcemia results from either parathyroid causes (primary hypoparathyroidism) or non-parathyroid causes, which include hypoalbuminemia, hypomagnesemia, decreased vitamin D, chronic renal failure, and hyperventilation. Hypocalcemia may produce numbness and tingling of the hands, feet, and lips or tetany (spontaneous tonic muscular contractions). Two clinical tests to demonstrate tetany are Chvostek's sign (tapping on the facial nerve produces twitching of the ipsilateral facial muscles) and Trousseau's sign (inflating a blood pressure cuff for several minutes produces painful carpal muscle contractions). Hypocalcemia produces tetany by the following pathomechanism. A low ionized calcium allows sodium ions to preferentially enter channels in the cell membranes of neurons. This depolarizes the nerve and causes tetanic spasms of muscle. Patients who hyperventilate develop respiratory alkalosis because they are blowing off CO_2. This increased pH increases the negative charge on albumin, which increases the amount of calcium bound to albumin. Although the total serum calcium levels are not changed, the ionized calcium is decreased and this produces tetany.

414. The answer is a. (*Kumar, pp 1184–1187. Chandrasoma, pp 857–863.*) Hyperparathyroidism is caused by excess production of parathyroid hormone (PTH). In patients with hyperparathyroidism, it is important to distinguish primary hyperparathyroidism from secondary hyperparathyroidism. Both forms may be associated with the development of bone lesions, but excess PTH production in primary hyperparathyroidism leads to different laboratory values than those seen with secondary hyperparathyroidism. Increased levels of PTH in primary hyperparathyroidism result in increased serum calcium (hypercalcemia) and decreased serum phosphorus. The serum calcium levels are elevated because of increased bone resorption and increased intestinal calcium absorption, the result of increased activity of vitamin D. PTH also increases calcium reabsorption in the distal renal tubule, but, because the filtered load of calcium exceeds the ability for reabsorption, calcium is increased in the urine (hypercalciuria). PTH also increases urinary excretion of phosphate. The excess calcium in the urine predisposes to renal stone formation, especially calcium oxalate or calcium phosphate stones. Urinary stones can produce flank pain and hematuria. This is the most common presentation for patients with hyperparathyroidism. The hypercalcemia of hyperparathyroidism may also cause peptic ulcer disease due to the stimulation of gastrin release and increased acid secretion from the parietal cells. The hypercalcemia also results in muscle weakness, fatigue, and hypomotility of the GI tract, which can lead to constipation and nausea. Alterations of mental status are also common.

In contrast to primary hyperparathyroidism, secondary hyperparathyroidism results from hypocalcemia. This causes secondary hypersecretion of PTH and produces the combination of hypocalcemia and increased PTH production. It is primarily found in patients with chronic renal failure. Patients with hypoparathyroidism develop hypocalcemia and hyperphosphatemia but have normal serum creatinine levels. Primary hypoparathyroidism and pseudohypoparathyroidism also result in decreased 24-h excretion of calcium and phosphate.

415. The answer is c. (*Kumar, pp 1187–1188. Rubin, pp 1180–1183.*) Parathyroid hyperplasia may be associated with either primary or secondary hyperparathyroidism. In contrast to primary hyperparathyroidism, secondary hyperparathyroidism results from hypocalcemia and causes secondary hypersecretion of parathyroid hormone (PTH). This results in the combination of hypocalcemia and increased PTH. This abnormality is principally found in patients with chronic renal failure, where phosphate retention is thought to cause hypocalcemia. Since the failing kidney is not able to synthesize 1,25-dihydroxycholecalciferol, the most active form of vitamin D, this deficiency leads to poor absorption of calcium from the gut and relative hypocalcemia, which stimulates excess PTH secretion. Chronic renal failure is the most important cause, but secondary hyperparathyroidism also occurs in vitamin D deficiency, malabsorption syndromes, and pseudohypoparathyroidism. In any of the causes of parathyroid hyperplasia, all four parathyroid glands are typically enlarged. Parathyroid hyperplasia can be differentiated from parathyroid adenomas by the fact that parathyroid hyperplasia, either primary or secondary, results in enlargement of all four glands, while a parathyroid adenoma or parathyroid carcinoma produces enlargement of only one gland. In most cases the other three glands are smaller than normal.

416. The answer is c. (*Kumar, pp 1188–1189. Chandrasoma, pp 857–863.*) To summarize the diseases of the parathyroid glands, since serum calcium levels are affected by serum PTH levels, plotting serum calcium levels and serum PTH on a graph will separate the different abnormalities of PTH functioning into different areas of the graph. Increased levels of PTH (hyperparathyroidism) may be either primary or secondary. Primary hyperparathyroidism is associated with increased PTH and increased calcium (area B), while secondary hyperparathyroidism is associated with increased PTH and decreased or normal calcium levels (boxes E and D, respectively). This can be seen in patients with a deficiency of 1-α-hydroxylase, because decreased active vitamin D levels produce decreased absorption of calcium, hypocalcemia, and resultant hyperparathyroidism.

Primary hypoparathyroidism refers to decreased levels of PTH and decreased levels of calcium (box C). Causes of primary hypoparathyroidism include iatrogenic factors, such as surgical accident during thyroidectomy, congenital abnormalities (DiGeorge's syndrome), and type I polyglandular autoimmune syndrome. Patients with the latter abnormality have at least two of the triad of Addison's disease, hypoparathyroidism, and mucocutaneous candidiasis. Pseudohypoparathyroidism refers to decreased levels of calcium and increased levels of PTH (box E, which is the same as hyperparathyroidism). Pseudohyperparathyroidism would theoretically refer to decreased levels of PTH and increased levels of calcium (box A). This combination does not occur with diseases of the parathyroid glands, but instead can be seen in patients with hypercalcemia as the result of production of a substance with parathyroid hormone like function (paraneoplastic syndrome). This substance is called parathyroid-hormone-related protein. In these patients, serum levels of PTH are decreased because of the high levels of calcium.

417. The answer is b. (*Kumar, pp 1188–1189. Rubin, pp 1179–1180.*) Hypoparathyroidism may be caused by either decreased secretion of parathyroid hormone (PTH) or end organ insensitivity to PTH (pseudohypoparathyroidism), both of which are associated with hypocalcemia and hyperphosphatemia. Many patients with pseudohypoparathyroidism have a defect in binding of many hormones to guanine nucleotide–binding protein (G protein). These hormones include PTH, thyroid-stimulating hormone, glucagon, and the gonadotropins follicle-stimulating hormone and luteinizing hormone. These patients have characteristic signs and symptoms including short stature, round face, short neck, reduced intelligence, and abnormally short metacarpal and metatarsal bones. In contrast to patients with hypothyroidism caused by decreased levels of PTH, patients with pseudohypoparathyroidism (Albright's hereditary osteodystrophy) have normal or increased levels of circulating PTH and in fact have hyperparathyroidism.

418. The answer is d. (*Kumar, pp 1211–1214. Rubin, pp 1184–1186.*) In the adrenal cortex, cholesterol is converted into either mineralocorticoids (aldosterone) in the zona glomerulosa, glucocorticoids (cortisol) in the zona fasciculata, or sex steroid precursors in the zona reticularis. Congenital adrenal hyperplasia (CAH) is a syndrome that results from a defect in the synthesis of cortisol. This leads to excess ACTH secretion by the anterior pituitary and resultant adrenal hyperplasia. The defect in the synthesis of cortisol is the result of a deficiency in one of the enzymes in the normal pathway of cortisol synthesis, such as 21-hydroxylase or 11-hydroxylase. Most cases of CAH result from a deficiency of 21-hydroxylase. Two forms of this deficiency include salt-wasting adrenogenitalism and simple virilizing adrenogenitalism. The salt-wasting syndrome results from a complete lack of the hydroxylase. There is no synthesis of mineralocorticoids or glucocorticoids in the adrenal cortex. Decreased mineralocorticoids cause marked sodium loss in the urine, hyponatremia, hyperkalemia, acidosis, and hypotension.

Because of the enzyme block there is increased formation of 17-hydroxyprogesterone, which is then shunted into the production of testosterone. This may cause virilism (pseudohermaphroditism) in female infants. That is, XX females with CAH develop ovaries, female ductal structures, and external male genitalia. Much more often there is only a partial deficiency of 21-hydroxylase, which leads to decreased production of both aldosterone and cortisol. The decreased cortisol levels cause increased production of ACTH by the pituitary, which results in adrenal hyperplasia, enough to maintain adequate serum levels of aldosterone and cortisol. In contrast to a complete deficiency of 21-hydroxylase, there is no sodium loss with a partial deficiency of 21-hydroxylase. The excess stimulation by ACTH, however, leads to increased production of androgens, which may cause virilism in female infants.

A deficiency of 11-hydroxylase, which is rare, also leads to decreased cortisol production and increased ACTH secretion. This in turn leads to the accumulation of deoxycorticosterone (DOC) and 11-deoxycortisol, both of which are strong mineralocorticoids. This results in increased sodium retention by the kidneys and hypertension. Patients also develop hypokalemia and virilization due to androgen excess. Patients with a deficiency of 17-hydroxylase also exhibit impaired cortisol production, increased ACTH, and secondary increased DOC. These patients, however, cannot synthesize normal amounts of androgens and estrogens. This is because the gene that codes for 17-hydroxylase is the same for the enzyme in the adrenal cortex and the gonads, and the deficiency is the same in both organs. Because of decreased sex hormones, genotypic females develop primary amenorrhea and fail to develop secondary sex characteristics, while genotypic males present as pseudohermaphrodites. Additionally, the plasma LH levels are increased due to decreased feedback inhibition.

419. The answer is d. (*Kumar, pp 1207–1210. McPhee, pp 588–597.*) The clinical effects of excess cortisol are called Cushing's syndrome. Many of the symptoms of Cushing's syndrome that result from excess cortisol production can be directly related to the normal function of cortisol. Because cortisol is a glucocorticoid, its major function involves the maintenance of normal blood glucose levels. In this regard cortisol increases gluconeogenesis and glycogen storage in the liver. To provide the protein for liver gluconeogenesis, muscle is broken down. Because muscle is primarily located in the extremities, patients lose muscle in the extremities. This produces muscle wasting and proximal muscle weakness. Cortisol, in contrast to insulin, inhibits glucose uptake by many tissues. Therefore, excess cortisol causes symptoms of glucose intolerance, hyperglycemia, and diabetes mellitus. Cortisol also stimulates the appetite and lipogenesis in certain adipose tissues (the face and trunk), while promoting lipolysis in the extremities. Therefore, excess cortisol is associated with truncal obesity, "moon" face, and "buffalo hump." Excess cortisol inhibits fibroblasts, which in turn leads to loss of collagen and connective tissue. This produces thinning of the skin and weakness of blood vessels, which in turn results in easy bruising (ecchymoses), purple abdominal striae, and impaired wound healing. Cortisol also decreases the intestinal absorption of calcium, decreases the renal reabsorption of calcium and phosphorus, and increases the urinary excretion of calcium (hypercalcinuria). The combination of decreased bone formation and increased bone resorption with excess cortisol produces osteoporosis (decreased bone mass). Hypertension also occurs in a majority of patients with Cushing's syndrome; the exact mechanism is unknown. Cortisol enhances erythropoietin function, resulting in secondary polycythemia, which is seen clinically as plethora. Cortisol also normally functions to inhibit many inflammatory and immune reactions. Hypercortisolism produces decreased neutrophil adhesion in blood vessels and increased destruction of lymphocytes and eosinophils. This results in an absolute neutrophilia, absolute lymphopenia, eosinopenia, and increased vulnerability to microbial infections. Patients with Cushing's syndrome also develop psychiatric symptoms that include euphoria, mania, and psychosis. Gonadal dysfunction also is frequent, which in premenopausal women leads to hirsutism, acne, amenorrhea, and infertility.

In contrast to Cushing's syndrome, which results from excess cortisol, Conn's syndrome results from excess aldosterone. Addison's disease results from hypofunctioning, not hyperfunctioning, of the adrenal cortex. It most commonly results from autoimmune destruction of the adrenal cortex. Finally, Schmidt's syndrome, which is a type of polyglandular autoimmune syndrome, is characterized by the combination of Hashimoto's disease, pernicious anemia, and type I diabetes mellitus.

420. The answer is e. (*Kumar, pp 1207–1210. Rubin, pp 1189–1194.*) Increased serum cortisol, which produces clinical symptoms of Cushing's syndrome, may be secondary to excess ACTH production or independent of ACTH production. Causes of increased cortisol levels that are independent of ACTH (box E in the diagram) may involve abnormalities of the adrenal gland itself, such as a cortical adenoma or cortical carcinoma, or they may involve exogenous (iatrogenic) corticosteroids. Increased cortisol levels that are dependent on ACTH are associated with excess ACTH production (box B in the diagram) and may result from an abnormality of the pituitary itself, such as a tumor of the anterior pituitary (Cushing's disease), or from the ectopic production of ACTH outside of the pituitary, such as paraneoplastic syndromes, one example being small cell carcinoma of the lung.

The high-dose dexamethasone suppression test is used to distinguish ACTH-induced Cushing's disease from the ACTH-independent type. Dexamethasone suppresses pituitary ACTH production, but has no effect on the adrenal gland. Therefore decreased cortisol levels with dexamethasone administration indicate the anterior pituitary as the cause of the ACTH-induced cortisol overproduction.

421. The answer is c. (*Kumar, pp 1207–1210. Rubin, pp 1189–1194.*) Excess aldosterone secretion may be due to an abnormality of the adrenal gland (primary aldosteronism) or an abnormality of excess renin secretion (secondary aldosteronism). Causes of primary hyperaldosteronism (Conn's syndrome), which is independent of the renin-angiotensin-aldosterone (RAA) system, include adrenal cortical adenomas (most commonly), hyperplastic adrenal glands, and adrenal cortical carcinomas. These diseases are associated with decreased levels of renin. The signs of primary hyperaldosteronism include weakness, hypertension, polydipsia, and polyuria. The underlying physiologic abnormalities include increased serum sodium and decreased serum potassium, the latter due to excessive potassium loss by the kidneys, which together with the loss of hydrogen ions produces a hypokalemic alkalosis. The elevated level of serum sodium causes expansion of the intravascular volume. In contrast to Conn's syndrome, secondary hyperaldosteronism results from conditions causing increased levels of renin, such as renal ischemia, edematous states, and Bartter's syndrome. Causes of renal ischemia include renal artery stenosis and malignant nephrosclerosis, while Bartter's syndrome results from renal juxtaglomerular cell hyperplasia.

422. The answer is c. (*Kumar, pp 1214–1217. Rubin, pp 1186–1189.*) Hypofunctioning of the cortex of the adrenal gland (adrenocortical insufficiency) may be the result of abnormalities involving either the adrenal gland itself (primary adrenocortical insufficiency) or the pituitary gland, which controls the adrenal (secondary adrenocortical insufficiency). Primary insufficiency may arise from either an acute process or a chronic process. Causes of primary acute adrenocortical insufficiency include acute hemorrhagic necrosis of the adrenals, seen in children as Waterhouse-Friderichsen syndrome. This syndrome is most commonly due to *Neisseria meningitidis* septicemia, which is characterized by meningitis, septicemia, DIC, and hypovolemic shock. Acute adrenocortical insufficiency may also occur with too rapid a withdrawal of steroid therapy if a patient has additional stress. Causes of primary chronic adrenocortical insufficiency (Addison's disease) include autoimmune adrenalitis, infections, amyloidosis, and metastatic cancer. Previously the most common cause of Addison's disease was tuberculosis of the adrenal gland, but now the majority of patients have adrenal autoantibodies and are thought to have autoimmune adrenalitis. Half of these cases involve other autoimmune endocrine diseases, the resulting syndromes being called polyglandular autoimmune (PGA) syndromes.

Secondary adrenocortical insufficiency, such as in decreased functioning of the pituitary or in prolonged suppression of the pituitary by exogenous glucocorticoid therapy, results in decreased ACTH and hypofunctioning of the adrenal. This produces symptoms similar to those of Addison's disease, such as weakness and weight loss. In contrast to the case with Addison's disease, secretion of aldosterone in patients with secondary adrenocortical insufficiency is normal, because aldosterone production is not controlled by the pituitary gland. Therefore these patients do not develop symptoms of aldosterone deficiency such as volume depletion, hypotension, hyperkalemia, or hyponatremia. Additionally, because ACTH levels are not elevated, there is no hyperpigmentation.

423. The answer is c. (*Kumar, pp 1215–1216. Rubin, pp 1187–1188.*) In 1855, when Thomas Addison first described primary adrenal insufficiency, the most common cause was tuberculosis of the adrenal gland. Now the majority of patients have adrenal autoantibodies and are thought to have autoimmune Addison's disease. Autoimmune adrenalitis may occur by itself (isolated autoimmune Addison's disease) or it may occur with other autoimmune endocrine diseases. Two major patterns of autoimmune polyendocrine syndromes have been described. In addition to autoimmune adrenitis, patients with autoimmune polyendocrine syndrome type 1 (APS1) have chronic mucocutaneous candidiasis and abnormalities of the skin, nails, and teeth (ectodermal dystrophy). APS1 is also known as APECED (autoimmune polyendocrinopathy, candidiasis, and ectodermal dystrophy). In addition patients have other autoimmune disorders including autoimmune hypoparathyroidism, idiopathic hypogonadism, and pernicious anemia. APS1 results from mutations of the autoimmune regulator (AIRE) gene, the product of which is expressed primarily in the thymus. Autoimmune polyendocrine syndromes type 2 (APS2) is not associated with candidiasis, ectodermal dysplasia, or autoimmune hypoparathyroidism. Instead, autoimmune adrenalitis is present with autoimmune thyroiditis (Hashimoto's thyroiditis) or type 1 diabetes mellitus.

Finally, do not confuse autoimmune polyendocrine syndromes with multiple endocrine neoplasia (MEN). Hyperplasia of the parathyroid glands is seen with both type I and type II MEN, while neoplasms of the anterior pituitary are seen with type I MEN only.

424. The answer is b. (*Kumar, pp 1221–1223. Rubin, pp 853–858, 1195–1196.*) Combinations of neoplasms affecting different endocrine organs in the same patient are referred to as multiple endocrine neoplasia (MEN) syndromes. There are several types of MEN syndromes. Patients with type 1 MEN syndrome (Wermer's syndrome) have pituitary adenomas, parathyroid hyperplasia (or adenomas), and neoplasms of the pancreatic islets. The latter most commonly are gastrinomas, which secrete gastrin and produce Zollinger-Ellison syndrome. Type 2A MEN syndrome (Sipple's syndrome) is characterized by the combination of medullary carcinoma of the thyroid, pheochromocytoma of the adrenal medulla, and hyper-parathyroidism. MEN type 2B syndrome (also known as type 3) is associ-ated with medullary carcinoma of the thyroid, pheochromocytoma of the adrenal medulla, and multiple mucocutaneous neuromas.

In contrast to the MEN syndromes, combinations of autoimmune dis-eases affecting different endocrine organs are called polyglandular syn-dromes. There are several types of polyglandular syndromes. Patients with type I polyglandular autoimmune syndrome have at least two of the triad of Addison's disease, hypoparathyroidism, and mucocutaneous candidia-sis. Type II polyglandular syndrome (Schmidt's syndrome) is not associated with either hypoparathyroidism or mucocutaneous candidiasis, but instead is associated with autoimmune thyroid disease (Hashimoto's thyroiditis) and insulin-dependent diabetes mellitus.

425. The answer is e. (*Kumar, pp 1219–1221. Rubin, pp 1195–1198.*) Tumors of the adrenal medulla include pheochromocytomas, ganglioneuromas, and neuroblastomas. Pheochromocytomas are composed of cells that contain membrane-bound, dense-core neurosecretory granules and have high cyto-plasmic levels of catecholamines. Secretion of these catecholamines produces the characteristic symptoms associated with pheochromocytomas, such as hypertension, palpitations, tachycardia, sweating, and glucose intolerance (dia-betes mellitus). Pheochromocytomas are associated with the urinary excretion of catecholamines or their metabolic breakdown products. The catecholamines include dopamine, norepinephrine, and epinephrine. These catecholamines are broken down by two enzymes, catecholamine orthomethyltransferase (COMT) and monoamine oxidase (MAO), into homovanillic acid, normetanephrine, metanephrine, or vanillylmandelic acid (VMA). Any of these metabolic products may be found in the urine of patients with pheochromo-cytomas; however, VMA is most common. The best screening tests are 24-h urinary metanephrine and VMA levels. Pheochromocytomas have been called the "10% tumor" as 10% are malignant, 10% are multiple (bilateral), 10% are extra-adrenal, 10% calcify, and 10% are familial. These familial tumors are associated with neurofibromatosis, MEN 2A, or MEN 2B.

426. The answer is b. (*Kumar, pp 178, 243, 565, 706. Rubin, pp 1200–1201.*) The branchial apparatus consists of the branchial clefts (ectoderm), the branchial arches (mesoderm and neural crest), and the branchial (pharyngeal) pouches (endoderm). The dorsal wings of the third pouch develop into the inferior parathyroid glands; the ventral wings of the third pouch develop into the thymus; the fourth pouch develops into the superior parathyroids; and the fifth pouch develops into the ultimo-branchial bodies, which in turn give rise to the C cells of the thyroid. DiGeorge's syndrome results from failure of the third and fourth pharyngeal pouches to develop. This abnormality is associated with tetany and an absence of T cells. The tetany results from the hypocalcemia caused by the lack of the parathyroid glands, while the absence of T cells is caused by the lack of the thymus gland.

427. The answer is c. (*Kumar, pp 706–707. Rubin, p 1201.*) The thymus, derived from the third pair of pharyngeal pouches and inconsistently from the fourth pair, is divided into an outer cortex and an inner medulla and is composed of lymphocytes and epithelial cells. The lymphocytes are mainly T cells, which are immature (thymocytes) in the cortex and are mature in the medulla, where they have phenotypic characteristics of peripheral blood T lymphocytes. The epithelial cells are mainly located in the medulla, forming Hassall's corpuscles. The thymus normally has a few neuroendocrine cells, which may give rise to carcinoid tumors or small cell carcinoma, and a few myoid cells, which are similar to striated muscle cells and may play a role in the autoimmune pathogenesis of myasthenia gravis. The appearance of lymphoid follicles with germinal centers is abnormal and is diagnostic of thymic hyperplasia.

428. The answer is a. (*Kumar, pp 707–708. Rubin, pp 1201–1203.*) Thymomas are tumors arising from thymic epithelial cells and are among the most common mediastinal neoplasms, especially in the anterosuperior mediastinum. Histologic sections reveal a proliferation of spindle-shaped cells. There is a scanty or rich lymphocytic infiltrate of T cells, which are not neoplastic, although their size and prominent nucleoli may cause histologic confusion with lymphoma. About 90% of thymomas are benign and occur at a mean age of 50 years. They are very rare in children. They may be asymptomatic or may cause pressure effects of dysphagia, dyspnea, or vena cava compression. Associated systemic disorders include myasthenia gravis, hematologic cytopenias, collagen vascular disease (lupus), and hypogammaglobulinemia. Malignant thymomas show infiltration and capsular invasion plus pleural implants or distant metastasis.

In contrast, the other type of cell found in the thymus, T lymphocytes, give rise to T-cell lymphoblastic lymphomas. Finally, recall that fibroblasts give rise to fibromas or fibrosarcomas, and mesothelial cells give rise to benign or malignant mesotheliomas.

Skin

Questions

DIRECTIONS: Each item below contains a question or incomplete statement followed by suggested responses. Select the **one best** response to each question.

429. A 25-year-old woman presents with diffuse pruritus that developed soon after she ate a small bag of salted peanuts. Physical examination finds diffuse pruritic wheals involving her trunk, abdomen, and arms. The clinical term "wheal" describes which of the following abnormalities?

a. Dry, horny, platelike crust caused by incomplete keratinization of the stratum corneum
b. Elevated areas of skin with erythematous borders caused by dermal edema
c. Raised areas of skin that are filled with purulent draining material
d. Thickening of the skin caused by hyperplasia of the stratum corneum
e. Traumatic breaks in the skin with irregular borders caused by deep scratching

430. A 35-year-old man presents with a 0.3-cm flat light brown lesion on his left forearm. The lesion is excised, and microscopy reveals nests of round nevus cells within the lower epidermis at the dermal-epidermal junction. There is no "fusion" present of adjacent nests of nevus cells. Cytologic atypia is not present, nor are nevus cells seen in the superficial or deep dermis. Which of the following is the most likely diagnosis?

a. Compound nevus
b. Dysplastic nevus
c. Halo nevus
d. Junctional nevus
e. Spitz nevus

431. A 68-year-old woman presents with a uniformly brown, round lesion that appears to be "stuck on" the right side of her face. The lesion is excised and histologic sections reveal hyperkeratosis with horn and pseudo-horn cyst formation within the epidermis. Which of the following is the most likely diagnosis?

a. Actinic keratosis
b. Bowen's disease
c. Keratoacanthoma
d. Seborrheic keratosis
e. Verruca vulgaris

432. A 23-year-old woman presents with a 0.4-cm nodule within the skin on the left side of her neck. The clinician removes the lesion and sends it to the pathology lab, calling it a "sebaceous cyst." Histologic sections reveal a cystic structure in the dermis that is filled with keratin and lined by a stratified squamous epithelium, which has a granular cell layer. This cyst is not ruptured, no adnexal structures are seen within the wall of the cyst, and no atypia is present. Which of the following is the most likely diagnosis?

a. Acrochordon
b. Cystic hygroma
c. Epithelial inclusion cyst
d. Intradermal nevus
e. Pilar cyst

433. A 65-year-old man who is a long-time farmer presents with a small, scaly erythematous lesion on the helix of his left ear. A biopsy from this lesion reveals marked degeneration of the dermal collagen (solar elastosis) along with atypia of the squamous epidermal cells. The atypia, however, does not involve the full thickness of the epidermis, and no invasion into the underlying tissue is seen. Which of the following is the most likely diagnosis?

a. Actinic keratosis
b. Bowen's disease
c. Keratoacanthoma
d. Seborrheic keratosis
e. Squamous cell carcinoma

434. A 54-year-old man presents with a recently enlarging, darkly pigmented lesion on his upper back. The lesion is biopsied and histologic sections reveal a lentiginous proliferation of atypical cells as seen in the picture. No invasion into the dermis is identified. Within the epidermis, however, these atypical cells, which stain positively with HMB45, infiltrate individually into the upper portions of the epidermis forming a "buckshot" appearance. Which of the following is the most likely diagnosis?

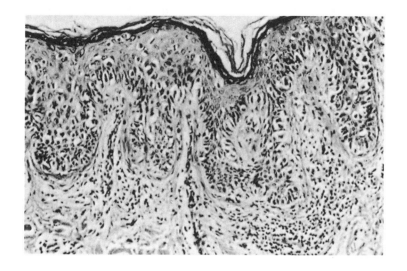

    a. Lentigo maligna melanoma
    b. Mycosis fungoides
    c. Paget's disease
    d. Squamous cell carcinoma in situ
    e. Superficial spreading malignant melanoma in situ

435. A 47-year-old man presents because of the recent enlargement of a pigmented lesion located on his left shoulder. Physical examination finds a pigmented, irregular skin lesion that measures 2.5 cm in greatest dimension. No cervical, axillary, or inguinal lymph nodes are palpable, and chest x-rays are unremarkable. The lesion is completely excised and histologic sections reveal malignant melanocytes infiltrating laterally within the epidermis and also into the dermis. Scattered Pagetoid cells are present in the epidermis and numerous mitoses are seen in the dermis. The intraepidermal radial growth phase is extensive and there is no maturation of the malignant cells at the base of the lesion, which extends into the reticular dermis. Numerous lymphocytes are seen at the periphery of the malignant cells. In the absence of metastases, the prognosis for this lesion is most dependent on which one of the following histologic features?

a. Degree of maturation of the malignant cells at the base of the lesion
b. Depth of invasion of the malignant cells into the dermis
c. Maximum diameter of the radial growth phase of the malignant cells
d. Number of mitoses present within the dermis
e. Number of Pagetoid cells present within the epidermis

436. A 72-year-old man presents with a slowly growing, ulcerated lesion located on the pinna of his right ear. The lesion is excised, and histologic sections reveal infiltrating groups of cells in the dermis. These cells have eosinophilic cytoplasm, intercellular bridges, and intracellular keratin formation. Which of the following is the most likely diagnosis?

a. Basal cell carcinoma
b. Dermatofibrosarcoma protuberans
c. Merkel cell carcinoma
d. Poorly differentiated adenocarcinoma
e. Squamous cell carcinoma

437. A 67-year-old man presents with a slowly growing lesion that involves the lower portion of his left lower eyelid. You examine the lesion and find it to be a pearly papule with raised margins and a central ulcer (rodent ulcer). Which one of the following histologic features would most likely be seen when examining histologic sections from this lesion?

a. Reactive epidermal cells surrounding a central superficial ulcer
b. Infiltrating groups of basaloid cells with peritumoral clefting
c. Infiltrating groups of eosinophilic cells with keratin formation
d. Dermal aggregates of small cells histologically similar to oat cell carcinoma
e. An in situ lesion with full-thickness epidermal atypia

438. A 65-year-old man presents with multiple plaque-like pruritic lesions scattered over his body. These lesions do not respond to topical steroid therapy. A biopsy of one of the lesions reveals a dermal infiltrate of atypical-appearing mononuclear cells, some of which occupy spaces within the epidermis. A periodic acid–Schiff (PAS) stain demonstrates areas of PAS-positive material in the cytoplasm of these cells. The peripheral smear exhibits similar atypical mononuclear cells, many of which have a prominent nuclear cleft. These malignant cells most likely originated from which one of the following cell types?

a. CD4-positive T cells
b. CD5-positive B cells
c. CD8-positive T cells
d. CD16-positive natural killer cells
e. CD21-positive B cells

439. A 23-year-old woman presents with a 0.4-cm firm brown lesion on her upper right thigh. Histologic sections from this lesion reveal an irregular area in the upper dermis that is composed of a mixture of fibroblasts, histiocytes, stromal cells, and capillaries. The majority of cells in this mixture are fibroblasts. The overlying epidermis reveals hyperplasia of the basal layers. Which of the following is the most likely diagnosis?

a. Dermatofibroma
b. Dermatofibrosarcoma protuberans
c. Fibroxanthoma
d. Pyogenic granuloma
e. Sclerosing hemangioma

440. A 26-year-old woman presents with multiple red-brown macules and papules, pruritus (itching), and flushing. Physical examination reveals that skin lesions can be produced by firm rubbing. A biopsy of one of these skin lesions reveals perivascular collections of mononuclear cells that stain positively with toluidine blue. Which of the following is the most likely diagnosis?

a. Mycosis fungoides
b. Merkel cell carcinoma
c. Weber-Christian disease
d. Letterer-Siwe disease
e. Urticaria pigmentosa

441. A 24-year-old woman presents with multiple skin lesions that developed soon after she took an oral sulfonamide for a urinary tract infection. Physical examination finds symmetrical located lesions on both of her hands and arms, many of which consist of red macules with pale vesicular centers. There is no involvement of her lips, conjunctiva, or oral mucosa. A biopsy of one of these lesions reveals epidermal spongiosus and necrosis with dermal vasculitis and edema. Which of the following is the most likely diagnosis?

a. Erythema infectiosum
b. Erythema marginatum
c. Erythema migrans
d. Erythema multiforme
e. Erythema nodosum

442. Histologic examination of a skin biopsy from an adult man reveals hyperkeratosis without parakeratosis, an increase in the granular cell layer, acanthosis, and a bandlike lymphocytic infiltrate in the upper dermis involving the dermal-epidermal junction. Which of the following describes the most likely clinical appearance of this patient's lesions?

a. Generalized skin eruptions with oval salmon-colored papules along flexure lines
b. Macules, papules, and vesicles on the trunk along with several target lesions
c. Pruritic purple papules and plaques on the flexor surfaces of the extremities
d. Red plaques covered by silver scales on the extensor surfaces of the elbows and knees
e. Soft yellow-orange plaques along the neck, axilla, and groin

443. A 34-year-old man presents with multiple large, sharply defined, silver-white scaly plaques on the extensor surfaces of his elbows and knees and on his scalp. Physical examination reveals discoloration and pitting of his fingernails. Lifting of one of the scales on his elbows produces multiple minute areas of bleeding (positive Auspitz sign). Which one of the following histologic changes would most likely be seen when examining histologic sections from one of these scaly plaques?

a. Subepithelial bullae
b. Regular elongation of the rete ridges
c. Liquefactive degeneration of the basal layer of the epidermis
d. Increased granular cell layer
e. Chronic inflammation below a zone of degenerated collagen

444. A 33-year-old man presents with signs of malabsorption and multiple pruritic red vesicles on his elbows and knees. A biopsy from his small intestines reveals villous atrophy, but no organisms are found. A biopsy from one of the skin lesions reveals subepidermal vesicles that contain scattered neutrophils. Aggregates of neutrophils are also found within the dermal papillae. Immunofluorescent staining of the skin biopsy reveals granular IgA deposits at the dermal-epidermal junction. Which of the following is the most likely diagnosis?

a. Pemphigus vulgaris
b. Bullous pemphigoid
c. Dermatitis herpetiformis
d. Chronic psoriasis
e. Lichen planus

445. The photomicrograph is from a small papillary lesion found on the dorsal surface of the left hand of an 18-year-old. Which of the following best describes the expected microscopic appearance of this lesion?

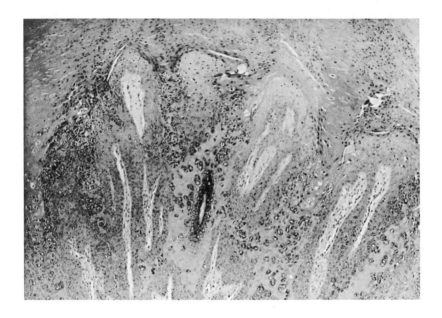

a. Acute necrotizing hemorrhagic vasculitis
b. Aggregates of epidermal cells with molluscum bodies
c. Dermal edema and mild superficial perivascular mixed inflammation
d. Hyperkeratosis, papillomatosis, and prominent keratohyalin granules
e. Intraepidermal vesicle, multinucleated giant cells, and Cowdry A inclusions

446. A 19-year-old man presents with a rash that involves a large, irregular portion of his trunk. Examination reveals several annular lesions that have a raised papulovesicular border with central hypopigmentation. Examination of this area under a Wood's lamp reveals a yellow fluorescence. A scraping of this area viewed under the microscope after KOH is added reveals the characteristic "spaghetti and meatball" forms of *Malassezia furfur*. A biopsy from this area would reveal these organisms to be located in which layer of the skin?

a. Stratum corneum
b. Stratum granulosum
c. Papillary dermis
d. Deep dermis
e. Subcutaneous fat

Skin

Answers

429. The answer is b. (*Kumar, pp 1229–1230.*) There are numerous terms used by clinicians to describe lesions of the skin. For example, pruritic, elevated areas of skin due to dermal edema are wheals, while traumatic breaks in the skin (such as produced by deep scratching) are called excoriations. A macule describes a flat, circumscribed area that has a different coloration from the surrounding skin. A macule is less than 1 cm, while a patch is greater than 1 cm in diameter. A papule describes an elevated area that is less than 1 cm in diameter (larger lesions are called nodules). If larger than 1 cm, it is called a plaque. Fluid-filled lesions less than 5 mm in diameter are called vesicles, while those greater than 5 mm are called bullae (the common term for both of these is blister). In contrast, a pustule is a raised area of skin that is filled with purulent material.

There are also numerous terms used by pathologists to histologically describe abnormalities of the epidermis and dermis. There may be hyperplasia of the entire epidermis (acanthosis), hyperplasia of the stratum corneum (hyperkeratosis), or hyperplasia of the papillary dermis (papillomatosis). Abnormalities of the normal maturation of keratinocytes include premature keratinization below the stratum granulosum (dyskeratosis) or retention of nuclei in the stratum corneum (parakeratosis). Intercellular abnormalities within the epidermis include edema (spongiosis) and loss of connections between keratinocytes (acantholysis).

430. The answer is d. (*Kumar, pp 1230–1234. Rubin, pp 1277–1280.*) Melanocytic hyperplasia, which causes hyperpigmentation of the skin, can be classified into several types of lesions. A lentigo consists of melanocytic hyperplasia in the basal layers of the epidermis along with elongation and thinning of the rete ridges. Two types of lentigines are lentigo simplex and lentigo senilis ("liver spots"). Increased numbers of melanocytes may form clusters located at the tips of the rete ridges in the epidermis (junctional nevus), within the dermis (intradermal nevus), or both at the tips of the rete ridges and within the dermis (compound nevus). A blue nevus is composed of highly dendritic melanocytes that penetrate more deeply into the dermis. This deep location gives the lesion its characteristic blue color. The

Spitz tumor (epithelioid cell nevus) is a benign lesion composed of groups of epithelioid and spindle melanocytes and is found in children and young adults. It may be mistaken histologically for a malignant melanoma. A freckle (ephelis) is a pigmented lesion caused by increased melanin pigmentation within keratinocytes of the basal layer of the epidermis. There is no increase in the number of melanocytes. These lesions fade with lack of sun exposure.

431. The answer is d. (*Kumar, pp 1237–1238. Rubin, pp 1288–1291.*) Keratosis refers to the proliferation of keratinocytes with excess keratin production. Seborrheic keratoses are very common, benign, elevated ("stuck-on") lesions that usually occur in older individuals. Histologically, these lesions reveal hyperkeratosis with horn and pseudohorn cyst formation. The sudden development of large numbers of seborrheic keratoses (Leser-Trelat sign) may occur in association with malignancy. This association with malignancies may also be seen with the malignant type of acanthosis nigricans, which consists of hyperpigmented areas of skin in the groin and axilla.

In contrast, keratoacanthomas (KAs) are rapidly growing lesions that microscopically reveal a cup-shaped lesion with a central keratin-filled crater surrounded by keratinocytes having eosinophilic ("glassy") cytoplasm. Atypia may be present, but these lesions are not considered to be malignant. The histologic appearance can make differentiating keratoacanthomas from squamous cell carcinomas on a histologic basis quite difficult. The clinical history of rapid development within several weeks is very helpful in making the correct diagnosis. Most cases of KA spontaneously resolve over several months. Human papillomavirus (HPV) causes several types of verrucae (warts), which are hyperkeratotic lesions. Verrucae vulgaris histologically reveal hyperkeratosis, papillomatosis, and koilocytosis. The latter term refers to large vacuolated cells with shrunken nuclei. Characteristically present are numerous enlarged keratohyalin granules. Finally, actinic (solar) keratoses, found on sun-damaged skin, microscopically show hyperkeratosis, parakeratosis, atypia of the epidermal keratinocytes, and degeneration of the elastic fibers in the dermis. The latter finding is referred to as solar elastosis. Clinically, actinic keratoses appear as irregular erythematous brown papules. When the atypia of the intraepidermal keratinocytes is extreme (full thickness), the lesion is referred to as Bowen's disease. These lesions are in fact carcinomas in situ since there is no invasion into the underlying dermis. If invasion were present, the lesion would be diagnostic of a squamous cell carcinoma.

432. The answer is c. (*Kumar, p 1238.*) Skin lesions may be polypoid or cystic. The most common polyp of the skin is called an acrochordon (skin tag), which histologically reveals a large polyp lined by squamous epithelium. Skin tags are polypoid or pedunculated. Epithelial cysts are also very common lesions, but are not pedunculated. Epidermal inclusion cysts are keratin-filled cysts that are lined by squamous epithelium having a granular cell layer. No adnexal structures are attached to this type of cyst. Clinically these very common cysts are called sebaceous cysts. This in fact is a misnomer, as these cysts have no sebaceous component. Other types of cysts include pilar cysts, which are keratin-filled cysts (lined by squamous epithelium not having a granular cell layer) found typically on the scalp, and dermoid cysts, which are similar to epidermal inclusion cysts with the addition of multiple adnexal structures, such as sebaceous glands or hair follicles.

433. The answer is a. (*Kumar, pp 1240–1241.*) Actinic (solar) keratoses, found on sun-damaged skin, microscopically show hyperkeratosis, parakeratosis, atypia of the epidermal keratinocytes, and degeneration of the elastic fibers in the dermis (referred to as solar elastosis). Clinically, actinic keratoses appear as irregular erythematous brown papules. When the atypia of the intraepidermal keratinocytes is extreme (full thickness), the lesion is referred to as Bowen's disease (carcinoma in situ). Obviously in this lesion there is no invasion into the underlying dermis, which, if present, would be diagnostic of a squamous cell carcinoma. Keratoacanthoma, a benign tumor, may resemble squamous cell carcinoma both clinically and histologically, but penetration of the dermis never extends deeper than adjacent hair follicles. The lesion is cup-shaped with central keratin; biopsy or excision excludes squamous carcinoma.

434. The answer is e. (*Kumar, pp 1234–1236. Rubin, pp 1281–1286.*) The photomicrograph shows a lentiginous (which means along the basal layer of the epidermis) proliferation of atypical cells some of which invade the upper levels of the epidermis. These individual cells resemble the cells of Paget's disease, but the clinical history, along with the fact that these cells stain positively with HMB45, make the diagnosis of malignant melanoma.

There are basically four types of invasive malignant melanoma, each of which may be confined to the epidermis (in situ) or may invade into the dermis. The most common type of malignant melanoma is superficial spreading melanoma, which is characterized by its lateral (radial) growth and upward infiltration of malignant cells within the epidermis, having a "buckshot" appearance (Pagetoid cells). The photomicrograph associated with this question reveals the basement membrane zone is intact. There are lymphocytes in the underlying dermis, but there is no invasion into the dermis. Therefore, the diagnosis for this lesion is superficial spreading malignant melanoma in situ.

In contrast to superficial spreading malignant melanoma, nodular melanomas are characterized by their dermal (vertical) growth and their minimal lateral (radial) growth. Acral lentiginous melanoma is an uncommon type of melanoma that is characterized by its unique location on the palm, sole, of subungual area. The last type of malignant melanoma, lentigo maligna melanoma, which is found in older individuals (mean age of 70 years), arises from a preexisting in situ lesion called a lentigo maligna (Hutchinson's freckle). Lentigo maligna are found on sun-exposed skin and clinically are seen as large, flat, irregularly pigmented lesions. Histologically, lentigo maligna reveal atypical melanocytes scattered throughout the basal layer of an atrophic epidermis with sun damage to the dermis. Since the lesion is in situ, no dermal invasion (vertical phase) is seen. When dermal invasion is present, the lesion is then invasive and is called a lentigo maligna melanoma.

435. The answer is b. (*Kumar, p 1236. Rubin, pp 1286–1288.*) In the absence of metastatic disease, the depth of invasion is the most important prognostic factor for a patient with a malignant melanoma. The Breslow's measurement is used to measure the depth of invasion. This measurement (in millimeters; determined using an ocular micrometer) is the distance from the granular cell layer to deepest tumor cell. Breakpoints at 0.75, 1.5, and 3.0 mm imply significant different prognoses. Another classification, Clark's levels, uses the anatomic layers of the skin and is divided into five levels as follows: level I is when tumor cells are located above the basement membrane zone only ("in-situ"); level II is when tumor cells invade, but do not expand the papillary dermis; level III is when tumor cells fill and expand the papillary dermis, but do not infiltrate into the reticular dermis; level IV is when tumor cells infiltrate the reticular dermis; and level V is when tumor cells infiltrate the subcutaneous tissue. The survival at 5 years is 90% if the tumor is Clark I or II and 0.76 mm or less in depth, but survival falls to 40 to 48% if the tumor is level III or IV and greater than 1.9 mm in depth.

436. The answer is e. (*Kumar, pp 1241–1242. Rubin, pp 1293–1294.*) Squamous cell carcinomas (SCCs) are one of the most common malignancies of the skin. They are usually found on sun-exposed skin of fair persons as a result of sun damage. This exposure to ultraviolet radiation with DNA damage is the most common etiology of SCCs, as indicated by the precursor lesion to SCC, actinic keratosis; however, SCCs are also associated with other conditions such as immunosuppression or inherited defects in DNA repair (xeroderma pigmentosa). SCCs may also develop in an area of chronic scarring, such as an osteomyelitis sinus tract or an old burn scar. An SCC arising in the latter is more likely to metastasize than an SCC occurring in sun-damaged skin. Basal cell carcinomas are also typically found in sun-damaged skin and are also associated with immunosuppression and xeroderma pigmentosa. Neither adnexal tumors nor Merkel cell carcinomas (a malignancy of small neural-crest-derived cells having neurosecretory cytoplasmic granules) are associated with old burn scars.

437. The answer is b. (*Kumar, pp 1242–1244. Rubin, pp 1291–1292.*) Basal cell carcinoma, arising from the pluripotential cells in the basal layer of the epidermis, is the most common tumor in patients with pale skin. This carcinoma is locally invasive and may be quite destructive. Metastasis, however, is quite rare. The classic clinical appearance is a pearly papule with raised margins and a central ulcer. Variants, which are not infrequent, include the superficial type (which may be multifocal), the morphea-like type (which has marked fibrosis and is difficult to eradicate locally), and the pigmented type (which may be mistaken clinically for malignant melanoma). Histologically the cells are deeply basophilic with palisading at the periphery of groups of tumor cells and peritumoral clefting. Abundant eosinophilic cytoplasm may be seen in squamous cell carcinomas, not basal cell carcinomas.

438. The answer is a. (*Kumar, pp 1249–1250. Rubin, pp 1296–1297.*) Mycosis fungoides is part of the spectrum of malignant T-cell lymphomas, mostly of the CD4+ T-cell subset, with a predilection for the skin. It is more common in males and the incidence increases with age. It arises primarily in the skin, but more than 70% of patients have extracutaneous spread, with the lymph nodes, spleen, liver, and lungs most often involved. Clinically mycosis fungoides presents as cutaneous patches, plaques, or nodules and is often misdiagnosed as psoriasis or other dermatitides. Histologically there is a bandlike infiltrate in the upper dermis of atypical lymphocytes with markedly convoluted nuclei—Sézary-Lutzner cells. These show epidermotropism and form characteristic intraepidermal clusters known as Pautrier's microabscesses. In some cases there is generalized erythroderma and Sézary-Lutzner cells in the peripheral blood. This is known as the Sézary syndrome.

439. The answer is a. (*Kumar, pp 1247–1248, 1320–1321. Rubin, pp 1294–1296.*) Two tumors that arise from fibroblasts in the dermis of the skin are the benign fibrous histiocytoma and the malignant dermatofibrosarcoma protuberans (DFSP). Benign fibrous histiocytomas are composed of a mixture of fibroblasts, histiocytes (some of which are lipid-laden), mesenchymal cells, and capillaries. Depending on which element predominates, these lesions have also been called dermatofibromas (mainly fibroblasts), fibroxanthomas (mainly histiocytes), and sclerosing hemangiomas (mainly blood vessels). Hyperplasia of the epidermis overlying a dermatofibroma is quite characteristic. In contrast, the lesions of dermatofibrosarcoma protuberans are cellular lesions composed of fibroblasts that form a characteristic pinwheel (storiform) pattern. They have irregular, infiltrative margins and are locally aggressive. They frequently extend into the underlying fat and complete excision is difficult. The overlying epidermis is characteristically thinned.

440. The answer is e. (*Kumar, pp 1250–1251. Rubin, pp 1093, 1245.*) Skin tumors may arise directly from epidermal or dermal cells, or may arise from cells that migrate to the skin, such as Langerhans cells (Langerhans cell histiocytosis, histiocytosis X), T lymphocytes (mycosis fungoides, cutaneous T-cell lymphoma), or mast cells (mastocytosis, urticaria pigmentosa). Mast cells contain numerous basophilic cytoplasmic granules that contain many different vasoactive substances, such as histamine and serotonin. In tissue sections, these granules are best seen with metachromatic stains, such as Giemsa stain or toluidine blue. Urticaria pigmentosa is caused by a local proliferation of mast cells within the dermis resulting in effects produced by histamine and heparin release, such as urticaria and flushing. These effects can be induced by firm rubbing (Darier's sign or dermatographism). Clinically, patients develop multiple red-brown macules and papules.

441. The answer is d. (*Kumar, pp 1255–1256. Rubin, pp 364, 414, 1245, 1264.*) There are several disorders of the skin that are easily confused as they have the word "erythema" (red lesion) in their name. Erythema multiforme (EM) is a hypersensitivity reaction to certain drugs (such as penicillin, sulfonamides, phenytoin) and infections. Clinically, patients develop lesions that are quite varied ("multiform") in appearance, such as macules, papules, vesicles, and bullae. The characteristic lesion, however, is a target lesion that consists of a red macule or papule having a pale vesicular center. Microscopic examination reveals epidermal spongiosis and necrosis with dermal vasculitis and edema. One variant of EM that is particularly severe is Stevens-Johnson syndrome. This occurs in children and produces hemorrhagic crusted lesions in multiple mucosal sites, such as the lips, oral mucosa, conjunctiva, and urethra. These lesions may become infected and may result in a fatal sepsis. Another variant of EM is toxic epidermal necrolysis, which produces extensive sloughing of the cutaneous and mucosal epithelium. This leads to clinical problems that are similar to severe burns.

In contrast to erythema multiforme, erythema infectiosum ("fifth disease"), which is caused by infection with parvovirus B19, can produce a "slapped cheek" appearance in children, while erythema migrans refers to the rash (active red, flat border with central clearing) associated with Lyme disease, erythema marginatum refers to the serpiginous, flat, nonscarring, painless rash associated with acute rheumatic fever, and erythema nodosum and erythema induratum are types of panniculitis.

442. The answer is c. (*Kumar, p 1258. Rubin, pp 1267–1268.*) Lichen planus is characterized by the formation of pruritic, purple, polygonal papules, usually on flexor surfaces of the extremities, such as the wrists and elbows. These lesions may also have white dots or lines within them, which are called Wickham's striae. The basic defect in lichen planus is a decreased rate of keratinocyte proliferation, which is the exact opposite of the increased rate of keratinocyte proliferation in psoriasis. Histologically, the skin reveals a characteristic bandlike lymphocytic infiltrate in the superficial dermis, which destroys the basal cell layer of the epidermis and causes a "saw tooth" appearance of the rete ridges. Anucleate, necrotic basal epidermal cells may be found in the inflamed papillary dermis. These cells are called colloid bodies or Civatte bodies. Because of the decreased rate of keratinocyte proliferation, there is an increase in the size of the granular cell layer, which is again the opposite of psoriasis.

Pityriasis rosea is a common idiopathic self-limited disease of the skin that is characterized by multiple oval salmon-pink papules that are covered by thin scales. The lesions typically follow flexure lines. Also present is a characteristic larger, sharply defined scaling plaque, which is called the "herald patch." Erythema multiforme (EM) is a hypersensitivity reaction to certain drugs and infections. Clinically, patients develop lesions that are quite varied (multiform) and include macules, papules, vesicles, and bullae. Psoriasis is a chronic skin disease characterized by large, sharply defined silver-white scaly plaques. These skin lesions are usually found on the extensor surfaces of the elbows and knees, the scalp, and the lumbosacral areas. Pseudoxanthoma elasticum is a hereditary disorder characterized by fragmented and thickened elastic fibers in the dermis and thickened, yellow-orange skin in the axillary folds and inguinal regions.

443. The answer is b. (*Kumar, pp 1256–1257. Rubin, pp 1251–1254.*) Psoriasis is a chronic skin disease characterized by large, sharply defined silver-white scaly plaques. These skin lesions are usually found on the extensor surfaces of the elbows and knees, the scalp, and the lumbosacral areas, but additionally about one-third of patients have nail changes including discoloration, pitting, and crumbling. The pathogenesis is not well understood, but about one-third of patients have a familial history. The pathogenesis involves a faster turnover time of the epidermal keratinocytes. The normal turnover time is about 28 days, but in patients with psoriasis this is decreased to about 3 days. Psoriasis is sometimes associated with other diseases, such as seronegative rheumatoid arthritis and AIDS. Clinically, if the scale of psoriasis is lifted, it forms multiple, minute areas of bleeding. This is referred to as an Auspitz sign and is due to increased, dilated vessels within the papillary dermis. The formation of new lesions at sites of trauma, referred to as the Koebner phenomenon, is also present. In patients with psoriasis, trauma may cause thickening of the epidermis (acanthosis), downward regular elongation of the rete ridges, hyperkeratosis, and parakeratosis. These changes may be related to faulty α-adrenergic receptors and decreased activity of adenyl cyclase in the lower epidermis. Because the keratinocyte turnover time is faster, there is no granular cell layer. Characteristically, neutrophils infiltrate the epidermis and form Munro's microabscesses in the stratum corneum or Kogoj spongiform pustules in the subcorneal region. These areas within the epidermis are slightly spongiotic, but no bullae are formed. Lymphocytes below a zone of degenerated collagen in the superficial dermis are found in lichen sclerosis, not psoriasis.

444. The answer is c. (*Kumar, pp 1259–1263. Rubin, pp 1254–1264.*) Numerous skin diseases result in the formation of vesicles and bullae (blisters) within the skin. These bullae have characteristic locations and microscopic appearances. Subcorneal blisters are seen with impetigo and pemphigus foliaceous; suprabasal blisters are seen with pemphigus vulgaris; and subepidermal blisters are seen with bullous pemphigoid and dermatitis herpetiformis (DH). The latter disorder is closely associated with gluten-sensitive enteropathy (celiac disease). In fact, the skin lesions of DH may improve with gluten-free diets. Early lesions show microabscesses at tips of dermal papillae with subepidermal vesicles, while immunofluorescent staining reveals granular deposits of IgA at tips of dermal papillae.

Pemphigus vulgaris is a chronic, severe, possibly fatal skin disease that is characterized by the formation of large bullae in the skin and oral mucosa. It is an autoimmune disease (type II hypersensitivity) caused by IgG antibodies to keratinocyte antigens involved in intercellular attachment. Immunofluorescence reveals a uniform "chicken-wire" appearance. Pemphigus vulgaris is characterized by acantholysis (separation of the keratinocytes) that produces intraepidermal (suprabasal) bullae. Clinically the bullae are large, flaccid, and easily ruptured because of their thin roof. Rupture produces denuded areas. Physical examination is positive for Nikolsky's sign (pressure extends the bullae). Systemic symptoms such as fever and weight loss are also present.

Bullous pemphigoid is caused by the presence of autoantibodies directed against the bullous pemphigoid antigen, which is normally found within hemidesmosomes at the dermal-epidermal junction. Biopsies from affected skin show nonacantholytic subepidermal bullae with eosinophilic infiltrate in surrounding dermis, while immunofluorescent staining reveals linear deposits of IgG and C3 in the lamina lucida. Bullous pemphigoid is a chronic recurring disorder that tends to be self-limited. It is less severe clinically than pemphigus vulgaris.

In contrast, psoriasis and lichen planus are two inflammatory disorders of the skin. Psoriasis is characterized by the production of red plaques that are covered by silver scales. These lesions are typically located on the extensor surfaces of the elbows and knees. The etiology of psoriasis is unknown, but it is associated with a faster turnover time of epidermal cells (3 days instead of normal 28 days). Microscopy typically reveals parakeratosis, loss of the granular cell layer, regular elongation of the rete ridges, and subcorneal microabscesses. Lichen planus is characterized by the production of "pruritic purple polygonal papules and plaques" that are typically located on the flexor surfaces of the extremities, oral cavity, and external genitalia. The etiology of lichen planus is unknown, but it is associated with a slower rate of cellular proliferation, which retains cells in the epidermis and increases keratin. Microscopy reveals a band-like lymphocytic infiltrated in the superficial dermis.

445. The answer is d. (*Weidner, p 1966. Kumar, pp 1265–1266. Rubin, pp 1288–1289.*) Verrucae (warts) are cutaneous lesions caused by human papillomaviruses (HPVs) that belong to the DNA-containing papovavirus group. Verrucae are classified according to their location and morphology. Verruca vulgaris, the most common type of wart, may occur anywhere on the body, but most commonly is located on the dorsal surfaces of the hands. The photomicrograph reveals characteristic features of verrucae vulgaris, including hyperkeratosis, papillary hyperplasia of the epidermis, and numerous large keratohyalin granules within the epidermal cells. Verrucae vulgaris have been associated with several types of HPV, including types 2 and 4. Plantar warts (hyperkeratotic lesions on the soles similar to a callus) are associated with HPV type 1, while verruca plana, typically found on the face, is associated with HPV type 3. Venereal warts, also called condyloma acuminata, are associated with HPV types 6 and 11. Carcinoma may develop in condyloma acuminata, in which case HPV types 16 and 18 are more frequently identified. Bowenoid papulosis (multiple hyperpigmented papules on the genitalia) is associated with HPV types 16 and 18. Epidermodysplasia verruciformis is an autosomal recessive disease associated with impaired cell-mediated immunity and the widespread development of multiple flat warts. These lesions have been associated with HPV types 5 or 8. Some of these lesions may develop into squamous cell carcinomas.

446. The answer is a. (*Kumar, pp 1267–1268. Rubin, p 444.*) Fungal infections of the skin can be classified into superficial mycoses, cutaneous mycoses, and subcutaneous mycoses. The superficial mycoses are characterized by infection of the stratum corneum of the epidermis. The most common type of superficial mycoses is pityriasis versicolor (tinea versicolor), an infection of the upper trunk that is caused by *Malassezia furfur* (*Pityrosporum orbiculare*). Clinically, there are multiple groups of macules (discolorations) with a fine peripheral scale. These macules are hyperpigmented (dark) in white-skinned races but hypopigmented (light) in dark-skinned races. These areas fluoresce yellow under a Wood's lamp. Potassium hydroxide (KOH) is used to identify fungal infections from scrapings of the skin. The KOH dissolves the keratin, and then the mycelial fungi can be seen. With tinea versicolor, KOH examination reveals a characteristic "spaghetti and meatball" appearance. The fragments of hyphae are the "spaghetti," and the round yeast cells are the "meatballs."

In contrast, the cutaneous mycoses infect the deeper epidermis, hair, or nails and are called the dermatophytes. Causative organisms include three genera: *Microsporum*, *Trichophyton*, and *Epidermophyton*. Clinically these infections are called tinea or ringworm. Different types of tinea include tinea capitis, tinea corporis, and tinea pedis (athlete's foot). Finally, the subcutaneous mycoses infect the dermis and subcutaneous tissue, an example of which is *Sporothrix schenkii*, a dimorphic fungus that causes sporotrichosis.

Musculoskeletal System

Questions

DIRECTIONS: Each item below contains a question or incomplete statement followed by suggested responses. Select the **one best** response to each question.

447. A young boy is being evaluated for a history of numerous fractures in the past. These fractures have resulted from minimal trauma. Examination of his peripheral blood reveals leukoerythroblastosis with numerous target cells. Which of the following abnormalities is most characteristic of this boy's disease process?

a. Abnormal "tunneling" of osteoclasts into bone trabeculae
b. Abnormal osteoclasts that lack the normal ruffled border
c. Decreased calcification of osteoid matrix
d. Decreased cartilage cell proliferation at epiphyseal plates of long bones
e. Defective synthesis of type I procollagen

448. A 4-year-old boy presents with a history of numerous fractures that are not related to excessive trauma. Physical examination reveals evidence of previous fractures along with abnormally loose joints, decreased hearing, and blue scleras. X-rays of the boy's arms reveal the bones to be markedly thinned. Which of the following is the most likely diagnosis?

a. Osteopetrosis
b. Osteoporosis
c. Osteomalacia
d. Osteogenesis imperfecta
e. Osteitis deformans

449. A 71-year-old woman presents with the sudden onset of severe lower back pain. Physical examination reveals severe kyphosis, while an x-ray of her back reveals a compression fracture of a vertebral body in the lumbar area along with marked thinning of the bones. Serum calcium, phosphorus, and alkaline phosphatase levels are all within normal limits. Which of the following is the most important factor in the pathogenesis of this woman's bone pathology?

a. High calcitonin levels
b. High prolactin levels
c. Low cortisol levels
d. Low estrogen levels
e. Low thyroid hormone levels

450. Sections of bone histologically show normal-sized trabeculae that are partially calcified and have enlarged seams of uncalcified osteoid. Which of the following is the most likely cause of these histologic changes?

a. Failure of bone remodeling
b. Failure of bone mineralization
c. Failure of osteoid formation
d. Reactive bone formation
e. Reduction in the amount of normally mineralized bone

451. A 61-year-old woman presents with increasing generalized bone pain. Physical examination documents hearing loss, while laboratory examination finds markedly elevated activity of alkaline phosphatase. Serum levels of calcium, phosphorus, and parathyroid hormone are all within normal limits. No masses are found, but a section of bone reveals prominent osteoid seams that form a mosaic pattern and very large osteoclasts with more than 12 hyperchromatic nuclei. Which one of the listed substances is most likely to be increased in the urine of this individual as a result of her disease?

a. Delta amino-levulinic acid
b. Formiminoglutamate
c. Hydroxy-indoleacetic acid
d. Hydroxyproline
e. Methylmalonic acid

452. A 5-year-old boy presents with the acute onset of fever, chills, and severe, throbbing pain over the metaphysis of his left femur. His peripheral leukocyte count is increased, and an x-ray of his left femur reveals a lytic focus of bone surrounded by a zone of sclerosis. Which of the following is the most likely diagnosis?

a. Avascular necrosis due to infarction of the femoral head
b. Acute pyogenic osteomyelitis due to infection with *Staphylococcus aureus*
c. Pott's disease due to infection with *Mycobacterium tuberculosis*
d. Chronic osteomyelitis due to infection with *Pasteurella multocida*
e. Osteitis deformans due to a viral infection of osteoclasts

453. Which of the following abnormalities is most likely to produce a spinal cord lesion that destroys both bone and the disk space (cartilage)?

a. Metastatic carcinoma
b. Multiple myeloma
c. Non-Hodgkin's lymphoma
d. Syringomyelia
e. Tuberculosis

454. A 25-year-old man presents with the acute onset of severe pain in his left leg. He denies any recent trauma to this area, but says the pain is such that he has trouble walking. Pertinent medical history is that he is a body builder and has been taking steroids for the past 2 years. After appropriate workup, surgery is performed and the femoral head of his left femur is resected. The pathologist examining this gross specimen makes the diagnosis of avascular necrosis. Which of the following gross changes is most likely to be present?

a. A yellow triangle-shaped area is present beneath the cartilage
b. An incomplete fracture is present causing subluxation of the femoral head
c. Multiple small, irregular, white deposits are present beneath the cartilage
d. The cortical bone is abnormally thick and black in color
e. The cortical bone is abnormally thin and the medullary cavity is absent

455. A 13-year-old boy presents with a slowly enlarging lesion that involves the distal portion of his right femur. He denies any history of trauma to this site. X-rays reveal a large destructive lesion that focally lifts the periosteum to form a triangular shadow between the cortex and the raised end of the periosteum (Codman's triangle). Laboratory examination reveals elevated serum levels of alkaline phosphatase. Which of the following histologic changes is most likely to be seen in a biopsy specimen taken from this bone lesion?

a. Multiple blood filled spaces that are not lined by endothelial cells
b. Haphazard arrangement of immature bony trabeculae forming "Chinese letters"
c. Lobules of hyaline cartilage with few cells
d. Malignant anaplastic cells secreting osteoid
e. Thick bone trabeculae with osteoclasts that lack a normal ruffled border

456. A 23-year-old woman presents with a nontender "bump" in her left leg. She states that this mass has been there for more than 5 years and has not changed in size. Workup reveals the presence of a cartilage-capped outgrowth of bone that is connected to the underlying skeleton by a bony stalk. Which of the following lettered locations in the figure is the most characteristic location for this tumor?

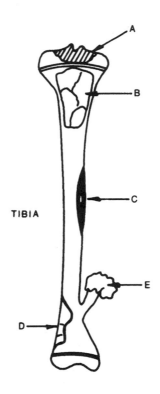

a. A
b. B
c. C
d. D
e. E

457. A 17-year-old man presents with nocturnal pain in the bone of his left leg. He relates that the pain is quickly relieved by taking aspirin. X-rays reveal a round, radiolucent area with central mineralization that is surrounded by thickened bone. The lesion measures approximately 1.2 cm in diameter. Which of the following is the most likely diagnosis?

a. Chondroma
b. Chondrosarcoma
c. Osteoblastoma
d. Osteoma
e. Osteoid osteoma

458. An incidental bone lesion was found in the femur of a 36-year-old woman. The lesion was excised and histologic sections revealed lobules of hyaline cartilage with very few cells. No bone formation was seen and no mitoses were present. Which one of the following statements best describes the most characteristic location and x-ray appearance for this benign bone tumor?

	Location	X-ray Appearance
a.	Cortex of metaphysis	Radiolucent area surrounded by thickened bone
b.	Medulla of diaphysis	Destructive lesion with concentric "onion-skin" layering
c.	Medulla of diaphysis	Radiolucent central cartilage surrounded by a thin layer of bone ("O-ring sign")
d.	Medulla of metaphysis	Bone destruction with subperiosteal elevation (Codman's triangle)
e.	Metaphysis or epiphysis	"Soap bubble" appearance

459. An 11-year-old boy presents with an enlarging, painful lesion that involves the medullary cavity of his left femur. X-rays reveal an irregular, destructive lesion that produces an "onion-skin" periosteal reaction. The lesion is resected surgically, and histologic sections reveal sheets of uniform small, round, "blue" cells. Most cases of this type of tumor are associated with which one of the listed translocations?

a. t(11;22)
b. t(14;18)
c. t(15;17)
d. t(8;14)
e. t(9;22)

460. A 65-year-old woman presents with pain, stiffness, and swelling of her knees. Physical examination of her knees reveals marked crepitus. Reconstructive surgery is performed on her knees. The resected bone reveals destruction of the articular cartilage and eburnation of the underlying exposed bone. Which one of the following best describes the etiology of this woman's disease?

a. "Wear and tear" destruction of articular cartilage
b. Anti-IgG autoantibodies
c. Deficient enzyme in the metabolic pathway involving tyrosine
d. Deposition of needle-shaped negatively birefringent crystals
e. Deposition of short, stubby, rhomboid-shaped positively birefringent crystals

461. A 36-year-old woman presents because of increasing pain in her hands and knees, which, she says, is worse in the morning. Physical examination finds her fingers to be swollen and stiff, and there is ulnar deviation of her metacarpophalangeal joints. A biopsy from her knee would likely show areas where histiocytes were palisading around irregular areas of necrosis, as seen in the picture. The biopsy would also likely show proliferation and hyperplasia of the synovium with destruction of the articular cartilage. Which one of the following terms best describes these pathologic changes?

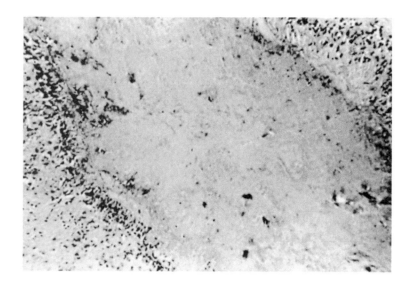

a. Eburnation
b. Gumma
c. Pannus
d. Spondylosis
e. Tophus

462. A 54-year-old man presents with chronic knee pain. Resection of the patella reveals chalky white deposits on the surface of intraarticular structures. Histologic sections reveal long, needle-shaped, negatively birefringent crystals. The photomicrograph was taken under polarized light. Which of the following is the most likely diagnosis?

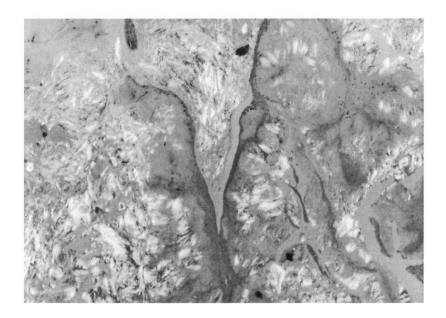

a. Osteoarthritis
b. Rheumatoid arthritis
c. Ochronosis
d. Gout
e. Pseudogout

463. A 4-month-old infant is being evaluated for progressive hypotonia and severe muscle weakness ("floppy infant"). Physical examination finds decreased deep tendon reflexes with fasciculations. A muscle biopsy reveals large numbers of small atrophic muscle fibers (panfascicular atrophy) along with scattered enlarged muscle fibers. Further workup finds deletions involving two genes located close together on chromosome 5. One of these deleted genes is the neuronal apoptosis inhibitory protein gene (NAIP). What is the other gene that is characteristically deleted in the autosomal recessive disease that this child has?

a. Myelin protein zero gene (MPZ)
b. Peripheral myelin protein 22 gene (PMP22)
c. Ryanodine receptor 1 gene (RYR1)
d. Sodium channel 4A gene (SCN4A)
e. Survival motor neuron gene (SMN1)

464. A 45-year-old man presents with rapidly progressive pain in his left leg over the past 3 days. Physical examination finds a low-grade fever with an increased heart rate. Examination of this man's left leg reveals a large necrotic area having crepitance and edema. There is a foul-smelling serosanguineous discharge from this necrotic tissue. A Gram's stain from this necrotic tissue reveals pleomorphic, gram-positive bacilli. Which of the following is the most likely diagnosis?

a. Gas gangrene
b. Necrotizing fasciitis
c. Opisthotonos
d. Tetanus
e. Trismus

465. A 34-year-old woman runner presents with pain in the plantar portion of her foot between the third and fourth metatarsal bones. Which of the following is the most likely cause of her foot pain?

a. Ganglion
b. Ganglioneuroma
c. Traumatic neuroma
d. Morton's neuroma
e. Schwannoma

466. A 5-year-old boy presents with clumsiness, a waddling gait, and difficulty climbing steps. Physical examination reveals that this boy uses his arms and shoulder muscles to rise from the floor or a chair. Additionally, his calves appear to be somewhat larger than normal. Which of the following is the most likely diagnosis?

a. Inclusion body myositis
b. Werdnig-Hoffmann disease
c. Polymyositis
d. Duchenne's muscular dystrophy
e. Myotonic dystrophy

467. A 59-year-old woman presents with difficulty swallowing, ptosis, and diplopia. Which of the following is the most likely cause of this woman's disease?

a. Antibodies to the acetylcholine receptor
b. Antibodies to the microvasculature of skeletal muscle
c. Lack of lactate production during ischemic exercise
d. Rhabdomyolysis
e. Corticosteroid therapy

468. An 8-year-old boy presents with weakness and pain over several of his proximal muscle groups. Physical examination reveals periorbital edema along with a lilac discoloration around his eyes and erythema over his knuckles. A muscle biopsy reveals atrophic fibers located primarily at the periphery of muscle fiber fascicles. Laboratory tests find the presence of antibodies directed against the microvasculature of skeletal muscle. Which of the following is the most likely diagnosis?

a. Ataxia-telangiectasia
b. Becker's muscular dystrophy
c. Charcot-Marie-Tooth disease
d. Dermatomyositis
e. McCardle's disease

Musculoskeletal System

Answers

447. The answer is b. (*Kumar, pp 1281–1282. Rubin, pp 1351–1352.*) Osteopetrosis (marble bone disease) is a rare inherited disease characterized by abnormal osteoclasts that histologically lack the usual ruffled borders and show decreased functioning. This abnormality results in reduced bone resorption and abnormally thickened bone. Long bones are widened in the metaphysis and diaphysis and have a characteristic "Erlenmeyer flask" appearance. In these patients multiple fractures are frequent as the bones are structurally weak and abnormally brittle, hence the name marble bone disease. The thickened bone can entrap cranial nerves and obliterate the marrow cavity, causing anemia and extramedullary hematopoiesis. The severe autosomal recessive form causes death in infancy, but the more common autosomal dominant adult form is relatively benign.

Osteopetrosis does not primarily affect the epiphyseal plate (growth plate), which is a layer of modified cartilage lying between the diaphysis and the epiphysis. This plate consists of the following zones: reserve (resting) zone, proliferating zone, zone of hypertrophy, zone of calcification, and zone of ossification. Disorders that do affect the growth plate include cretinism, achondroplasia, scurvy (vitamin C deficiency), and Hurler's syndrome. Cretinism (congenital hypothyroidism) results in mental retardation and dwarfism. The skeletal abnormalities result in defects in cartilage maturation of the epiphyseal plate. In achondroplasia, the most common inherited form of dwarfism, the zone of proliferating cartilage is either absent or greatly thinned. This in turn causes the epiphyseal plate to be thin. Vitamin C is essential for the normal synthesis and structure of collagen. In scurvy (vitamin C deficiency) there is a lack of osteoblastic synthesis of collagen (causing excess growth of chondrocytes at the epiphyseal plate) and fragility of the basement membrane of capillaries (causing periosteal hemorrhage). Many of the mucopolysaccharidoses (MPSs) involve skeletal deformities. Hurler's syndrome (MPS IH) is associated with increased tissue stores and excretion of dermatan sulfate and heparan sulfate. These mucopolysaccharides also accumulate in the chondrocytes of the growth plate, resulting in dwarfism.

448. The answer is d. (*Kumar, pp 1279–1281. Rubin, pp 1352–1353.*) Osteogenesis imperfecta (OI), or brittle bone disease, constitutes a group of disorders often inherited as autosomal dominant traits and caused by genetic mutations involving the synthesis of type I collagen, which comprises about 90% of the osteoid, or bone matrix. Very early perinatal death and multiple fractures occur in OI type II, which is often autosomal recessive. The major variant of OI, type I, is compatible with survival; after the perinatal period fractures occur in addition to other signs of defective collagen synthesis such as thin, translucent, blue scleras; laxity of joint ligaments; deafness from otosclerosis; and abnormal teeth. A hereditary defect in osteoclastic function with decreased bone resorption and bone overgrowth, which sometimes narrows or obliterates the marrow cavity, is characteristic of osteopetrosis, or marble bone disease. Osteomalacia is seen in adults due to vitamin D deficiency, while osteitis deformans is Paget's disease of bone.

449. The answer is d. (*Kumar, pp 1282–1284. Chandrasoma, pp 963–966.*) Osteoporosis is characterized by qualitatively normal bone that is decreased in amount. Histologic bone sections reveal thin trabeculae that have normal calcification and normal osteoblasts and osteoclasts. Osteoporosis predisposes patients to fractures of weight-bearing bones, such as the femurs and vertebral bodies. Patients typically have normal serum levels of calcium, phosphorus, alkaline phosphatase, and parathyroid hormone. Clinically significant osteoporosis is related to the maximum amount of bone a person has (peak bone mass), which is largely genetically determined.

Osteoporosis is classified as being primary or secondary. Primary osteoporosis, the most common type of osteoporosis, occurs most often in postmenopausal women. Decreased estrogen levels, secondary to ovarian failure, is the major factor producing postmenopausal osteoporosis. Also factors in the pathogenesis of postmenopausal osteoporosis are increased levels of interleukin-1 and interleukin-6. These cytokines stimulate osteoclasts by increasing RANK and RANKL. Secondary osteoporosis develops secondary to many conditions such as corticosteroid administration, hyperthyroidism, and hypogonadism.

450. The answer is b. (*Kumar, p 1287. Rubin, pp 1369–1372.*) Osteomalacia (soft bones) is a disorder of adults characterized by inadequate mineralization of newly formed bone matrix and is most often associated with abnormalities of vitamin D metabolism (such as dietary deficiency or intestinal malabsorption of vitamin D), hypoparathyroidism, or chronic renal diseases. Rickets is a similar condition that occurs in children. Defective mineralization results in an increase in the thickness of the osteoid seams. In contrast, vitamin C deficiency (scurvy), which results from failure of osteoid formation, is characterized by thin osteoid seams. Osteopetrosis (marble bone) is a bone modeling abnormality related to hypofunction of the osteoclasts. Osteoporosis results from a reduction in the mass of bone, which still has the normal ratio of mineral to matrix. Reactive bone formation occurs in bone or soft tissue in response to such conditions as tumors, infections, or trauma.

451. The answer is d. (*Kumar, pp 1284–1286, 1229. Rubin, pp 1376–1379.*) Paget's disease (osteitis deformans) is characterized by an uncoupling of osteoblastic and osteoclastic activity and is divided into three phases: an initial osteoclastic (osteolytic) resorptive stage, a mixed osteoblastic and osteoclastic activity stage, and a late sclerotic, burnt-out stage. Histologically, prominent osteoid seams separate irregular islands of bone into a mosaic ("jigsaw") pattern. The osteoclasts of Paget's disease are characteristically large with an increased number of hyperchromatic nuclei and viral inclusions. It is currently thought that Paget's disease is caused by a slow viral infection with a *paramyxovirus*. Because of the high bone turnover, the serum alkaline phosphatase level is markedly increased, and amounts of collagen breakdown products, such as hydroxyproline and hydroxylysine, are increased in the serum and the urine.

In contrast, high urine levels of delta amino-levulinic acid are seen with lead poisoning or porphyria, increased formiminoglutamate (FIGlu) with folate deficiency, increased hydroxy-indoleacetic acid (HIAA) with carcinoid syndrome, and increased methylmalonic acid with vitamin B_{12} deficiency.

452. The answer is b. (*Rubin, pp 1359–1360. Kumar, pp 1290–1291.*) Osteomyelitis refers to inflammation of bone caused by an infectious organism. Most commonly the organism is *Staphylococcus aureus* (but remember patients with sickle cell anemia are prone to develop Salmonella osteomyelitis). Cat bites are associated with *Pasteurella multocida*; human bites are associated with anaerobes; foot puncture wound with pseudomonas; and hip replacement with *S. epidermidis*. Pott's disease of the spine is caused by tuberculous infection of the lower thoracic vertebrae, usually from hematogenous spread from a primary site elsewhere, usually the lungs. Typical granulomatous infections produce caseous necrosis of the bone and bone marrow leading to destruction and collapse of vertebral bodies.

Clinically patients with osteomyelitis develop an acute illness with malaise, fever, chills, and severe, throbbing pain over the affected portion of bone. The peripheral blood reveals increased numbers of neutrophils (neutrophilia), and blood cultures are usually positive. X-rays may reveal a lytic focus of bone destruction surrounded by a peripheral zone of sclerosis. The new osteoblastic periosteal bone is called the involucrum; the trapped necrotic bone is the sequestrum. The abscess may drain through the bone (the hole formed in the bone being called the cloaca) forming a draining sinus. An area of infection may be walled off and contained, but may still be a nidus of chronic infection (Brodie's abscess).

The most common site of infection varies with age: kids at metaphysis and adults at epiphysis and subchondral. Organisms may be introduced into the bone by direct penetration or hematogenous spread. Recall that nutrient arteries to long bones divide to supply the metaphyses and diaphyses. In the metaphyses, the arteries become arterioles and finally form capillary loops adjacent to epiphyseal plates. This anatomic feature allows bacteria to settle in the region of the metaphysis and makes it the site initially involved in hematogenous osteomyelitis.

453. The answer is e. (*Kumar, pp 1291–1292. Rubin, pp 1360–1363.*) Pott's disease of the spine is caused by tuberculous infection of the lower thoracic and the lumbar vertebrae. Destruction of the intervertebral disks and adjacent vertebral bodies is characteristic of tuberculosis. This destruction causes the bone to collapse, and these compression fractures may result in angular kyphosis or scoliosis. Caseous material may extend from the vertebrae into paravertebral muscles and along the psoas muscle sheath to form a psoas abscess in the inguinal regions. Tuberculous osteomyelitis occurs most often in the long bones and spine and via hematogenous spread from a primary site elsewhere.

454. The answer is a. (*Damjanov, p 2624. Kumar, pp 1289–1290. Rubin, pp 1356–1357.*) Avascular necrosis (osteonecrosis) refers to infarction of bone and marrow. Osteonecrosis may be either medullar infarcts or subchondral infarcts. Medullary infarcts produce geographic necrosis of the cancellous bone and marrow only; the cortical bone is not involved. Subchondral infarcts are characterized by a wedge-shaped pale area of necrosis that has the subchondral bone as the base and the center of the epiphysis as the apex. For example, avascular necrosis of the femoral head will be seen grossly as a wedge-shaped yellow infarct. X-ray may show a crescent sign or space between cartilage and underlying infarct. Avascular necrosis (AVN) of bone is a moderately frequent complication of high-dose systemic corticosteroid therapy—the usual cause of bilateral segmental infarction or AVN of the femoral head. Clinical features include the sudden onset of severe pain and difficulty in walking. Avascular necrosis of the femoral head in children is called Legg-Calve-Perthes disease. Children develop pain in the groin that radiates to the knee. Compare this to Osgood-Schlatter disease, which results from avascular necrosis of the anterior tibial tuberosity where the patellar tendon inserts. Individuals will develop intermittent swelling and pain below the knee at the tibial tuberosity.

In contrast to the abnormal yellow area of avascular necrosis, irregular white deposits in joints may suggest pseudogout (chondrocalcinosis), while bone that is grossly black in color is suggestive of alkaptonuria (ochronosis). This disorder is caused by the excess accumulation of homogentisic acid, which results from a deficiency of homogentisic oxidase. Finally abnormally thin bone trabeculae is seen with osteoporosis.

455. The answer is d. (*Kumar, pp 1294–1296. Rubin, pp 1384–1385.*) Osteosarcoma is the most common primary malignant bone tumor except for multiple myeloma and lymphoma. It is the most common bone cancer of children. Osteosarcomas usually arise in the metaphyses of long bones of the extremities, although they may involve any bone. They are composed of malignant anaplastic cells, which are malignant osteoblasts that secrete osteoid. There may be marked variation histologically depending on the amount of type I collagen, osteoid, and spicules of woven bone produced. Osteosarcomas produce a characteristic sunburst x-ray pattern due to calcified perpendicular striae of reactive periosteum adjacent to the tumor. They may also show periosteal elevation at an acute angle (Codman's triangle) or penetrate cortical bone with extension into the adjacent soft tissue. Two-thirds of cases are associated with mutations of the retinoblastoma (Rb) gene. Patients with retinoblastoma are at an increased risk for developing osteogenic sarcoma. In older patients, there is an association with multifocal Paget's disease of bone, radiation exposure (as in painters of radium watch dials), fibrous dysplasia, osteochondromatosis, and chondromatosis. Osteosarcomas metastasize hematogenously and usually spread to the lungs early in the course of the disease. With surgery, radiation, and chemotherapy the 5-year survival rate is now about 60%.

In contrast to the histologic appearance of osteogenic sarcoma, aneurysmal bone cysts are composed of multiple blood filled spaces that are not lined by endothelial cells. They are not true neoplasms. Fibrous dysplasia displays a haphazard arrangement of immature bony trabeculae forming "Chinese letters," while benign chondromas display lobules of hyaline cartilage with few cells. Finally, osteopetrosis is characterized clinically by thick bone trabeculae with osteoclasts that lack a normal ruffled border.

456. The answer is e. (*Damjanov, p 2532. Kumar, pp 1296–1297.*) Cartilage-forming tumors include osteochondromas, chondromas, and chondroblastomas. Osteochondromas (exostoses) usually occur at the cortex of the metaphysis near the growth plates of long tubular bones. They are thought to occur as a result of the displacement of the lateral portion of the growth plate. Histologically benign hyaline cartilage caps a stalk of mature bone. In contrast, chondromas usually occur at the diaphysis and may be found either within the medullary cavity (enchondromas) or on the surface of the bone, while chondroblastomas usually occur at epiphyses of the distal femur and proximal tibia or humerus. Histologically chondroblastomas are characterized by the presence of sheets of chondroblasts within a background of "chicken-wire" mineralization and occasional non-neoplastic osteoclast-type giant cells.

457. The answer is e. (*Kumar, pp 1293–1294. Rubin, p 1383.*) Many benign tumors of bone are capable of producing either bone or cartilage. Bone-producing tumors include osteomas, osteoid osteomas (OOs), and osteoblastomas. OOs are bone tumors that are typically found in the cortex of the metaphysis. OOs occurs predominantly in children or young adults in the second and third decades of life as a benign osteoblastic (bone-forming) lesion of small size, which by definition is less than 3 cm. In OO malignant change does not occur, unlike the case for the closely related but larger osteoblastoma, in which there is occasional malignant change. OOs are often located in the diaphyseal cortex of the tibia or femur, unlike osteoblastomas, which occur in the spine (vertebral arch) or medulla of long bones. OOs are characteristically painful because of the excess production of prostaglandin E_2. The pain occurs at night and is promptly relieved by aspirin. X-rays typically reveal a radiolucent area (the tumor itself) surrounded by thickened (reactive) bone. Histologic sections reveal an oval mass, the central nidus of which consists of interconnected trabeculae of woven bone containing numerous osteoblasts and uncalcified osteoid. This central nidus is surrounded by a rim of sclerotic bone. Treatment is complete excision of the nidus to prevent recurrence.

A histologic picture that is identical to the central nidus of an osteoid osteoma is seen with the osteoblastoma. Osteoblastomas are sometimes called giant osteoid osteomas. They differ from OOs by their larger size (greater than 2 cm) and lack of a decreased pain response to aspirin. Osteoblastomas also lack the surrounding sclerotic bone formation of OOs and are found in the medulla of bone rather than the cortex. Osteomas are usually solitary and clinically silent. They may be multiple in patients with Gardner's syndrome (familial colonic adenomatous polyposis with mesenchymal lesions). Osteomas are composed of a circumscribed mass of dense sclerotic bone and are typically found in flat bones, such as the skull and facial bones.

458. The answer is c. (*Kumar, pp 1296–1297. Rubin, pp 1381–1384.*) Chondromas usually occur at the diaphysis and may be found either within the medullary cavity (enchondromas) or on the surface of the bone. Histologically they are composed of lobules of hyaline cartilage with very few cells. Importantly no mitoses are present. Chondromas are usually solitary lesions, but may be multiple (Ollier's disease). If they are associated with soft-tissue hemangiomas, the syndrome is called Maffucci's syndrome. X-rays reveal a characteristic "O-ring sign" (radiolucent central cartilage surrounded by a thin layer of bone). Solitary enchondromas are not associated with malignant transformation. There is, however, an increased risk of chondrosarcoma in patients with Ollier's disease. In contrast to benign chondromas, chondrosarcomas show a peak incidence in the sixth and seventh decades. Most chondrosarcomas (85%) arise de novo, but the peripheral type, unlike the central type, may arise in benign tumors of cartilage, especially if they are multiple. Frequent sites of origin include the pelvic bones (50%), humerus, femur, ribs, and spine. Although a fairly common form of bone cancer, chondrosarcoma is preceded in frequency by metastatic carcinoma, multiple myeloma, and osteosarcoma. Histologic grading is most important in prognosis, since grade I and grade II lesions present very good 5-year survival rates following surgery, unlike grade III poorly differentiated tumors, which invade quickly and metastasize to the lungs.

Finally, a radiolucent area surrounded by thickened bone describes the x-ray appearance of osteoid osteoma (found in the cortex of metaphysis); a destructive lesion with concentric "onion-skin" layering describes Ewing's sarcoma (found in the medulla of diaphysis); bone destruction with subperiosteal elevation (Codman's triangle) describes osteogenic sarcoma (found in the medulla of the metaphysis); and a "soap bubble" appearance describes giant cell tumor (found in the metaphysis or epiphysis).

459. The answer is a. (*Rubin, pp 1387–1389. Kumar, pp 1301–1302.*) Ewing's sarcoma (primitive neuroectodermal tumor; PNET) is an uncommon tumor primarily affecting patients younger than 20 years of age that usually is located in the diaphysis or metaphysis of the long bones. With Ewing's sarcoma, reactive new bone formation may cause concentric "onion-skin" layering in half of the cases. With a combination of chemotherapy, radiation, and surgery, the 5-year survival rate is now 75%.

Histologically, the tumor is composed of a diffuse proliferation of small, uniform, round cells. Occasionally the tumor cells form rosettes around central blood vessels (Homer-Wright pseudorosettes), indicating neural differentiation. These small round "blue" cells are similar in appearance to the neoplastic cells of lymphoma, rhabdomyosarcoma, neuroblastoma and small cell (oat cell) carcinoma. To differentiate this lesion from these other malignancies, PAS staining of glycogen-positive, diastase-sensitive cytoplasmic granules within the tumor cells of Ewing's sarcoma is characteristic. Also useful in differentiation from neuroblastoma is the fact that Ewing's sarcoma is associated with the translocation t(11;22). This results in fusion of the EWS gene on chromosome 22 to a member of the ETS family of transcription factors, most commonly FLT1. That is, the most common result of the t(11;22) is the formation of the fusion gene EWS-FLI1.

In contrast to the t(11;22), the t(14;18) is characteristic of follicular non-Hodgkin's lymphoma; the t(15;17) is seen with acute promyelocytic leukemia; the t(8;14) with some cases of Burkitt's lymphoma, and the t(9;22) is characteristic of chronic myelocytic leukemia.

460. The answer is a. (*Kumar, pp 1304–1305. Rubin, pp 1392–1396.*) Osteoarthritis (degenerative joint disease), the single most common form of joint disease, is a "wear and tear" disorder that destroys the articular cartilage, resulting in smooth subchondral bone (eburnated, "ivory-like"). This loss of cartilage results in formations of new bone, called osteophytes, at the edges of the bone. Osteophytes located over the distal interphalangeal (DIP) joints are called Heberden's nodes, while osteophytes located at the proximal interphalangeal (PIP) joints are called Bouchard's nodes. Fragments of cartilage may also break free into affected joint spaces, producing loose bodies called "joint mice." Patients develop pain, stiffness, and swelling of the affected joints without acute inflammation. A characteristic clinical appearance is the presence of crepitus, a grating sound produced by friction between adjacent areas of exposed subchondral bone.

In contrast, anti-IgG autoantibodies (rheumatoid factor) are seen with rheumatoid arthritis, deficient enzyme in the metabolic pathway involving tyrosine (homogentisic acid oxidase) is seen with alkaptonuria, deposition of needle-shaped negatively birefringent crystals (uric acid) is seen with gout, and deposition of short, stubby, rhomboid-shaped positively birefringent crystals (calcium pyrophosphate) is seen with pseudogout.

461. The answer is c. (*Damjanov, pp 2630–2634. Kumar, pp 1305–1309.*) Pannus is the name given to describe the classic destructive joint lesion found in individuals with rheumatoid arthritis. This lesion is characterized by proliferation of the synovium (hyperplasia) along with numerous chronic inflammatory cells. The thickened synovial membrane may develop villous projections, which can destroy the joint cartilage. Nodular collections of lymphocytes resembling follicles are characteristically seen along with numerous plasma cells. Palisades of proliferating cells may surround areas of necrosis. This latter histologic appearance can be seen in subcutaneous nodules (rheumatoid nodules), but rheumatoid arthritis most frequently affects the small joints of the hands and feet. Larger joints are involved later. In contrast to a pannus, gummas are seen with syphilis, while tophi are found with gout. Finally, eburnation describes the "polished" appearance of the bone affected by degenerative joint disease, while spondylosis refers to a degenerative process of the vertebrae that can compress the spinal cord and its nerve roots.

462. The answer is d. (*Kumar, pp 1311–1314. Rubin, pp 1402–1406.*) Gout is associated with increased serum levels of uric acid, even though less than 15% of all persons with elevated serum levels of uric acid develop symptoms of gout. Gout may be classified as primary or secondary. Secondary gout may result from increased production of uric acid or from decreased excretion of uric acid. Primary (idiopathic) gout usually results from impaired excretion of uric acid by the kidneys. Most patients present with pain and redness of the first metatarsophalangeal joint (the great toe). Needle-shaped, negatively birefringent crystals of sodium urate precipitate to form chalky white deposits. Urate crystals may precipitate in extracellular soft tissue, such as the helix of the ear, forming masses called tophi. Pseudogout is caused by deposition of calcium pyrophosphate dihydrate (CPPD) in synovial membranes, which also forms chalky white areas on cartilaginous surfaces. CPPD crystals are not needle-shaped like urate crystals, but are short, stubby, and rhomboid; they are also birefringent. The degenerative joint disease osteoarthritis is the single most common form of joint disease. It is a "wear and tear" disorder that destroys the articular cartilage, resulting in smooth (eburnated, "ivory-like") subchondral bone. Rheumatoid arthritis, a systemic disease frequently affecting the small joints of the hands and feet, is associated with rheumatoid factor. Rheumatoid factors are antibodies—usually IgM—that are directed against the Fc fragment of IgG. In the joints, the synovial membrane is thickened by a granulation tissue (a pannus) that consists of many inflammatory cells, mainly lymphocytes and plasma cells. Ochronosis, caused by a defect in homogentisic acid oxidase, is associated with deposition of dark pigment in the cartilage of joints and degeneration of the joints.

463. The answer is e. (*Kumar, pp 1336, 1339–1340. Rubin, pp 1437–1438.*) Spinal muscular atrophy (SMA) refers to a group of autosomal recessive motor neuron diseases that begin in childhood or adolescence. (Motor neuron diseases are progressive disorders that affect the cells of the anterior horn of the spinal cord.) Most cases of SMA have deletions of the survival motor neuron gene (SMN1) and the nearby neuronal apoptosis inhibitory protein gene (NAIP). The most common form of SMA is Werdnig-Hoffman disease (type I spinal muscular atrophy). Degeneration of the anterior horn (motor) neurons produces severe flaccid paralysis and hypotonia. Histologic examination of a muscle biopsy from a patient with Werdnig-Hoffman disease will reveal the combination of large numbers of small atrophic muscle fibers (panfasicular atrophy) along with scattered enlarged muscle fibers and fiber type grouping. The prognosis for a child with Werdnig-Hoffman disease is poor. The disease begins in the first couple of months of life and progresses to death by the age of 3.

Numerous different genes are abnormal with muscle diseases. The peripheral myelin protein 22 (PMP22) gene and the myelin protein zero (MPZ) gene are both associated with hereditary motor sensory neuropathy type I (Charcot-Marie-Tooth disease), while the ryanodine receptor 1 gene (RYR1) and the sodium channel 4A gene (SCN4A) are two of the many different genes involved in the pathogenesis of malignant hyperthermia, a rare clinical syndrome that is triggered by induction of anesthesia. The sodium channel 4A gene is also abnormal in patients with hyperkalemic periodic paralysis.

464. The answer is a. (*Kumar, pp 393–394. Rubin, pp 397–401.*) Gas gangrene (myonecrosis) is caused by the large, gram-positive, spore-forming bacilli *Clostridium perfringens* or *Clostridium septicum.* These organisms secrete a myotoxin, which is a phospholipase capable of destroying the membranes of muscle cells. *C. perfringens* also produces a lecithinase, hyaluronidase, collagenase, and hemolysins. The lecithinase (alpha toxin) destroys the plasma membranes of erythrocytes, leukocytes, and endothelial cells. These enzymes cause extensive necrotizing spreading inflammation; gas production is due to fermentation of sugars by the bacteria within tissue. In contrast to gas gangrene, tetanus is due to infection with *Clostridium tetani*, a gram-positive, motile, nonencapsulated, anaerobic, spore-bearing bacillus, which produces tetanospasmin, a neurotoxin that blocks the release of the inhibitory neurotransmitter glycine in anterior horn cells. Clinical signs of tetanus include stiffness of jaw (trismus) and muscle spasms of face, abdomen, and back (opisthotonos). Finally necrotizing fasciitis is a rapidly progressive and spreading infection of the deep fascia and subcutaneous tissue. The bacterial cause of necrotizing fasciitis is varied and includes aerobic, anaerobic, and mixed flora.

465. The answer is d. (*Kumar, pp 1335, 1411. Rubin, p 1532.*) Peripheral nerve trauma may result in specific symptoms and pathologic changes at specific sites. Transection of a peripheral nerve may result in the formation of a traumatic neuroma if the axonal sprouts grow into scar tissue at the end of the proximal stump. Sometimes peripheral nerves may be compressed (entrapment neuropathy) due to repeated trauma. Carpal tunnel syndrome is the most common entrapment neuropathy and results from compression of the medial nerve within the wrist by the transverse carpal ligament. Symptoms include numbness and paresthesias of the tips of the thumb and second and third digits. Another type of compression neuropathy is associated with a painful swelling of the plantar digital nerve between the second and third or the third and fourth metatarsal bones. This lesion, called a Morton's neuroma, is most often found in females.

466. The answer is d. (*Kumar, pp 1336–1338. Rubin, 1420–1423.*) Duchenne's muscular dystrophy (DMD) is a noninflammatory inherited myopathy that causes progressive, severe weakness, and degeneration of muscles, particularly the proximal muscles, such as the pelvic and shoulder girdles. The defective gene is located on the X chromosome and codes for dystrophin, a protein found on the inner surface of the sarcolemma. Histologically, muscle fibers in patients with DMD show variations in size and shape, degenerative and regenerative changes in adjacent myocytes, necrotic fibers invaded by histiocytes, and progressive fibrosis. There are rounded, atrophic muscle fibers mixed with hypertrophied fibers. These muscle changes cause creatine kinase levels in the serum to be elevated. The weak muscles are replaced by fibrofatty tissue, which results in pseudohypertrophy. In Duchenne's muscular dystrophy, symptoms begin before the age of 4, are progressive and lead to difficulty in walking, and are eventually followed by involvement of respiratory muscles, which causes death from respiratory failure before the age of 20. The classification of the muscular dystrophies is based on the mode of inheritance and clinical features. X-linked inheritance characterizes Duchenne's muscular dystrophy, autosomal dominant inheritance characterizes both myotonic dystrophy and the fascioscapulohumeral type, and limb-girdle dystrophy is autosomal recessive. Sustained muscle contractions and rigidity (myotonia) are seen in myotonic dystrophy, the most common form of adult muscular dystrophy.

In contrast, dermatomyositis is an autoimmune disease that is one of a group of idiopathic inflammatory myopathies. The inflammatory myopathies are characterized by immune-mediated inflammation and injury of skeletal muscle and include polymyositis, dermatomyositis, and inclusion-body myositis. These diseases are associated with numerous types of autoantibodies, one of which is the anti-Jo-1 antibody. The capillaries are the principle target in patients with dermatomyositis. Damage is by complement-mediated cytotoxic antibodies against the microvasculature of skeletal muscle. In addition to proximal muscle weakness, patients typically develop a lilac discoloration around the eyelids with edema. Patients may also develop erythema over their knuckles (Gorton's sign). Histologically, examination of muscles from patients with dermatomyositis reveals perivascular inflammation within the tissue around muscle fascicles. This is in contrast to the other types of inflammatory myopathies, where the inflammation is within the muscle fascicles (endomysial inflammation). In particular, inclusion-body myositis is characterized by basophilic granular inclusions around vacuoles ("rimmed" vacuoles). Werdnig-Hoffmann disease is a severe lower motor neuron disease that presents in the neonatal period with marked proximal muscle weakness ("floppy infant").

467. The answer is a. (*Kumar, pp 1334–1335. Rubin, pp 141–142, 1430–1431.*) Myasthenia gravis is an acquired autoimmune disease with circulating antibodies to the acetylcholine receptors at the myoneural junction. These antibodies cause abnormal muscle fatigability, which typically involves the extraocular muscles and leads to ptosis and diplopia. Other muscles may also be involved, and this may cause many different symptoms, such as problems with swallowing. Two-thirds of patients with myasthenia gravis have thymic abnormalities; the most common is thymic hyperplasia. A minority of patients have a thymoma. Lack of lactate production during ischemic exercise is seen in metabolic diseases of muscle caused by a deficiency of myophosphorylase. Dermatomyositis is an autoimmune disease produced by complement-mediated cytotoxic antibodies against the microvasculature of skeletal muscle. Rhabdomyolysis is destruction of skeletal muscle that releases myoglobin into the blood. This may cause myoglobinuria and acute renal failure. Rhabdomyolysis may follow an influenza infection, heat stroke, or malignant hyperthermia. Corticosteroid therapy may cause muscle weakness and selective type 2 atrophy.

468. The answer is d. (*Kumar, pp 1342–1343. Rubin, pp 1426–1430.*) Dermatomyositis is an autoimmune disease that is one of a group of idiopathic inflammatory myopathies. The inflammatory myopathies are characterized by immune-mediated inflammation and injury of skeletal muscle and include polymyositis, dermatomyositis, and inclusion-body myositis (the most common type of myositis in the elderly). These disorders are associated with numerous types of autoantibodies, one of which is the anti-Jo-1 antibody. The capillaries are the principal target in patients with dermatomyositis. Damage is by complement-mediated cytotoxic antibodies against the microvasculature of skeletal muscle. In addition to proximal muscle weakness, patients typically develop a lilac discoloration around the eyelids with edema. Patients may also develop erythema over their knuckles (Gorton's sign). Histologically, examination of muscles from patients with dermatomyositis reveals perivascular inflammation within the tissue that surrounds muscle fascicles. This is in contrast to the other types of inflammatory myopathies, where the inflammation is within the muscle fascicles (endomysial inflammation). In particular, inclusion-body myositis is characterized by basophilic granular inclusions around vacuoles ("rimmed" vacuoles).

Nervous System

Questions

DIRECTIONS: Each item below contains a question or incomplete statement followed by suggested responses. Select the **one best** response to each question.

469. A 50-year-old man presents with headaches, vomiting, and weakness of his left side. Physical examination reveals his right eye to be pointing "down and out" along with ptosis of his right eyelid. His right pupil is fixed and dilated and does not respond to accommodation. Marked weakness is found in his left arm and leg. Swelling of the optic disk (papilledema) is found during examination of his retina. Which of the following is most likely present in this individual?

a. Aneurysm of the vertebrobasilar artery
b. Arteriovenous malformation involving the anterior cerebral artery
c. Subfalcine herniation
d. Tonsillar herniation
e. Uncal herniation

470. A newborn infant is being evaluated for a cystic mass found in his lower back at the time of delivery. Physical examination reveals a large mass in the lumbosacral area that transilluminates. Workup finds flattening of the base of the skull along with a decrease in the size of the posterior fossa. Clinically it is thought that this infant might have an Arnold-Chiari malformation and would therefore be at the greatest risk for developing which one of the following within the first few days after delivery?

a. Holoprosencephaly
b. Hydrocephalus
c. Aplasia of the cerebellar vermis
d. Facial angiofibromata
e. Hemangioblastoma of the cerebellum

471. A 23-year-old woman is being evaluated for the development of polyhydramnios during the 15th week of her first pregnancy. Laboratory testing finds increased α-fetoprotein in her serum, and an ultrasound finds an abnormal shape to the head of the fetus with an absence of the skull. Which of the following therapies would most decrease the probability of this abnormality occurring in subsequent pregnancies for this individual?

a. Completely avoid alcohol
b. Decrease dietary caffeine
c. Vaccinate against rubella
d. Increase dietary folate
e. Increase dietary vitamin A

472. An 18-year-old male high school baseball player gets hit in the head with a fastball in the temporal area. He does not lose consciousness, but afterward develops a slight headache. He is not taken to the emergency room. By evening he develops severe headache with vomiting and confusion. At that time he is taken to the emergency room, where, after being examined by a neurosurgeon, he is taken to the operating room for immediate surgery for an epidural hematoma. Which of the following is most likely present in this individual?

a. Transection of a branch of the middle meningeal artery
b. Bleeding from torn bridging veins
c. Rupture of a preexisting berry aneurysm
d. Rupture of an arteriovenous malformation
e. Cortical bleeding occurring opposite the point of a traumatic injury

473. A 27-year-old woman presents with the acute onset of severe headaches and vomiting. She describes these headaches as being the "worst headaches" she has ever had. There is no history of trauma. She is afebrile, and her blood pressure is within normal limits. Physical examination reveals stiffness in her neck, but papilledema is not present. A lumbar puncture reveals blood within the cerebrospinal fluid, but the cell count and the glucose levels are within normal limits. The signs and symptoms in this individual are most likely the result of an abnormality located at which one of the following anatomic sites?

a. Anterior thalamic nucleus
b. Circle of Willis
c. Medial inferior pons
d. Superior cerebellar artery
e. Superior sagittal sinus

474. A 25-year-old man fell out of a kayak on a rain-swollen river and remained underwater for approximately 5 minutes before being rescued. He was immediately taken to the hospital and put on a ventilator, but never regained consciousness. The next day he was pronounced dead after an electroencephalogram did not detect brain activity, and deep tendon reflexes and a respiratory drive were not found. At autopsy his brain was found to be swollen with side gyri and narrow sulci. No gross area of acute infarction was identified. Histologic sections from which of the following areas are most likely to show the earliest changes of acute neuronal injury, such as the formation of red neurons?

a. Dorsomedial nucleus of the hypothalamus
b. Nucleus ambiguus of the lateral medulla
c. Sommer sector of the hippocampus
d. Substantia gelatinosa of the spinal cord
e. Ventral posterolateral nucleus of the thalamus

475. A 63-year-old man presents with progressive uncontrolled movements of his left hand. He states that his hand "has a mind of its own." Physical examination finds apraxia (inability to make a requested voluntary movement) with rigidity. He is admitted to the hospital but dies suddenly 2 days after admission. An autopsy finds cortical atrophy involving the motor and premotor cortex. Tau positive inclusions were found in astrocytes and neurons in these atrophic regions. Which of the following is the most likely diagnosis?

a. Corticobasal degeneration
b. Déjérine-Roussy syndrome
c. Gerstmann's syndrome
d. Parinaud's syndrome
e. Wallenberg syndrome

476. A 79-year-old woman who lived alone and had a medical history of poorly controlled chronic hypertension died while at home. During the autopsy the pathologist finds a recent intracerebral hemorrhage involving the putamen. Histologic sections from this area reveal lipid and hyaline material to be deposited in the walls of cerebral arterioles, an abnormality that is associated with the formation of which of the following types of aneurysm?

a. Atherosclerotic aneurysm
b. Berry's aneurysm
c. Charcot-Bouchard aneurysm
d. Mycotic aneurysm
e. Saccular aneurysm

477. Histologic examination of the brain from a 39-year-old man who died from encephalitis finds numerous microglial nodules composed of mononuclear cells, microglia, and scattered multinucleated giant cells. Which one of the following is most likely to be present within the cells of these microglial nodules?

a. Cytomegalovirus
b. Herpes simplex virus
c. Human immunodeficiency virus
d. Poliovirus
e. Rabies virus

478. A lumbar puncture is performed on a patient with headaches, photophobia, clouding of consciousness, and neck stiffness. If these symptoms are the result of bacterial infection of the meninges, which of the following would examination of the cerebrospinal fluid (CSF) most likely reveal?

	Pressure	Gross Appearance	Protein	Glucose	Inflammation
a.	Increased	Cloudy	Increased	Decreased	Neutrophils
b.	Increased	Clear	Increased	Normal	Lymphocytes
c.	Increased	Clear	Increased	Normal	Mononuclear cells
d.	Decreased	Clear	Decreased	Normal	Lymphocytes
e.	Increased	Clear	Increased	Normal	Mixed

479. A 42-year-old immunosuppressed man presents with rapidly progressive neurologic symptoms including mental deterioration, visual loss, abnormal speech, and ataxia. Radiographic studies demonstrate multifocal lesions in the white matter without mass effect (no shift in the cerebral hemispheres is seen). A stereotactic brain biopsy reveals irregular areas of demyelination at the periphery of which are oligodendrocytes with markedly enlarged nuclei that have a "ground-glass" appearance. What is the best diagnosis?

a. Cysticercosis
b. Neuroborreliosis
c. Neurosyphilis
d. Progressive multifocal leukoencephalopathy
e. Subacute sclerosing panencephalitis

480. A 62-year-old man presents with rapidly progressive dementia and dies. At autopsy, marked spongiform degeneration of the brain is found. The familial form of this disorder is associated with mutations of what gene?

a. FGFR3
b. PRNP
c. PTEN
d. SOD1
e. UBE3A

481. Physical examination of a 34-year-old woman with the new onset of an intention tremor finds medial rectus palsy on attempted lateral gaze in the adducting eye and monocular nystagmus in the abducting eye with convergence. Which of the following is the most likely cause of these clinical findings?

a. An apical lung cancer
b. A pituitary adenoma
c. Diabetes mellitus
d. Multiple sclerosis
e. Tertiary syphilis

482. A 45-year-old man presents with weakness and cramping that involves both of his hands. Physical examination reveals atrophy of the muscles of both hands, hyperactive reflexes and muscle fasciculations involving the arms and legs, and a positive Babinski reflex. Sensation appears normal in the arms and legs. Which of the following is the most likely diagnosis?

a. Metachromatic leukodystrophy
b. Amyotrophic lateral sclerosis
c. Guillain-Barré syndrome
d. Huntington's disease
e. Wilson's disease

483. A 73-year-old woman presents with progressive memory loss. Her family relates several recent episodes where she left home by herself, got lost in her own neighborhood, and could not find her way back. Neurologic examination was unremarkable except for severe cognitive deficits. Within 2 years she had to be admitted to a nursing home, where she died 3 years later. Autopsy revealed bilateral, symmetrical atrophy of the frontal lobes with wide sulci and narrow gyri. Microscopic examination of tissue taken from this area revealed bundles of filaments in the cytoplasm of neurons and focal collections of neuritic processes surrounding central amyloid cores. Which one of the listed enzymes is responsible for the production of these abnormal amyloid cores?

a. Adenosine deaminase
b. Alpha-reductase
c. Beta-secretase
d. PROTO oxidase
e. Xanthine oxidase

484. A 65-year-old man presents with bradykinesia, tremors at rest, and muscular rigidity. Physical examination reveals the patient to have a "masklike" facies. In this patient, from which one of the following sites would biopsies most likely reveal intracytoplasmic eosinophilic inclusions within neurons?

a. Basal ganglia
b. Caudate nucleus
c. Hippocampus
d. Midbrain
e. Substantia nigra

485. Shy-Drager syndrome, a Lewy body disease, is characterized by orthostatic hypotension, impotence, abnormal sweating, increased salivation, and pupil abnormalities. What is the major component of Lewy bodies?

a. Alpha-synuclein
b. Beta-amyloid
c. Hamartin
d. Parkin
e. Ubiquitin

486. A 41-year-old man presents with involuntary rapid jerky movements and progressive dementia. He soon dies, and gross examination of his brain reveals marked degeneration of the caudate nucleus. Which of the following is the most likely cause of this individual's symptoms?

a. Decreased functioning of GABA neurons
b. Increased functioning of dopamine neurons
c. Relative increased functioning of acetylcholine neurons
d. Relative decreased functioning of acetylcholine neurons
e. Decreased functioning of serotonin neurons

487. A 5-year-old boy presents with projectile vomiting and progressive ataxia. Workup finds obstructive hydrocephalus due to an infiltrative tumor located in the posterior fossa and originating from the midline of the cerebellum. What is the most likely diagnosis for a tumor located in this location in this child?

a. Glioblastoma multiforme
b. Dysembryoplastic neuroepithelial tumor
c. Primary CNS lymphoma
d. Primary germ cell tumor
e. Primitive neuroendocrine tumor

488. A 55-year-old woman presents with the onset of seizure activity. Computed tomography (CT) scans and skull x-rays demonstrate a mass in the right cerebral hemisphere that is markedly calcific. The mass is removed and histologic sections reveal sheets of cells with clear halos ("fried-egg" appearance) and scattered calcification. The presence of which one of the listed abnormalities within this type of tumor is associated with a better response to chemotherapy?

a. Deletion of region 12 on chromosome 22
b. Disruption of the p16/CDKNZA gene
c. Duplication of the long arm of chromosome 17
d. Loss of heterozygosity for chromosomes 1p and 19q
e. Overexpression of PDGF-A and its receptor

489. A 44-year-old woman presents with the new onset of seizures along with increasing frequency of severe headaches. Her medical history is otherwise unremarkable. Physical examination finds bilateral neurologic defects. Workup reveals a large, ill-defined, necrotic mass that involves both the right and left cerebral cortex. Histologic sections from this lesion reveal a hypercellular tumor with pseudopalisading of tumor cells around large areas of serpentine necrosis. Marked vascular endoneural proliferation is present. Numerous atypical nuclei and mitoses are seen. This tumor is best classified as what type of high-grade neoplasm?

a. Astrocytoma
b. Lymphoma
c. Medulloblastoma
d. Oligodendroglioma
e. Schwannoma

490. A 38-year-old woman presents with increasing frequency of severe headaches. The previous day she had a seizure that lasted several minutes. Her past medical history is otherwise unremarkable, and she has no previous history of seizure activity. She is admitted to the hospital and a CT scan of her head finds a 2-cm mass attached to the dura in her right frontal area. Which of the following histologic changes is most likely to be seen in a biopsy specimen taken from this tumor?

a. Antoni A areas with Verocay bodies
b. A whorled pattern with psammoma bodies
c. Endothelial proliferation with serpentine areas of necrosis
d. "Fried-egg" appearance of tumor cells without necrosis
e. True rosettes and pseudorosettes

491. A 63-year-old woman is hospitalized secondary to markedly decreased vision. She has no history of polydipsia or nocturia. Physical examination finds bilateral sluggish light reflexes and a bitemporal hemianopsia. No papilledema is present, and her urine specific gravity is within normal limits. A CT scan of the head finds a suprasellar mass with calcification. Which of the following is the most likely diagnosis?

a. Craniopharyngioma
b. Germinoma
c. Juvenile pilocytic astrocytoma
d. Medulloblastoma
e. Meningioma

492. Juvenile pilocytic astrocytoma is the most likely diagnosis for which one of the following clinical situations?

a. A poorly defined cystic calcified tumor in the hypothalamus of an adult
b. A well-circumscribed cystic tumor in the cerebellum of a child
c. A well-circumscribed noncystic tumor attached to the dura of an adult
d. An infiltrative noncystic tumor in the cerebellum of a child
e. An infiltrative necrotic tumor that crosses the midline in an adult

493. A 45-year-old woman presents with unilateral tinnitus and unilateral hearing loss. Physical examination reveals facial weakness and loss of corneal reflex on the same side as the tinnitus and hearing loss. Where would a tumor need to be located to produce these clinical signs and symptoms?

a. Anterior horn of the spinal cord
b. Anterior pituitary
c. Cerebellopontine angle
d. Frontal cortex
e. Lateral ventricle

494. The combination of facial angiofibromas, seizures, mental retardation, and central nervous system hamartomas is most characteristic of which neurocutaneous syndrome (phakomatosis)?

a. Neurofibromatosis type 1
b. Neurofibromatosis type 2
c. Peutz-Jeghers syndrome
d. Tuberous sclerosis
e. von Hippel-Lindau disease

495. A 9-year-old boy presents with progressive severe headaches along with signs of precocious puberty. Physical examination finds paralysis of upward gaze and increased intracranial pressure due to a mass of the pineal gland producing an obstructive hydrocephalus. Which of the following is the most likely diagnosis?

a. Benedikt's syndrome (paramedian midbrain syndrome)
b. Jugular foramen syndrome (abnormality affecting CN IX, X, and XI)
c. Parinaud's syndrome (dorsal midbrain syndrome)
d. Subclavian steal syndrome
e. Weber's syndrome (medial midbrain syndrome)

496. Wallenberg syndrome is characterized by a large constellation of clinical findings that include nystagmus, vertigo, ataxia, ipsilateral laryngeal paralysis, loss of gag reflex, contralateral loss of pain and temperature from the trunk and extremities, ipsilateral loss of pain and temperature from the face, and ipsilateral Horner syndrome. Wallenberg syndrome is most likely to result from occlusion of what artery?

a. Anterior cerebral artery supplying the medial portion of the cerebral hemisphere
b. Lenticulostriate artery supplying the posterior limb of the internal capsule
c. Middle cerebral artery supplying the lateral portion of the cerebral hemisphere
d. Posterior cerebral artery supplying the occipital lobe
e. Posterior inferior cerebellar artery supplying the cerebellum

497. A 47-year-old man presents with increasing back pain and is found to have bilateral loss of pain and temperature sensations in both arms. His sense of touch and position is within normal limits. Which of the following clinical tests is most likely to make a definitive diagnosis in this individual?

a. CT scan of the lower spinal cord
b. MRI of the cervical spinal cord
c. Conduction studies on the sural nerve
d. Protein electrophoresis on cerebrospinal fluid
e. Viral cultures of cerebrospinal fluid

498. A 33-year-old man presents with acute onset of weakness involving the left side of his face. He says he cannot completely close his left eye, and he notes increased formation of tears from this eye. Physical examination finds facial asymmetry characterized by flattening of the entire left side of his face, but no abnormalities are seen on the right side. It is noted that when he tries to forcefully close his left eye, it rotates up and out. Which of the following abnormalities is the most likely cause of these signs and symptoms?

a. A lower motor neuron lesion involving the facial nerve
b. A lower motor neuron lesion involving the trigeminal nerve
c. An upper motor neuron lesion involving the accessory nerve
d. An upper motor neuron lesion involving the glossopharyngeal nerve
e. An upper motor neuron lesion involving the vagus nerve

499. After recovering from a viral respiratory tract infection, a 23-year-old woman presents with weakness in her distal extremities that rapidly ascends to involve proximal muscles. Physical examination reveals absent deep tendon reflexes, and a lumbar puncture reveals the CSF protein to be increased, but very few cells are present. A biopsy of a peripheral nerve reveals inflammation and demyelination (radiculoneuropathy). Which of the following is the most likely diagnosis?

a. Brown-Séquard's syndrome
b. Charcot-Marie-Tooth disease
c. Diabetes mellitus
d. Guillain-Barré syndrome
e. Syringomyelia

500. Carpal tunnel syndrome, produced by damage to or pressure on the median nerve deep to the flexor retinaculum, is best characterized by which one of the following clinical signs?

a. Hyperextension of fingers at metacarpophalangeal joints and flexion at interphalangeal joints (claw hand)
b. Numbness in fifth finger and medial portion of ring finger
c. Pain in thumb, index finger, middle finger, and lateral half of ring finger
d. Adduction, extension, and internal rotation of upper limb ("porter's tip" sign)
e. Weakness of extensors of wrist and fingers (wristdrop)

Nervous System

Answers

469. The answer is e. (*Kumar, pp 1352–1353.*) Increased intracranial pressure can result from mass lesions in the brain, cerebral edema, or hydrocephalus. Increased intracranial pressure can cause swelling of the optic nerve (papilledema), headaches, vomiting, or herniation of part of the brain into the foramen magnum or under a free part of the dura.

Brain herniations are classified according to the area of the brain that is herniated. Subfalcine herniations are caused by herniation of the medial aspect of the cerebral hemisphere (cingulate gyrus) under the falx, which may compress the anterior cerebral artery. Transtentorial herniation, which occurs when the medial part of the temporal lobe (uncus) herniates over the free edge of the tentorium, may result in compression of the oculomotor nerve, which results in pupillary dilation and ophthalmoplegia (the affected eye points "down and out"). Tentorial herniation may also compress the cerebral peduncles, within which are the pyramidal tracts. Ipsilateral compression produces contralateral motor paralysis (hemiparesis), while compression of the contralateral cerebral peduncle against Kernohan's notch causes ipsilateral hemiparesis. Further caudal displacement of the entire brainstem may cause tearing of the penetrating arteries of the midbrain (Duret hemorrhages). This caudal displacement may also stretch the trochlear nerve (cranial nerve VI), causing paralysis of the lateral rectus muscle (the abnormal eye turns inward). Masses in the cerebellum may cause tonsillar herniation, in which the cerebellar tonsils are herniated into the foramen magnum. This may compress the medulla and respiratory centers, causing death. Tonsillar herniation may also occur if a lumbar puncture (LP) is performed in a patient with increased intracranial pressure. Therefore, before performing an LP, check the patient for the presence of papilledema.

470. The answer is b. (*Kumar, pp 1353–1355. Rubin, pp 1452–1453.*) Developmental abnormalities of the brain include the Arnold-Chiari malformation, the Dandy-Walker malformation, and the phakomatoses, which include tuberous sclerosis, neurofibromatosis, von Hippel-Lindau disease, and Sturge-Weber syndrome. The Arnold-Chiari malformation consists of herniation of the cerebellum and fourth ventricle into the foramen magnum, flattening of the base of the skull, and spina bifida with meningomyelocele. Newborns with this disorder are at risk of developing hydrocephalus within the first few days of delivery secondary to stenosis of the cerebral aqueduct. In contrast, severe hypoplasia or absence of the cerebellar vermis occurs in the Dandy-Walker malformation. There is cystic distention of the roof of the fourth ventricle, hydrocephalus, and possibly agenesis of the corpus callosum. Tuberous sclerosis may show characteristic firm, white nodules (tubers) in the cortex and subependymal nodules of gliosis protruding into the ventricles ("candle drippings"). Other signs of tuberous sclerosis include the triad of seizures, mental retardation, and congenital white spots or macules (leukoderma). Facial angiofibromata (adenoma sebaceum) may also occur. In von Hippel-Lindau disease, multiple benign and malignant neoplasms occur, including hemangioblastomas of the retina, cerebellum, and medulla oblongata; angiomas of the kidney and liver; and renal cell carcinomas. Patients with Sturge-Weber syndrome, a nonfamilial congenital disorder, display angiomas of the brain, leptomeninges, and ipsilateral face, which are called port-wine stains (nevus flammeus).

471. The answer is d. (*Kumar, pp 1353–1354. Rubin, pp 1449–1451.*) Neural tube developmental defects are caused by defective closure of the neural tube. These defects, which may occur anywhere along the extent of the neural tube, are classified as either caudal or cranial defects. Failure of development of the cranial end of the neural tube results in anencephaly, while failure of development of the caudal end of the neural tube results in spina bifida. Anencephaly, which is not compatible with life, is characterized by the absence of the forebrain. Instead, there is a mass of disorganized glial tissue with vessels in this area called a cerebrovasculosa. Ultrasound examination will reveal an abnormal shape to the head of the fetus with an absence of the skull. Note that neural tube defects are associated with increased maternal serum levels of α-fetoprotein (AFP), which is a glycoprotein synthesized by the yolk sac and the fetal liver. Increased serum levels are also associated with yolk sac tumors of the testes and liver cell carcinomas (note that decreased AFP is associated with Down syndrome). Neural tube defects are associated with maternal obesity and decreased folate during pregnancy (folate supplementation in diet decreases the incidence of these developmental defects).

472. The answer is a. (*Kumar, pp 1359–1360. Damjanov, pp 2733–2736.*) Epidural hemorrhages result from hemorrhages into the potential space between the dura and the bone of the skull. These hemorrhages result from severe trauma that typically causes a skull fracture. The hemorrhage results from rupture of one of the meningeal arteries, as these arteries supply the dura and run between the dura and the skull. The artery involved is usually the middle meningeal artery, which is a branch of the maxillary artery, as the skull fracture is usually in the temporal area. Since the bleeding is of arterial origin (high pressure), it is rapid and the symptoms are rapid in onset, although the patient may be normal for several hours (lucid interval). Bleeding causes increased intracranial pressure and can lead to tentorial herniation and death.

473. The answer is b. (*Kumar, pp 1366–1367. Rubin, p 1461.*) Subarachnoid hemorrhage, which is much less common than hypertensive intracerebral hemorrhage, most often results from the rupture of a berry aneurysm. These aneurysms are saccular aneurysms that result from congenital defects in the media of arteries. They are typically located at the bifurcations of arteries. They are not the result of atherosclerosis. Instead, berry aneurysms are called congenital, although the aneurysm itself is not present at birth. Berry aneurysms are most commonly found in the circle of Willis, typically either at the junction of the anterior communicating artery with the anterior cerebral artery or at the junction of the middle cerebral artery and the posterior communicating artery. The chance of rupture of berry aneurysms increases with age (rupture is rare in childhood). Rupture causes marked bleeding into the subarachnoid space and produces severe headaches, typically described as the "worst headache ever." Additional symptoms include vomiting, pain and stiffness of the neck (due to meningeal irritation caused by the blood), and papilledema. Death may follow rapidly.

474. The answer is c. (*Kumar, pp 1361–1363. Rubin, pp 1470–1475.*) Decreased brain perfusion may be generalized (global) or localized. Global ischemia results from generalized decreased blood flow, such as with shock, cardiac arrest, or hypoxic episodes (e.g., near drowning or carbon monoxide poisoning). The gross changes produced by global hypoxia include watershed (border zone) infarcts, which typically occur at the border of areas supplied by the anterior and middle cerebral arteries, and laminar necrosis, which is related to the short, penetrating vessels originating from pial arteries. The microscopic changes produced by global hypoxia are grouped into three categories. The earliest histologic changes, occurring in the first 24 h, include the formation of red neurons (acute neuronal injury), characterized by eosinophilia of the cytoplasm of the neurons, followed in time by pyknosis and karyorrhexis. The Purkinje cells of the cerebellum and the pyramidal neurons of Sommer's sector in the hippocampus are particularly sensitive to ischemic damage and are most likely to demonstrate these early changes. The last two microscopic categories of global hypoxic change are subacute changes, which occur at 24 h to 2 weeks, and repair, which occurs after 2 weeks. Subacute changes include tissue necrosis, vascular proliferation, and reactive gliosis, while repair is characterized by the removal of the necrotic tissue.

475. The answer is a. (*Kumar, pp 1390–1391. Goldman, p 2140. Goetz, pp 416, 945, 949–950. Young, pp 275, 277.*) The "alien hand" syndrome is an unusual neurologic disorder in which one of the patient's hands seems to have a life of its own; that is, the patient does not recognize their hand as being a part of his own body and they can't control movement of the hand or arm. There are many different causes of the "alien hand," such as damage to the anterior part of the corpus callosum. However, the combination of "alien hand" along with extrapyramidal rigidity, sensory cortical dysfunction, and tau-positive inclusions in astrocytes, oligodendroglia, and neurons, is most suggestive of corticobasal degeneration. The cortical dysfunction seen in this syndrome includes disorders of language and apraxia, which is the inability to carry out learned movements.

Disorders of speech and language usually involve the dominant cerebral hemisphere, usually the left side in right-handed individuals. This dominant hemisphere is also involved with calculation, while the nondominant side is involved with three-dimensional or spatial perception, perception of social cues, and nonverbal ideation, such as music and poetry. Damage to the dominant parietal lobe can produce apraxia. Furthermore, damage to this area can produce the Gerstmann's syndrome, which is characterized by right-left confusion, finger agnosia (problems naming and identifying fingers), agraphia (problems writing), and dyscalculia (problems with simple math calculations).

In contrast to these clinical findings, Déjérine-Roussy syndrome refers to the clinical combination of contralateral loss of sensory with contralateral dysthesia (pain); while Parinaud's syndrome refers to large impaired conjugate vertical gaze, pupillary abnormality, and absence of accommodation reflex due to compression of upper midbrain and pretectal areas. Finally, Wallenberg syndrome is the lateral medullary syndrome and results from occlusion of the vertebral artery or occlusion of the posterior inferior cerebellar artery (hence its other name, PICA syndrome).

476. The answer is c. (*Kumar, pp 1368–1369. Rubin, pp 1466–1470.*) Hypertension is a common cause of intracerebral hemorrhage. Hypertension aggravates and extends atherosclerosis into distal, smaller branches of blood vessels. Hypertension also causes lipid and hyaline material to be deposited in the walls of cerebral arterioles, this being called lipohyalinosis. This weakens the wall and forms small Charcot-Bouchard aneurysms, which may eventually rupture. Hypertensive hemorrhage shows a predilection for the distribution of the lenticulostriate arteries (branch of middle cerebral artery) with small (lacunar) hemorrhages, or large hemorrhages obliterating the corpus striatum, including the putamen and internal capsule. Hypertensive hemorrhages also commonly occur in cerebellum and pons and are often fatal. In contrast to Charcot-Bouchard aneurysms, berry aneurysms (small saccular aneurysms) are the result of congenital defects in the media of blood vessels and are located at the bifurcations of arteries. Atherosclerotic aneurysms are fusiform (spindle-shaped) aneurysms usually located in the major cerebral vessels. They rarely rupture, but may become thrombosed. Mycotic (septic) aneurysms result from septic emboli, most commonly from subacute bacterial endocarditis.

477. The answer is c. (*Kumar, pp 1372–1377. Rubin, pp 1481–1483, 1486–1489.*) Microglial nodules within the brain that are composed of mononuclear cells, microglia, and scattered multinucleated giant cells are characteristic of meningoencephalitis caused by HIV (human immunodeficiency virus). Previously most patients with AIDS at some time during their illness developed neurologic symptoms, but the incidence of this has markedly decreased following the use of antiretroviral therapy.

In contrast, herpes simplex virus produces characteristic Cowdry type A intranuclear inclusions in neurons and glial cells, while rabies forms characteristic inclusions within neurons called Negri bodies. Rabies, caused by a single-stranded RNA rhabdovirus, is transmitted by the bite of a rabid animal, usually a dog, and travels to the brain via peripheral nerves. Symptoms caused by destruction of neurons in the brainstem include irritability, difficulty in swallowing and spasms of the throat (these two resulting in "hydrophobia"), seizures, and delirium. The illness is almost uniformly fatal. Enlarged cells (cytomegaly) with intranuclear and intracytoplasmic inclusions are seen with cytomegalovirus infection. Finally, poliovirus does not infect the brain but rather it invades the anterior horn motor neurons of the spinal cord, where it causes muscular paralysis.

478. The answer is a. (*Kumar, pp 1369–1371. Goldman, pp 1649, 2125.*) Meningitis [inflammation of the arachnoid and the cerebrospinal fluid (CSF)] may be classified as acute pyogenic, aseptic, or chronic. The etiology and CSF findings vary in these three groups. The CSF in acute pyogenic meningitis, which is usually caused by bacteria, is grossly cloudy (not bloody, which is suggestive of a subarachnoid hemorrhage) and displays increased pressure, increased neutrophils, increased protein, and decreased glucose. With chronic meningitis, such as that caused by Mycobacterium tuberculosis, the CSF is clear grossly, with only a slight increase in leukocytes (either mononuclear cells or a mixed infiltrate), a markedly increased protein level, increased pressure, and moderately decreased or normal amounts of sugar. Both brain abscesses and subdural empyemas, which are parameningeal infections rather than direct meningeal infections, cause increased CSF pressure (more marked with abscess because of mass effect) along with increased inflammatory cells (lymphocytes and polys) and increased protein but a normal glucose level. The CSF is clear. Encephalitis, also not a direct infection of the meninges, results in clear CSF, increased pressure, increased protein, normal glucose, and possibly increased lymphocytes.

479. The answer is d. (*Kumar, pp 406–407, 1372, 1376–1377. Rubin, pp 1484–1491.*) Progressive multifocal leukoencephalopathy (PML) is a demyelinating disease of the central nervous system that results from infection of oligodendrocytes by the JC polyomavirus. Signs and symptoms of PML are varied but include dementia and ataxia along with abnormal vision and speech. The pathognomonic feature of PML is the oligodendrocytes in areas of demyelination, which have a "ground-glass" appearance of their nuclei due to infection with the viral particles. PML occurs as a terminal complication in immunosuppressed individuals, especially individuals with AIDS.

Neurosyphilis, a tertiary stage of syphilis, includes syphilitic meningitis, paretic neurosyphilis, and tabes dorsalis. Syphilitic meningitis is characterized by perivascular infiltrates of lymphocytes and plasma cells that cause obliterative endarteritis and meningeal fibrosis. Tabes dorsalis is the result of degeneration of the posterior columns of the spinal cord. This is caused by compression atrophy of the posterior spinal sensory nerves, which produces impaired joint position sensation, ataxia, loss of pain sensation (leading to joint damage, i.e., Charcot joints), and Argyll Robertson pupils (pupils that react to accommodation but not to light).

Finally, subacute sclerosing panencephalitis (SSPE) is caused by infection of the CNS by an altered measles virus; neuroborreliosis refers to infection of the CNS by *Borrelia burgdorferi*, the causative agent of Lyme disease; and cysticercosis results from ingestion of the eggs of *Taenia solium*.

480. The answer is b. (*Kumar, pp 1380–1382. Rubin, pp 1492–1495.*) The spongiform encephalopathies include Creutzfeldt-Jakob disease (CJD), Gerstmann-Sträussler-Scheinker syndrome (GSS), fatal familial insomnia, and kuru. Patients with CJD initially have subtle changes in memory and behavior, which are followed by a rapidly progressive dementia and death within several months. Microscopically, there is characteristic spongiform change in the gray matter ("cluster of grapes" vacuolation) without inflammation.

All of the spongiform encephalopathies are associated with abnormal forms of a prion protein (PrP). The term prion stands for infectious particle and was coined by Prusiner in 1982. Disease results from alternate folding of the normal α-helix (called PrP^c) to an abnormal β-pleated sheet form (called PrP^{sc} or PrP^{res}). This conformational change can occur spontaneously at a very slow rate. Once formed, however, PrP^{sc} can combine with PrP^c to much more quickly form many more PrP^{sc} particles, which can "crystallize" and form plaques. PrP^c can also form PrP^{sc} at much higher rates if mutations are present in PrP^c, which can result from mutations in the gene that codes for PrP^c called PRNP. Mutations in this gene have been identified in patients with the familial forms of CJD, GSS, and fatal familial insomnia. In contrast, SOD1 mutations are seen with amyotrophic lateral sclerosis (ALS), FGFR3 mutations with achondroplasia, UBE3A mutations with Angelman's syndrome, and PTEN mutations with endometrial and prostate cancers.

481. The answer is d. (*Ayala, pp 269, 297. Kumar, pp 1382–1385. Henry, pp 793, 1013.*) In primary CNS demyelination there is loss of myelin sheaths with relative preservation of axons. Primary demyelination is seen predominately in multiple sclerosis, in the perivenous encephalomyelopathies, and in progressive multifocal leukoencephalopathy (PML). Multiple sclerosis (MS), a disease of unknown etiology, causes disseminated but focal plaques of primary demyelination anywhere in the CNS, but often in the white matter near the angles of the lateral ventricles. It primarily affects young adults between 20 and 40 years of age, with the onset of symptoms such as abnormalities of vision, tremors, paresthesias, and incoordination. The course is typically remitting and relapsing. Early findings include weakness of the lower extremities and visual abnormalities with retrobulbar pain. The classic (Charcot) triad in patients with MS consists of scanning speech, intention tremor, and nystagmus (mnemonic is SIN). Also pathognomonic for MS is internuclear ophthalmoplegia (INO), also known as the MLF syndrome, which results from demyelination of the medial longitudinal fasciculus. It results in medial rectus palsy on attempted lateral gaze and monocular nystagmus in abducting eye with convergence. Examination of the CSF in patients with MS reveals increased T lymphocytes, increased protein, and normal glucose. Protein electrophoresis of the CSF reveals oligoclonal bands (individual monoclonal spikes), although this latter finding is not specific for MS.

482. The answer is b. (*Kumar, pp 1396–1397. Rubin, pp 1495, 1504–1506.*) Amyotrophic lateral sclerosis (ALS), also known as Lou Gehrig's disease, is a degenerative disorder of motor neurons, principally the anterior horn cells of the spinal cord, the motor nuclei of the brainstem, and the upper motor neurons of the cerebral cortex. Clinically, this disease is a combination of lower motor neuron (LMN) disease with weakness and fasciculations and upper motor neuron (UMN) disease with spasticity and hyperreflexia. Early symptoms include weakness and cramping and then muscle atrophy and fasciculations. Reflexes are hyperactive in upper and lower extremities, and a positive extensor plantar (Babinski) reflex develops because of the loss of upper motor neurons. The triad of atrophic weakness of hands and forearms, slight spasticity of the legs, and generalized hyperreflexia—in the absence of sensory changes—suggests the diagnosis. The clinical course is rapid, and death may result from respiratory complications. There is no effective treatment for ALS. Theories about the etiology of ALS include viral infections, immunologic causes, or oxidative stress. The latter is related to a defect in zinc-copper binding superoxide dismutase (SOD) on chromosome 21. Decreased SOD activity leads to apoptosis of spinal motor neurons.

In contrast, metachromatic leukodystrophy is an autosomal recessive disorder of sphingomyelin metabolism that results from deficiency of cerebroside sulfatase (aryl-sulfatase A). Sulfatides accumulate in lysosomes and stain metachromatically with cresyl violet. Diagnostic measures include amniocentesis, enzyme analysis, and measuring decreased urinary aryl-sulfatase A. Demyelination is widespread in the cerebrum and peripheral nervous system. Acute inflammatory demyelinating polyradiculoneuropathy (Guillain-Barré syndrome) is a life-threatening disease of the peripheral nervous system. The disease usually follows recovery from an influenza-like upper respiratory tract infection and is characterized by a motor neuropathy that leads to an ascending paralysis that begins with weakness in the distal extremities and rapidly involves proximal muscles. Sensory changes are usually minimal. The disease is thought to result from immune-mediated segmental demyelination. Huntington's disease is characterized by choreiform movements and progressive dementia that appear after the age of 30. Wilson's disease (hepatolenticular degeneration) is an autosomal recessive disorder of copper metabolism in which the total circulating copper is decreased, but the free copper is increased. This leads to athetoid movements, cirrhosis of the liver, and copper deposits in the limbus of the cornea that produce the Kayser-Fleischer ring.

483. The answer is c. (*Kumar, pp 1386–1389. Rubin, pp 1509–1512.*) Alzheimer's disease (AD) is the most common cause of dementia in elderly (followed by vascular multi-infarct dementia and diffuse Lewy body disease). AD often begins insidiously with impairment of memory and progresses to dementia. Histologically, AD is characterized by numerous neurofibrillary tangles and senile plaques with a central core of amyloid alpha-protein. Both tangles and plaques are found to a lesser extent in other conditions, for example, neurofibrillary tangles in Down syndrome. Silver stains demonstrate tangles and plaques and Congo red shows amyloid deposition in plaques and vascular walls (amyloid angiopathy). In AD there are also numerous Hirano bodies, and granulovacuolar degeneration is found in more than 10% of the neurons of the hippocampus. Grossly, brain atrophy (narrowed gyri and widened sulci) is predominant in the frontal and superior temporal lobes.

The etiology of AD is not well understood (age is the main risk factor), but it is clear that there are multiple etiologic pathways to this disease state. Alzheimer's disease has been linked to abnormalities involving four specific genes. The gene for beta-amyloid (A-beta) is located on chromosome 21 (note the high incidence of Alzheimer's disease in individuals with trisomy 21). Cleavage of the beta-amyloid precursor protein (beta-APP) by alpha-secretase precludes beta-A formation; but cleavage of beta-APP at a site N-terminal to the start of the transmembrane domain by beta-secretase (BACE-1) or within the transmembrane by gamma-secretase produces fragments that tend to aggregate into the pathogenic amyloid fibrils. Beta-amyloid deposition is necessary but not sufficient for the development of Alzheimer's disease. Early-onset familial Alzheimer's is also related to mutations in presenilins. The presenilin 1 (PS1) gene is located on chromosome 14, while the presenilin 2 (PS2) gene is located on chromosome 1.

In contrast to beta-secretase, 5-alpha-reductase is the enzyme that normally converts testosterone to DHT. A deficiency of this enzyme produces male pseudohermaphroditism. Xanthine oxidase catalyzes the oxidation of hypoxanthine to xanthine. Levels of this enzyme are increased in patients with liver disease. Finally a deficiency of adenosine deaminase is seen with the autosomal recessive form of SCIDs, while a deficiency of PROTO oxidase is seen with variegate porphyria.

484. The answer is e. (*Kumar, pp 1391–1393. Rubin, pp 1502–1504.*) The degenerative diseases of the CNS are diseases that affect the gray matter and are characterized by the progressive loss of neurons in specific areas of the brain. In Parkinson's disease, characterized by a masklike facial expression, coarse tremors, slowness of voluntary movements, and muscular rigidity, there is degeneration and loss of pigmented cells in the substantia nigra, resulting in a decrease in dopamine synthesis. Lewy bodies (eosinophilic intracytoplasmic inclusions) are found in the remaining neurons of the substantia nigra. The decreased synthesis of dopamine by neurons originating in the substantia nigra leads to decreased amounts and functioning of dopamine in the striatum. This results in decreased dopamine inhibition and a relative increase in acetylcholine function, which is excitatory in the striatum. The effect of this excitation, however, is to increase the functioning of GABA neurons, which are inhibitory. The result, therefore, is increased inhibition or decreased movement. The severity of the motor syndrome correlates with the degree of dopamine deficiency. Therapy may be with dopamine agonists or anticholinergics.

485. The answer is a. (*Kumar, pp 1393, 1391–1392.*) Lewy bodies are intracytoplasmic eosinophilic inclusions that are composed of fine filaments, which are densely packed in the core but loose at their rim. These filaments are composed of neurofilament antigens, parkin, and ubiquitin, but the major component of the Lewy body is alpha-synuclein. The histologic presence of Lewy bodies can be seen in several disorders (Lewy body disorders) that differ in the location where the Lewy bodies are found. In classic Parkinson's disease, Lewy bodies are found in the nigrostriatal system (producing extrapyramidal movement disorder). In Lewy body dementia, Lewy bodies are found in the cerebral cortex (producing dementia; this is the third most common cause of dementia). In Shy-Drager syndrome, Lewy bodies are found in sympathetic neurons in the spinal cord (causing autonomic dysfunction, including orthostatic hypotension, impotence, abnormal sweat and salivary gland secretion, and pupillary abnormalities). Unlike Parkinson's disease, however, no mutations in the gene that codes for alpha-synuclein have been found with the Shy-Drager syndrome.

In contrast, hamartin and tuberin are proteins associated with tuberous sclerosis, while beta-amyloid is a component of the core of cerebral plaques seen with Alzheimer's disease.

486. The answer is a. (*Kumar, pp 1393–1394. Rubin, pp 1506–1507.*) Huntington's disease, an autosomal dominant disorder that results from an abnormal gene on chromosome 4, involves the extrapyramidal system and atrophy of the caudate nuclei and putamen. Choreiform movements and progressive dementia appear after the age of 30. There is degeneration of GABA neurons in the striatum, which leads to decreased function (decreased inhibition) and increased movement. Huntington's disease is one of four diseases that are characterized by long repeating sequences of three nucleotides (the other diseases being fragile X syndrome, myotonic dystrophy, and spinal and bulbar muscular atrophy). Therapy for excessive movement (hyperkinetic) disorders can be attempted with dopamine antagonists. Decreased dopamine in the striatum theoretically causes a relative increase in acetylcholine and an increase in excitation in the striatum. This causes increased GABA function, which leads to increased inhibition of movement. The same result could theoretically be achieved with inhibition of acetylcholine breakdown (cholinesterase inhibitors). Compare this to the same treatment of hypokinetic (Parkinsonian) disorders. Dopamine agonists increase the inhibition in the striatum, leading to decreased GABA in the striatum and decreased inhibition of movement (increased movement). The same result could theoretically be achieved with anticholinergics.

487. The answer is e. (*Kumar, pp 1406–1409. Rubin, p 1519.*) Primitive neuroectodermal tumors (PNETs) are a type of malignant embryonal tumor that can be found at sites within or outside of the central nervous system. An example of a PNET located outside of the CNS is Ewing's sarcoma of bone. PNETs of the CNS can be divided into supratentorial tumors (sPNET) and infratentorial tumors (iPNET). The latter are also called medulloblastomas, these tumors being the most common tumor located in the posterior fossa of a child. They usually arise in the midline of the cerebellum (the vermis) but in adults, where the incidence is much less than in children, they are more apt to arise in the cerebellar hemispheres in a lateral position. Medulloblastomas grow by local invasive growth and may block cerebrospinal fluid circulation (CSF block) via compression of the fourth ventricle. Recently, aggressive treatment with the combined modalities of excision, radiotherapy, and chemotherapy has improved survival rates.

Dysembryoplastic neuroepithelial tumor (DNT) and primary brain germ cell tumor (PBGCT) are also tumors that are more common in children. DNT is a low-grade tumor that is most commonly located in the superficial portions of the temporal lobe, while PBGCTs are located most often in the pineal and suprasellar region. Neither glioblastoma multiformes nor primary CNS lymphomas are CNS tumors of childhood.

488. The answer is d. (*Kumar, pp 1401–1410. Rubin, p 1518.*) Oligodendrogliomas, which most commonly involve the cerebrum (hemispheres) in adults, are slow-growing tumors that have a high recurrence rate. Some oligodendrogliomas do proliferate in a rapid and aggressive fashion and may be associated with a malignant astrocytoma component. Histologically, oligodendrogliomas consist of sheets of cells with clear halos ("fried-egg" appearance) and various amounts of calcification (which can be seen on x-ray). Cytogenetic abnormalities have therapeutic significance for this type of tumor, as only tumors with deletion involving 19q or 1p respond to chemotherapy.

In contrast, deletion of region 12 on chromosome 22 is the most common cytogenetic abnormality of meningiomas, while duplication of the long arm of chromosome 17 is the most common genetic abnormality seen in medulloblastomas. Finally some cases of glioblastoma multiforme result from the progression of low grade astrocytoma to a higher grade (secondary glioblastoma multiforme). This progression is associated with several genetic abnormalities, such as disruption of the p16/CDKNZA gene or overexpression of PDGF-A and its receptor.

489. The answer is a. (*Kumar, pp 1401–1404. Rubin, pp 1515–1518.*) The features listed in the question are characteristic of a high-grade astrocytoma, which is commonly called a glioblastoma multiforme. Astrocytomas, the most common primary brain tumors in adults, range from low grade to very high grade (glioblastoma multiforme). These grades of astrocytomas include grade I (the least aggressive and histologically difficult to differentiate from reactive astrocytosis), grade II (some pleomorphism microscopically), grade III (anaplastic astrocytoma, characterized histologically by increased pleomorphism and prominent mitoses), and grade IV (glioblastoma multiforme). Glioblastoma multiforme is a highly malignant tumor characterized histologically by endothelial proliferation and serpentine areas of necrosis surrounded by peripheral palisading of tumor cells. It frequently crosses the midline ("butterfly tumor").

In contrast to the highly malignant glioblastoma, schwannomas are benign tumors that generally appear as extremely cellular spindle cell neoplasms, sometimes with metaplastic elements of bone, cartilage, and skeletal muscle. Medulloblastomas, however, are malignant tumors that occur exclusively in the cerebellum and microscopically are highly cellular with uniform nuclei, scant cytoplasm, and, in about one-third of cases, rosette formation centered by neurofibrillary material. Oligodendrogliomas, which are marked by foci of calcification in 70% of cases, commonly show a pattern of uniform cellularity and are composed of round cells with small dark nuclei, clear cytoplasm, and a clearly defined cell membrane.

490. The answer is b. (*Kumar, pp 1409–1410. Rubin, pp 1519–1520.*) A tumor that is attached to the dura is most likely to be a meningioma. This type of tumor arises from the arachnoid villi of the brain or spinal cord. Although they usually occur during middle or later life, a small number occur in persons 20 to 40 years of age. They commonly arise along the venous sinuses (parasagittal, sphenoid wings, and olfactory groove). Although meningiomas are benign and usually slow-growing, some have progesterone receptors and rapid growth in pregnancy occurs occasionally. The rare malignant meningioma may invade or even metastasize. The typical case, however, does not invade the brain, but displaces it, causing headaches and seizures. Histologically, many different patterns can be seen, but psammoma bodies and a whorled pattern of tumor cells are somewhat characteristic. In contrast to this histologic appearance, Antoni A areas with Verocay bodies are seen in schwannomas, endothelial proliferation and serpentine areas of necrosis are seen in glioblastoma multiformes, a "fried-egg" appearance of tumor cells is characteristic of oligodendrogliomas, and true rosettes and pseudorosettes can be seen in medulloblastomas.

491. The answer is a. (*Kumar, p 1164. Rubin, p 1518.*) Both oligodendroglioma and craniopharyngioma show calcification fairly frequently; oligodendroglioma is often located in the frontal lobe, whereas craniopharyngioma occurs around the third ventricle and demonstrates suprasellar calcification. CT scan and particularly MRI are essential in diagnosis. Patchy intracerebral calcification may develop in tuberous sclerosis, an autosomal dominant disease characterized by the triad of epilepsy, mental retardation, and facial skin lesions (multiple angiofibromas). In addition, subependymal gliosis, cardiac rhabdomyoma, renal angiomyolipoma, and periungual fibroma occur. Calcification of the basal ganglia occurs in about 20% of patients with chronic hypoparathyroidism, which sometimes leads to a Parkinsonian syndrome.

492. The answer is b. (*Kumar, pp 1403–1404. Weidner, pp 2062–2073.*) The location of a tumor and the age of the patient are both very important in the differential diagnosis of tumors of the central nervous system. Astrocytomas occur predominately in the cerebral hemispheres in adult life and old age, in the cerebellum and pons in childhood, and in the spinal cord in young adults. The pilocytic astrocytoma is a subtype that is the most common brain tumor in children, and therefore it is also called a juvenile pilocytic astrocytoma. It is characterized by its location in the cerebellum and better prognosis. Meningiomas, found within the meninges, have their peak incidence in the fourth and fifth decades. The highly malignant glioblastoma multiforme is also found primarily in adults. Oligodendrogliomas also involve the cerebrum in adults. Ependymomas are found most frequently in the fourth ventricle, while the choroid plexus papilloma, a variant of the ependymoma, is found most commonly in the lateral ventricles of young boys. The medulloblastoma is a tumor that arises exclusively in the cerebellum and has its highest incidence toward the end of the first decade. In children medulloblastomas are located in the midline, while in adults they are found in more lateral locations.

493. The answer is c. (*Kumar, pp 1411–1412. Rubin, pp 1532–1533.*) Schwannomas (neurilemomas) are single, encapsulated tumors of nerve sheaths, usually benign, occurring on peripheral, spinal, or cranial nerves. The acoustic neuroma is an example of a schwannoma that arises from the vestibulocochlear nerve (CN VIII). These tumors are typically located at the cerebellopontine angle or in the internal acoustic meatus. Initially, when they are small, these tumors produce symptoms by compressing CN VIII and CN VII (facial). CN VIII symptoms include unilateral tinnitus (ringing in the ear), unilateral hearing loss, and vertigo (dizziness). Involvement of the facial nerve produces facial weakness and loss of corneal reflex. Histologically, an acoustic neuroma consists of cellular areas (Antoni A) and loose edematous areas (Antoni B). Verocay bodies (foci of palisaded nuclei) may be found in the more cellular areas.

494. The answer is d. (*Kumar, pp 859, 862, 1413–1414. Rubin, pp 1524–1525. Inoki, pp 19–24.*) Tuberous sclerosis is an autosomal dominant syndrome characterized by the clinical triad of angiofibromas ("adenoma sebaceum"), seizures, and mental retardation. Patients develop hamartomas in the central nervous system including "tubers," which are firm areas with haphazardly arranged neurons and glia with stout processes. The syndrome is associated with the development of several different types of tumors, including subependymal giant cell tumor, rhabdomyoma of the heart, and angiomyolipoma of the kidney. Mutations at several loci have been associated with tuberous sclerosis including the TSC1 locus, which codes for hamartin, and the TSC2 locus, which codes for tuberin. These two proteins inhibit mTOR, which is the mammalian target for rapamycin. mTOR plays a central role in the regulation of cell growth. Dysregulation of mTOR activity is associated with several hamartoma syndromes, including the tuberous sclerosis, von Hippel-Lindau syndrome, Peutz-Jeghers syndrome, and the PTEN-related hamartoma syndromes. In von Hippel-Lindau disease, a rare autosomal dominant disorder, multiple benign, and malignant neoplasms occur. These include hemangioblastomas of retina and brain (cerebellum and medulla oblongata), angiomas of kidney and liver, and renal cell carcinomas (multiple and bilateral) in 25 to 50% of cases. Peutz-Jeghers syndrome is characterized by the combination of hamartomatous polyps of the GI tract and pigmentation around the lips.

Classic neurofibromatosis (NF-1) is characterized by café-au-lait skin macules, axillary freckling, multiple neurofibromas, plexiform neurofibromas, and Lisch nodules (pigmented iris hamartomas). Lisch nodules are found in 95% of patients after age 6. Hamartomas of the iris are not present in central or acoustic neurofibromatosis (NF-2), though both types of neurofibromatosis produce café-au-lait macules and neurofibromas. Only the central, or acoustic, form produces bilateral acoustic neuromas; the classic form may produce unilateral acoustic neuroma. There is increased risk of developing meningiomas or even pheochromocytoma. A major complication of NF-1 is the malignant transformation of a neurofibroma to a neurofibrosarcoma. The gene for the classic form (NF-1) is located on chromosome 17. It encodes for neurofibromin, a protein that regulates the function of p21 ras oncoprotein.

495. The answer is c. (*Young, pp 266, 275–276. Goetz, pp 160–161.*) Lesions of the midbrain in general produce partial ophthalmoplegia and contralateral hemiplegia. In particular, the dorsal midbrain syndrome (Parinaud's syndrome) affects the superior colliculus and pretectal areas (producing paralysis of upward and downward gaze) and obstructs the cerebral aqueduct (producing a noncommunicating hydrocephalus). Parinaud's syndrome is frequently the result of a tumor of the pineal. Primary tumors of the pineal gland are very uncommon but are of interest, especially in view of the mysterious and relatively unknown functions of the pineal gland itself. The gland secretes neurotransmitter substances such as serotonin and dopamine, with the major product being melatonin. Tumors of the pineal gland include germ cell tumors of all types, including embryonal carcinoma, choriocarcinoma, teratoma, and various combinations of germinomas. Germ cell tumors may arise extragonadally within the retroperitoneal space and the pineal gland, with the only commonality being that these structures are in the midline. Primary tumors of the pineal gland occur in two forms: the pineoblastoma and the pineocytoma. Pineoblastomas occur in young patients and consist of small tumors having areas of hemorrhage and necrosis with pleomorphic nuclei and frequent mitoses. Pineocytomas occur in older adults and are slow-growing; they are better differentiated and have large rosettes. In contrast, the medial midbrain syndrome (Weber's syndrome) affects the oculomotor nerve roots, the corticobulbar tracts (producing contralateral weakness of the lower face (CN VII), the tongue (CN XII), the palate (CN X), and the corticospinal tracts (producing contralateral spastic paralysis of the trunk and extremities).

496. The answer is e. (*Young, pp 275, 277. Goetz, pp 156, 203, 220, 261, 269, 357, 416.*) The lateral medullary syndrome (Wallenberg syndrome) results from occlusion of the posterior inferior cerebellar artery (hence its other name, PICA syndrome). The signs and symptoms produced are related to the structures of the caudal medulla normally supplied by this vessel. These structures include the vestibular nuclei (nystagmus, nausea, vomiting, vertigo), the inferior cerebellar peduncle (ipsilateral cerebellar signs), the nucleus ambiguus (ipsilateral laryngeal, pharyngeal, and palatine paralysis), the glossopharyngeal nerve roots (loss of gag reflex), the vagal nerve roots (same signs as the nucleus ambiguus), the spinothalamic tracts (contralateral loss of pain and temperature sensation from trunk and extremities), the spinal trigeminal nucleus (ipsilateral loss of pain and temperature sensation from the face), and the descending sympathetic tract (ipsilateral Horner syndrome), which passes through the lateral aspects of the medulla in the dorsal longitudinal fasciculus.

497. The answer is b. (*Kumar, pp 1356–1357. Goldman, p 2077.*) Bilateral loss of pain and temperature sensations in both arms is most likely to be caused by syringomyelia, which is a chronic myelopathy that results from formation of a cavity (syrinx) involving the central gray matter of the spinal cord. This is the location where pain fibers cross to join the contralateral spinothalamic tract. Interruption of the lateral spinothalamic tracts results in segmental sensory dissociation with loss of pain and temperature sense, but preservation of the sense of touch and pressure or vibration, usually over the neck, shoulders, and arms. Since the most common location of a syrinx is the cervicothoracic region, the loss of pain and temperature sensation affects both arms. The diagnosis of syringomyelia is best made with MRI of the spine, and since the most common location is the cervical region, this is the area that should be examined first. Other features of syringomyelia include wasting of the small intrinsic hand muscles (claw hand) and thoracic scoliosis. The cause of syringomyelia is unknown, although one type is associated with a Chiari malformation with obstruction at the foramen magnum.

498. The answer is a. (*Young, pp 52, 290–294. Ayala, pp 30–31.*) The physical finding of facial asymmetry is suggestive of an abnormality involving the facial nerve (CN VII). The facial nucleus, which is located within the pons, is divided in half; the upper neurons innervate the upper muscles of the face, while the lower neurons innervate the lower portion of the face. It is important to realize that each half receives input from the contralateral motor cortex, while only the upper half receives input from the ipsilateral motor cortex. Therefore an upper motor neuron (UMN) lesion will produce a defect involving only the contralateral lower half of the face. Causes of UMN lesions involving the facial nerve include strokes that involve the cortex or the internal capsule. In contrast, lesions that affect the facial nerve from the facial nucleus to the remaining length of the nerve result in lower motor neuron (LMN) lesions. Patients present with facial asymmetry involving the ipsilateral upper and lower quadrants. Lesions to the facial nerve within the facial canal (frequently due to cold weather) cause Bell's palsy. Patients present with paralysis of all muscles of facial expression. Bell's phenomenon refers to the finding of the affected eye looking up and out when patients try to close their eyes. Because the lacrimal punctum in the lower eyelid moves away from the surface of the eye, lacrimal fluid does not drain into the nasolacrimal duct. This produces "crocodile tears."

In contrast to a LMN lesion of the facial nerve producing Bell's palsy, a LMN lesion involving the trigeminal nerve (CN V) can produce tic douloureux (trigeminal neuralgia). This disorder is characterized by recurrent episodes of sharp, stabbing pain in the distribution of branches of the trigeminal nerve on one side of the face, usually in the area supplied by the second and third divisions. The cause of trigeminal neuralgia is usually unknown, but one possible cause of this syndrome is a redundant loop of the superior cerebellar artery that impinges on the trigeminal root. An upper motor neuron lesion involving the accessory nerve (CN XI) will produce weakness in shrugging shoulder and turning the head toward the opposite side. Finally, the glossopharyngeal nerve (CN IX) and the vagus nerve (CN X) are usually clinically examined together by testing the gag reflex and swallowing. Upper motor neuron lesions affecting either of these cranial nerves will produce dysphagia and problems with the gag reflex.

499. The answer is d. (*Kumar, p 1331. Rubin, p 1528.*) Inflammatory polyneuropathies may be acute or chronic. Acute inflammatory demyelinating polyradiculoneuropathy (Guillain-Barré syndrome) is a life-threatening disease of the peripheral nervous system. The disease usually follows recovery from an influenza-like upper respiratory tract infection and is characterized by a motor neuropathy that leads to an ascending paralysis that begins with weakness in the distal extremities and rapidly involves proximal muscles. Sensory changes are usually minimal. The disease is thought to result from immune-mediated segmental demyelination. In rare patients, instead of an acute course, Guillain-Barré syndrome takes a chronic course with remissions and relapses. This process is called chronic inflammatory demyelinating polyradiculoneuropathy (CIDP).

500. The answer is c. (*Kumar, p 1335. Rubin, p 1530.*) Peripheral neuropathy is a clinical term that generally refers to nontraumatic diseases of the peripheral nerves. Peripheral neuropathies may either be focal or diffuse. Focal peripheral neuropathies may involve one nerve (mononeuropathy) or multiple nerves (multiple mononeuropathy or monoradiculopathy). An example of a mononeuropathy is compression of the median nerve, which produces carpal tunnel syndrome. The median nerve provides sensory information from the palmar surface of the lateral three and one-half digits and the lateral portion of the palm. Also innervated by the median nerve are the major pronators (pronator teres and pronator quadratus), the thumb flexors (flexor pollicus longus and flexor pollicus brevis), and the opponens pollicis. The median nerve does not innervate any muscles in the forearm. Damage to the median nerve at the wrist as it lies deep to the flexor retinaculum results in burning sensations in the thumb, index, and middle fingers, and lateral half of the ring finger (carpal tunnel syndrome). This syndrome is found in people who use their hands a lot, such as jackhammer operators, typists, and tailors. Treatment may involve cutting the transverse carpal ligament to decompress the nerve.

Bibliography

Abenhaim L, Moride Y, Brenot F, et al: Appetite-suppressant drugs and the risk of primary pulmonary hypertension. *N Engl J Med* 335(9):609–616, 1996.

Alberts B, et al: *Molecular Biology of the Cell*, 4/e. New York, Garland, 2002.

Angulo P: Nonalcoholic fatty liver disease. *N Engl J Med Apr* 18;346(16): 1221–1231, 2002.

Ayala C, Spellberg B: *Pathophysiology for the Boards and Wards*, 4/e. Malden, MA, Blackwell, 2003.

Behrman RE, Kliegman RM, Jenson HB: *Nelson's Textbook of Pediatrics*, 17/e. Philadelphia, Saunders, 2004.

Braunwald E, et al (eds): *Harrison's Manual of Medicine*, 15/e. New York, McGraw-Hill, 2002.

Carson, FL: *Histology A Self-Instructional Text*, 2/e. Chicago, ASCP Press, 1997.

Champe PA, Harvey RA: *Biochemistry*, 2/e. Philadelphia, Lippincott, 1994.

Chandrasoma P, Taylor CR: *Concise Pathology*, 3/e. Stamford, CT, Appleton & Lange, 1998.

Connolly HM, Crary JL, et al: Valvular heart disease associated with fenfluramine-phentermine. *N Engl J Med* 337(9):581–588, 1997.

Damjanov I, Linder J (eds): *Anderson's Pathology*, 10/e. St. Louis, Mosby, 1996.

Duchin JS, et al: Hantavirus pulmonary syndrome: a clinical description of 17 patients with a newly recognized disease. *N Engl J Med* 330:949–955, 1994.

Fawcett DW: *A Textbook of Histology*, 12/e. New York, Chapman & Hall, 1997.

Feldman M, Friedman LS: *Sleisenger and Fordtran's Gastrointestinal and Liver Disease*, 7/e. Philadelphia, Saunders, 2002.

Flake AW, Roncarolo MG, et al: Brief report: treatment of x-linked severe combined immunodeficiency by in utero transplantation of paternal bone marrow. *N Engl J Med* 335(24):1806–1810, 1996.

Goetz CG (ed): *Textbook of Clinical Neurology*, 2/e. Philadelphia, Saunders, 2003.

Goetz CG (ed): *Textbook of Clinical Neurology*, 2/e. Philadelphia, Saunders, 2003.

Goldman L, Bennett JC: *Cecil's Textbook of Medicine*, 22/e. Philadelphia, Saunders, 2004.

Henry JB, et al (eds): *Clinical Diagnosis and Management by Laboratory Methods*, 20/e. Philadelphia, Saunders, 2001.

Hoffman R, Benz EJ, Shattil SJ: *Hematology: Basic Principles and Practice*, 4/e. New York, Churchill Livingstone, 2005.

Inoki K, Corradetti MN, Guan KL: Dysregulation of the TSC-mTOR pathway in human disease. *Nature Genetics* 37:19–24, 2005.

Joklik WK, et al (eds): *Zinsser Microbiology*, 20/e. Norwalk, CT, Appleton & Lange, 1992.

Jorde LB, et al: *Medical Genetics*, 3/e. St. Louis, Mosby, 2003.

Kumar V, Abbas AK, Fausto N: *Robbins and Cotran Pathologic Basis of Disease*, 7/e. Philadelphia, Saunders, 2004.

Lekstrom-Himes JA, Gallin JI: Advances in immunology: Immunodeficiency diseases caused by defects in phagocytes. *N Engl J Med* 343(23): 1703–1714, 2000.

Mandell GL, et al (eds): *Principles and Practice of Infectious Diseases*, 5/e. New York, Churchill Livingstone, 1998.

McPhee SJ, et al: *Pathophysiology of Disease*, 4/e. Stamford, CT, Appleton & Lange, 2002.

Ravel R: *Clinical Laboratory Medicine*, 6/e. St. Louis, Mosby-Year Book, 1995.

Rubin E, Farber JL: *Pathology*, 3/e. Philadelphia, Lippincott, 1999.

Sadler TW: *Langman's Medical Embryology*, 9/e. Philadelphia, Lippincott, 2004.

Schneider AS, Szanto PA: *Pathology*, 3/e. Philadelphia, Lippincott, 2006.

Townsend CM, et al: *Sabiston's Textbook of Surgery*, 16/e. Philadelphia, WB Saunders, 2001.

Warren MP: Health issues for women athletes: exercise-induced amenorrhea. *J Clin Endo & Met* 84(6):1892–1896, 1999.

Weidner N (ed): *Modern Surgical Pathology*, 1/e. Philadelphia, WB Saunders, 2003.

Wilson JD, Larsen PR, Shlomo M: *Williams Textbook of Endocrinology*, 10/e. Philadelphia, WB Saunders, 2002.

Young PA, Young PH: *Basic Clinical Neuroanatomy*, 1/e. Philadelphia, Lippincott, 1997.

Index